Techniques of Plastic Surgery

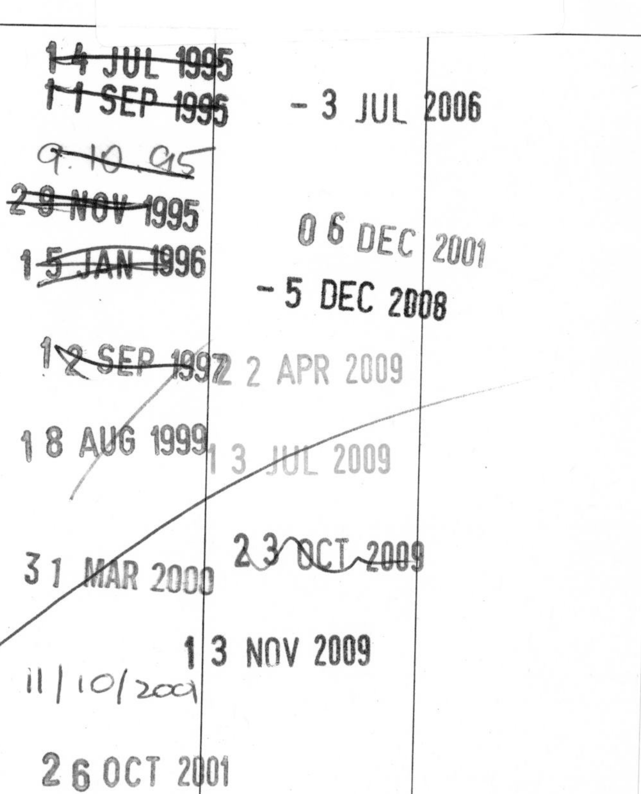

The authors

Ian A. McGregor
Formerly Director,
West of Scotland Regional Plastic Surgery Unit,
Canniesburn Hospital,
Bearsden, Glasgow, UK

Alan D. McGregor
Professor of Reconstructive Plastic Surgery,
University of Wales;
Consultant Plastic Surgeon,
Morriston Hospital,
Swansea, South Wales

Foreword by

The late **Sir Charles Illingworth CBE**
Formerly Emeritus Regius Professor of Surgery,
University of Glasgow

For Churchill Livingstone

Commissioning Editor: Sheila Khullar
Copy Editor: Robin Watson
Indexer: Liz Granger
Design Direction: Erik Bigland
Project Manager: Mark Sanderson
Sales Promotion Executive: Caroline Boyd

Fundamental Techniques of Plastic Surgery

AND THEIR SURGICAL APPLICATIONS

Ian A. McGregor
DSc ChM FRCS (Eng) FRCS (Glasg) Hon FRACS Hon FRCSI Hon FRCS (Ed) Hon FACS

Alan D. McGregor
MD FRCS (Glasg) FRCS (Plast Surg)

FOREWORD BY
The late Sir Charles Illingworth CBE
MD ChM FRCS (Glasg) FRCS (Ed) Hon FACS Hon FRCS (Eng)

ARTWORK BY
Ian Ramsden

Churchill Livingstone

EDINBURGH
LONDON
MADRID
MELBOURNE
NEW YORK
AND
TOKYO
1995

NINTH EDITION

CHURCHILL LIVINGSTONE
Medical Division of Longman Group Limited

Distributed in the United States of America by Churchill Livingstone Inc., 650 Avenue of the Americas, New York, N.Y. 10011, and by associated companies, branches and representatives throughout the world.

First edition 1960
Second edition 1962
Third edition 1965
Fourth edition 1968
Fifth edition 1972
Sixth edition 1975
Seventh edition 1980
Eighth edition 1989
Translated into Spanish, Japanese, Italian, German
Ninth edition 1995

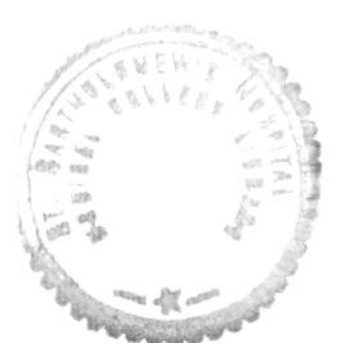

ISBN 0 443 05028 7

British Library Cataloguing in Publication Data
A catalogue record for this book is available from the British Library.

Library of Congress Cataloging in Publication Data
A catalog record for this book is available from the Library of Congress.

Produced by Longman Singapore Publishers (Pte) Ltd.
Printed in Singapore

The publisher's policy is to use **paper manufactured from sustainable forests**

Contents

Foreword

Like other surgical specialties, Plastic Surgery originated through the efforts of a small group of enthusiasts who, by utilising a particular refinement of technique, soon raised the standards of surgical craftsmanship within a narrow field to a high pitch of efficiency.

Then came the war, and the techniques primarily evolved for hiding facial blemishes and correcting visible deformities were applied with immense success to the treatment of wounds in general. Since then, as a natural sequel, plastic surgeons have widened still further their range of interests, notably in casualty work, in hand injuries and in burns. In doing so, they have implicitly ceased to regard themselves as a class apart, exclusive authorities in a chosen field, but rather as expert advisers and helpful collaborators in a wide range of surgery.

Mr McGregor is emphatically of this latter class, trained in the Glasgow School of Plastic Surgery, broadened in experience by the responsibility of a busy casualty department, and with a particular interest in the surgery of the hand. His book reflects these interests and this experience, being designed not for specialists but for all those who are concerned with the healing of wounds. Its approach is essentially practical, dealing as it does with the choice of incisions, with stitchcraft, avoidance of ugly scars, methods of skin grafting, and similar matters, and with their application to casualty surgery, orthopaedics and general surgery. It will assuredly receive a warm welcome.

Glasgow, 1960 C. F. W. Illingworth

Preface to the Ninth Edition

In this edition, Alan McGregor, contributor to the eighth edition, is a co-author and responsibility for the text is a joint one.

Since the previous edition, changes in the basic techniques have varied with each, and this has been reflected in the revision required — least with the Z-plasty, greatest with the flaps. Before discussing the various flap types, it has seemed logical to provide a general account of the perfusion patterns of the skin in the various sites used as flap sources and, in describing the range of flap types, we have omitted any reference to the tube pedicle. One of the authors never having raised one, while the other had not raised one in the last 25 years, it seemed sensible, though it was salutary to realise just how many of the techniques developed for use with tube pedicles are still used in pedicled flap practice generally.

Decisions had to be made as to which individual flaps to describe and, in making them, it was apparent that, since publication of the eighth edition, there have been winners and losers. Fashion plays a significant role in current usage, and we have endeavoured to tread a judicious path through the minefield. The problem of selection is greatest when the various flaps are discussed in different therapeutic contexts, given that some surgeons with microvascular expertise see free flaps as a near universal solution, while others take a more balanced view, seeing a place for the more traditional techniques. The needs of the group who have to practise without an operating microscope also have to be catered for. We can only hope that we have achieved a reasonable compromise.

Liposuction and the use of the laser have been introduced as new topics, and tissue expansion has been given more extended coverage. With all three, the aim has been to discuss principles of usage and clinical role rather than provide a detailed exposition of each technique.

Plastic surgery is based on surgical techniques rather than on an anatomical system or on a specific pathological sequence, and this creates problems in discussing its surgical applications. In previous editions, the appropriate surgical specialties provided the framework; in this edition, the groupings have been more pragmatic, anatomy providing the common factor with some, pathology with others.

In response to the preference expressed in market surveys carried out by the publishers, many of the photographic illustrations from the eighth edition have been replaced by line drawings, in the belief that this would make them clearer. The new drawings, as with those in the previous edition, are the work of Ian Ramsden, and most have been converted directly from the previous photographs with his usual clarity and economy of line.

Thanks are due for help which we received in the preparation of this edition, particularly from Philip Sykes, whose constructive criticism and advice was so valuable in the chapter on hand surgery. We would also acknowledge our debt to the Bibliotheque Nationale in Paris in providing the microfiche of *Artères de la Peau* by Michel Salmon, from which Figure 4.1 was prepared, and to Professor Wayne Morrison for permission to use illustrations from *Reconstructive Microsurgery* as the basis for Figure 4.56.

In preparing a new edition, the author has to look afresh at current practice, note changes in mainstream thinking, and assess the directions in which basic and applied research are moving, particularly in the fields of cell and molecular biology. None has made a real impact on surgical practice as yet, but the speed with which microsurgical techniques have moved from the laboratory to the patient is perhaps a portent for the future.

Glasgow and
Swansea, 1995

Ian A. McGregor
Alan D. McGregor

Preface to the First Edition

Plastic surgical methods are being used increasingly often by surgeons who have received no formal training in plastic surgery and who are looking for guidance on the basic techniques. Advanced textbooks of plastic surgery are apt to pass over those elementary but nonetheless fundamental methods while the sections on plastic surgery in textbooks of surgery describe its scope and results without giving enough detail of actual technique to be of practical use. This book I hope may help to fill the gap.

The first part describes the basic techniques of plastic surgery in detail and the second considers their application to the situations which surgeons in other specialties are likely to encounter. A difficulty in the second part has been that of deciding what material to include and what to leave out. The deciding factor generally has been to include such topics and techniques as it was felt a surgeon in the particular field might reasonably wish to deal with himself without necessarily referring the patient to a plastic surgeon.

The book makes no attempt to describe all possible methods of repair and reconstruction. To include a multiplicity of methods in a book of this nature would merely confuse and I have preferred instead of describe those methods which I have found work best in practice.

In discussing the basic techniques I have tried to stress the difficulties of each and to describe the complications, how they can be avoided and how to cope with them when they do occur. I have endeavoured too, to bring out the principles of the various methods in the hope that an understanding of these principles may weld the technical details into a coherent, rational pattern and prevent them from being a mere jumble of empirical instructions.

A difficult decision has been whether or not to use the eponyms in which plastic surgery abounds. Eponyms are an essential part of everyday surgical shorthand and they recall men who have stood as signposts along the way of an advancing specialty. But often they lack precise meaning and they are liable to cause confusion, firstly because they sometimes have different meanings in different countries, secondly because they are frequently used loosely so that in some instances a name has even come to be applied to a procedure different from that described by its owner. The Thiersch graft is an example of this latter category, being nowadays applied to a graft of quite different thickness from that originally described by Thiersch. For these reasons I have regretfully avoided eponyms altogether.

References have purposely not been introduced into the text. Instead I have listed a few papers and monographs at the end of each chapter under suitable subject headings to provide a starting point for anyone wishing to pursue a particular subject further.

I must acknowledge my debt to many who have helped me in preparing this book. To Professor C. F. W. Illingworth who encouraged me at the outset in its writing and Mr J. S. Tough who was responsible for my training in Plastic Surgery and gave me free access to the photographic records of the Unit I am deeply grateful. I am greatly in debt of Mr Douglas R. K. Reid for his constructive criticism of the text and for the pains he has taken to make it as lucid as possible without sacrificing brevity in the process. To Professor Roland Barnes and Dr J. C. J. Ives who read and criticised parts of the text I express my thanks.

The illustrations are all-important in a book largely concerned with surgical techniques. Mr Robin Callander made all the drawings and I find it difficult to convey fully the care and trouble he has taken to portray visually what I wished to express. Any usefulness which the book may have is due in no small way to his illustrations. The photographs are the work of Mr T. Meikle and Mr R. Macgregor of the Plastic Surgery Units at Ballochmyle Hospital and Glasgow Royal Infirmary; Mr R. McLean, Department of Medical Illustration, Western Infirmary; Mr P. Kelly, Photographic Department and Mr E. Towler, Department of Surgery, Glasgow Royal Infirmary. For the care and trouble which each has taken I am most grateful. I am also indebted to Messrs Chas. F. Thackray for permission to use illustrations of their instruments.

The typing and retyping of the manuscript was carried out with patience and good humour by Mrs A. M. Drummond.

I should like lastly to record my thanks to Mr Charles Macmillan and Mr James Parker of Messrs E. and S. Livingstone for the advice and help which they have given me throughout.

Glasgow, 1960 Ian A. McGregor

PART

1

Basic techniques

CHAPTER

1 Wound management

Given accurate approximation of the wound edges, and freedom from infection and haematoma, epidermal healing of a wound occurs extremely rapidly, but the healing processes which go on in the dermis are much more prolonged and, as far as the ultimate appearance of the resulting scar is concerned, much more important. The transition from fibrin, formed between the two surfaces of the wound as the first stage of healing, through the phase of diminishing reaction, to the quiescent relatively avascular scar takes place slowly over a period of months.

Early on, the scar tends to be red and the immediate surroundings are indurated. Gradually the induration and redness diminish and disappear, leaving a soft scar, generally paler than the surrounding skin. The degree of redness and induration is extremely variable, as is the time taken for the reaction to subside. The appearance of a scar can be expected to improve for a year and more.

This gradually diminishing induration constitutes normal progress to quiescence, but such a sequence is not invariable. Instead, the fibrous tissue of the dermis may become hypertrophic giving rise clinically to a raised, red, **hypertrophic** scar or, when the reaction is more florid, to a **keloid** scar. These conditions are discussed in Chapter 6.

The tensile strength of the wound gradually increases during the healing phase. The sutures take what little strain there is until they are removed, and if the scar is going to stretch thereafter it does so gradually over the next few weeks. Support of the wound for as long as is feasible appears to have little effect. A scar is more likely to stretch badly when there is obvious wound tension, but often stretching occurs when there is no apparent tension other than that deriving from the normal elasticity of the skin.

Nevertheless in many parts of the body the direction of the scar appears to influence the amount of stretching which takes place, and in certain body sites the directions which result in minimal stretching can be systematised into **lines of election** for scars.

In the *face and neck*, the lines of election lie at right angles to the direction of the resultant pull of the muscles of facial expression. With the loss of elasticity that goes with ageing they become set into a pattern of wrinkles (Fig. 1.1). In the *vicinity of the flexures*, the lines of election are parallel to the skin creases which are clearly present in the region of the flexure. In the *skin surfaces between the flexures*, the evidence for a specific line of election is less clear cut, and the placing of an incision there is determined more often by considerations other than the eventual appearance of the scar.

There is great and uncontrollable individual variation in healing characteristics. Examples of factors beyond the surgeon's control are the age of the patient, the site and often the direction of the wound or incision. Scars in children generally remain harder and redder for longer than in the adult, and the end result is poorer, this quite apart from the greater tendency of scars in children than in adults to develop hypertrophic change or even keloid. One of the compensations of age is the fact that the more wrinkled the skin the more rapidly a scar settles and the better is its final appearance, hidden amongst the wrinkles.

Scars also behave very differently in different individuals and different parts of the body. Outside the face and neck, scars are apt to stay conspicuous despite careful surgical technique, and stretching even of the most meticulously handled incision is frequent. In the face too, different sites and different skins vary greatly in the way they behave. Coarse, oily skin tends to produce more than the usual reaction to sutures and suture marks are more common as a result. The problem arises most strikingly in the nose where the skin can be very thick, with active sebaceous glands, most markedly towards the tip. In hairless skin sites, such as the red margin of the lips and the palms and soles, scars are usually less conspicuous. Probably the best example of the influence of site is the upper sternal area where scars almost always become keloid.

These unavoidable factors may set a limit to what can be achieved by pure surgical technique, but it is true nonetheless that to produce the best result in a given set of circumstances a meticulous technique is essential. It must also be emphasised that failure in a single aspect may be enough to give a poor result.

PLACING THE SCAR

Use of natural lines

Incisions should be placed wherever possible so that the scar will lie in a **line of election**, or at least parallel to it (Fig. 1.1), so that in the course of time it will settle in to look like another wrinkle. Even if wrinkling is not actually present, the site and line of the wrinkles likely to develop in the future can often be found by getting the patient to simulate the appropriate facial expression, e.g. smiling, frowning, closing the eyelids tightly, etc. This brings the more obvious potential wrinkle lines into being.

The most generally useful wrinkles are the *nasolabial fold*, the *glabellar wrinkle pattern*, the *lateral canthal 'crow's foot'*, the *forehead wrinkles*, each a site which overlies one of the main concentrations of the muscles of facial expression. Where these are absent, as over the masseter, the wrinkle pattern is less clear cut, and in the ear and nasal tip it is completely lacking.

In the older patient, additional wrinkling results from the effect of gravity on a background of skin slackness. In many ageing faces the criss-cross of fine wrinkling is a mixture of gravity wrinkling and expression lines.

The smooth skin of the child can make it extremely difficult, especially away from the eyes and mouth, to select the best line for an incision. Fortunately, the need to make the choice is rare.

The use of a **natural junction line** has the effect of distracting the eye from a scar and can be used to good effect. Examples are the *junction lines between nose and face* especially around the base of the ala, the *nostril rim*, the margin between the *red border of the lip and the skin*, the junction line between the *ear and the masseteric region*, and in the *lower eyelid just below the line of the eyelashes*. These and others are used routinely to distract the eye of the observer and render the scar less conspicuous.

Placing the scar where it will not be visible

The obvious examples are inside the hairline or in the eyebrow. In these sites the incision, instead of being perpendicular to the skin surface, should be made parallel to the hair follicles. This avoids the creation of the hairless scar line which results from sectioning of the hair follicles. A practical point to note in making a scalp incision is the possibility of subsequent baldness revealing a scar previously hidden. In this, account should be

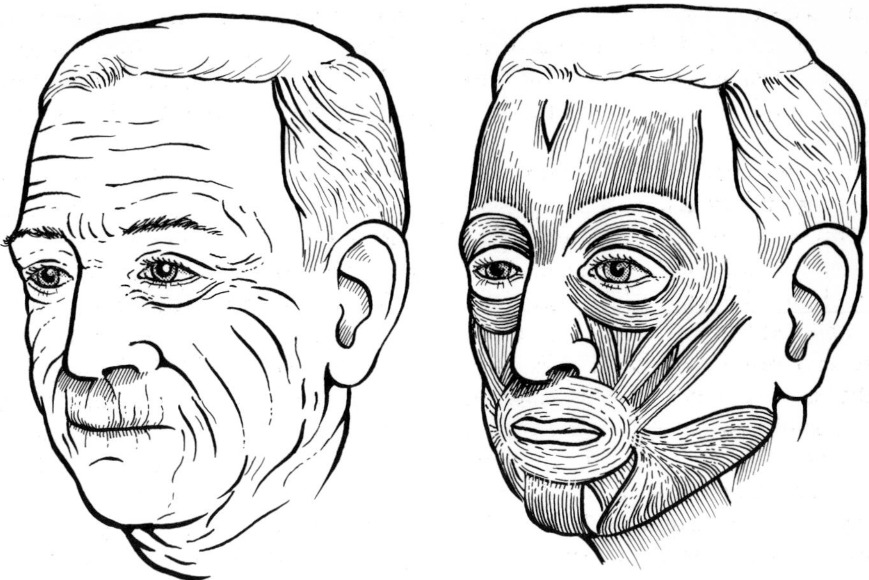

Fig. 1.1 The lines of election for the placing of scars in the face and neck, indicated by the pattern of wrinkling of the skin, and their relation to the line of the underlying muscles of facial expression.

taken of the patient's sex, and any hereditary factors, in the potential pattern of baldness.

Use of the Z-plasty

The Z-plasty has a potentially significant role as an adjunct to other methods designed to improve the appearance of scars. The technical aspects of design are described in Chapter 2, but the general point to be made at this juncture is that the Z-plasty is unsuitable for use in the initial management of a wound resulting from trauma. It should be reserved for possible use in subsequent scar revision, and even then it calls for careful judgment, skill in design, and scrupulous technique.

PREPARATION OF THE WOUND

The presence or absence of damaged tissue determines whether or not a wound needs to be excised. It is axiomatic that all dirt and other foreign material must be removed, and when the dirt is ingrained this may entail the vigorous use of a sharp spoon or wire brush to ensure that removal is demonstrably complete. The apparent coarseness of the methods involved may seem inappropriate, but total removal of grit and dirt at this stage takes priority.

Excisional policy

Where the cosmetic result is of paramount importance, as in the face, a conservative policy to excision of wound margins is desirable, only obviously non-viable tissue being removed, the limited objective being to replace structures in their normal position and suture them there. This policy is particularly necessary in the more extensive wounds (Fig. 1.2). It recognises that an optimum result cannot be expected from the healing of such a wound, and accepts at the outset the probable need for subsequent revisional surgery. It also permits the salvage of tissue whose viability is felt to be in doubt, and which might otherwise be excised, tissue which may be of considerable value later.

It is often important to know when a piece of traumatised tissue is viable and should be conserved or whether it should be excised. The decision is made on the basis of evidence of an active circulation. The relevant signs are the presence of blanching of the skin on pressure with return of the original colour on release, and

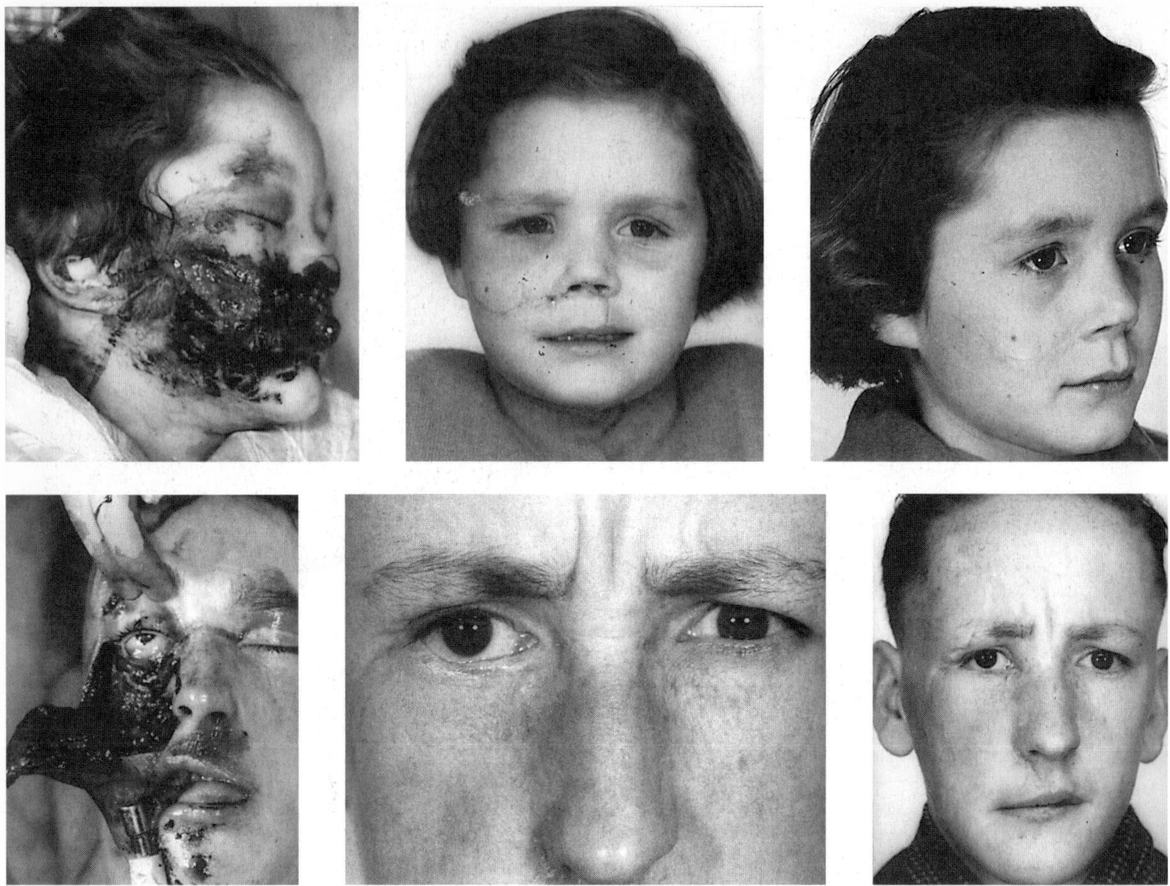

Fig. 1.2 Examples of the conservative treatment of severe soft tissue injuries of the face involving the eyelids, nose and mouth, where there has been no skin loss, showing the results of accurate tissue replacement with careful matching.

the presence of bleeding from the cut edge of the tissue concerned. Where there is doubt, the anatomy of the region and its known vascularity, together with the size and content of the pedicle, help in making a decision (Fig. 1.3). The problem arises most acutely in the face, ear and scalp. The vascularity of these sites is on the side of survival, and flaps with even a small pedicle should not be excised lightly.

In the case of the scalp and the ear, the possibility exists of a totally detached flap being replanted using microvascular techniques, but for success immediate referral to a Unit with the necessary expertise is essential.

Quite apart from its use in judging viability in the context of trauma, skin colour has to be assessed frequently and accurately in most plastic surgical procedures, and for this reason the agents chosen for skin cleansing and sterilisation should be ones which do not stain the skin or tissues. Satisfactory from this point of view are Cetrimide and an aqueous solution of Chlorhexidine (Hibitane).

Wound closure

In suturing an irregular wound the secret lies in looking first for landmarks on either side to match. With two points which definitely fit sutured together, fresh parts of the jigsaw fall into place until enough key points have been matched to allow the intervening sutures to be placed readily. Time spent fitting a jigsaw of tissue accurately at the time of original suture is never wasted. The

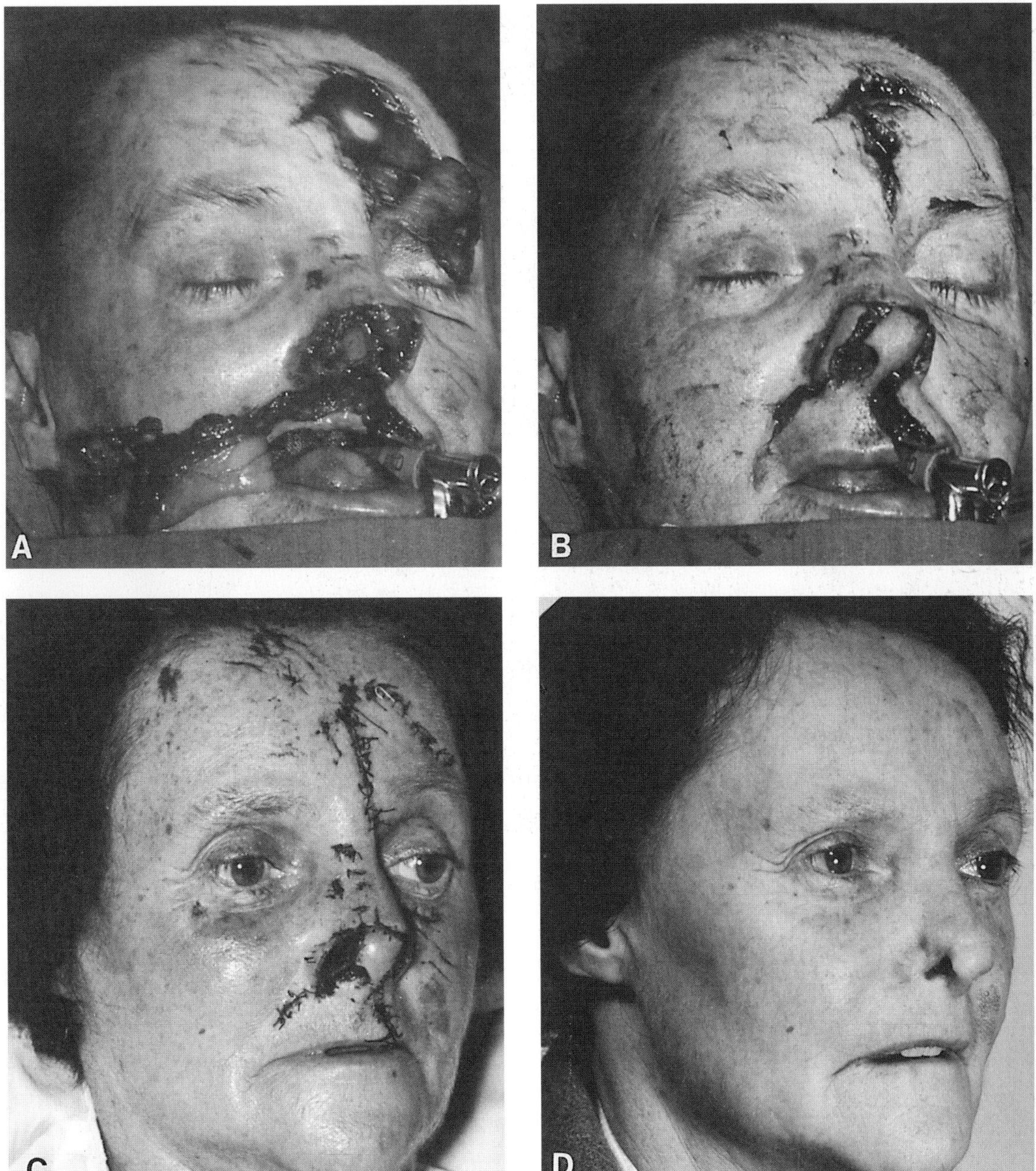

Fig. 1.3 Survival and non-survival of traumatic flaps in the face, treated conservatively.

A, B Flaps before suture, showing the extent of the injury.
C Survival and non-survival of flaps.
D The late result prior to reconstruction of the ala of the nose.

chance comes only once, and if it is missed the results can be difficult to correct. As already stressed, it may be apparent that Z-plasties will be required later, but these should not be used at the primary operation.

When tissue has been lost the governing principle is that surviving tissues should be replaced in their correct position so that the defect can be properly displayed and assessed in terms of the tissues lost. The experienced plastic surgeon might

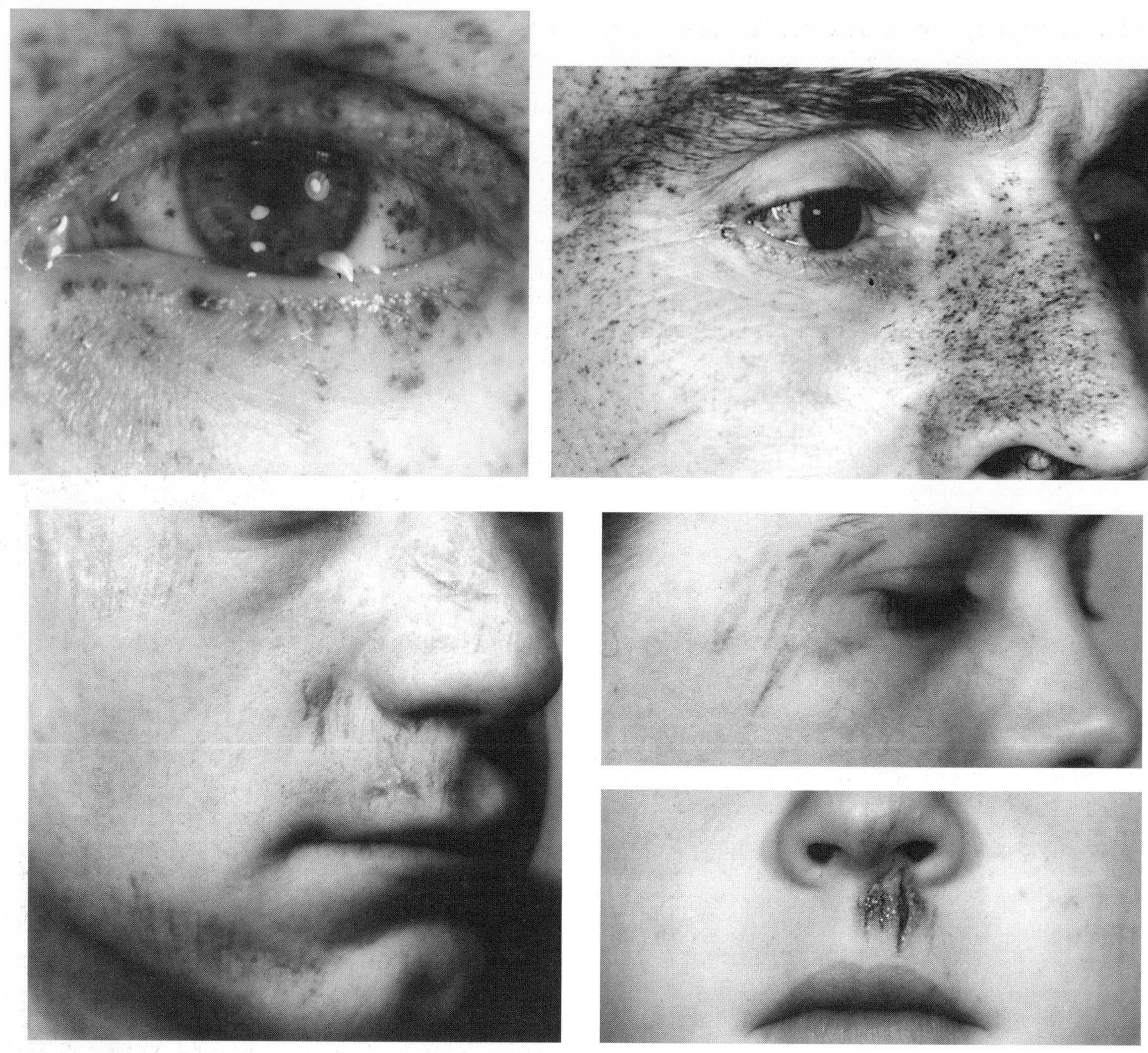

Fig. 1.4 Tattooed scarring, – the result of failure to remove ingrained dirt and grit from the wound at the time of primary treatment.

then consider the possibility of a definitive primary reconstruction, though probably only to discard the thought. The less experienced surgeon should certainly have a more modest target and, if the defect cannot be closed directly without creating distortion, he should apply a split skin graft in most instances. Such an approach has the merit of allowing healing to occur quickly with minimal scarring and leaves conditions suitable for a definitive repair or reconstruction subsequently.

Ideally, wound edges being sutured together should be vertical if the best scar result is to be achieved, and accurate suturing is also very much easier when the faces of tissue brought together are of the same thickness. In the case of facial injuries, particularly those resulting from windscreen trauma, neither may be present, shelving lacerations being the norm. A compromise from the ideal situation is then unavoidable. Excision to create vertical wound margins would involve unacceptable sacrifice of viable tissue in many instances, and then only sufficient of the wound edges are excised to remove clearly devitalised tissue. The residual shelving makes suturing more difficult, but it has to be accepted as the lesser of two evils. In practice the best result is achieved by using a large number of very fine sutures, and even then the need for possible revision or dermabrasion of the resulting scar subsequently has to be accepted.

Errors in wound management

The common errors made in treating facial wounds at this stage are *failure to remove all dirt from the wound, creation of a scar with gross suture marks*, and *failure to suture the various wound edges in the precise position which they occupied relative to one another before the injury.*

The effect of failure to remove all dirt from the wound is to leave foci of tattooed scarring in the dermis (Fig. 1.4). These are always difficult, and often impossible, to eradicate completely later once healing has taken place. Suture marks along the line of a scar result from the use of coarse suture material and/or failure to remove sutures sufficiently early, allowing the sutures to cut into the tissues. The coarser the suture material the broader and more obtrusive is the linear scar which it creates (Fig. 1.5). Such marks are virtually impossible to eradicate subsequently. Failure to suture the wound margins in the position which they occupied prior to the injury leaves irregularities (Fig. 1.6), which are especially obvious when the lip margin, eyelid, eyebrow or nostril have been imperfectly matched.

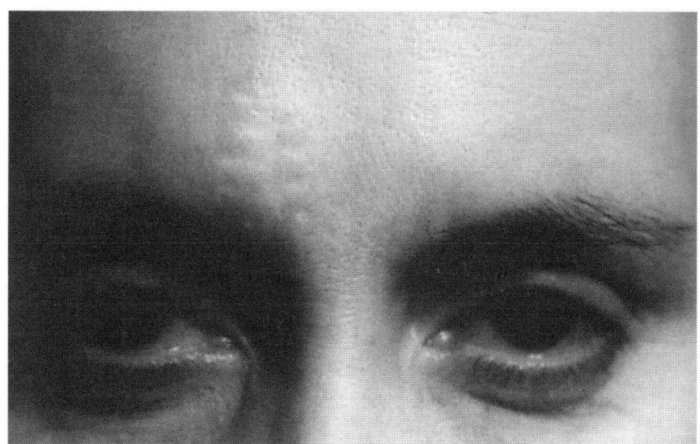

Fig. 1.5 Suture marks resulting from the use of coarse suture material left in position for too long.

Use of undercutting

When the presence of tension adds to the difficulty of wound closure, the use of undercutting of the wound margins to allow a degree of advancement is frequently recommended. Before this can even be considered the vascular state of the skin has to be assessed, and the potential effect of tension on its viability, particularly if the injury has involved an element of degloving. Personal experience has been that the amount of advancement achieved in practice is often disappointingly small.

The levels at which such undercutting is carried

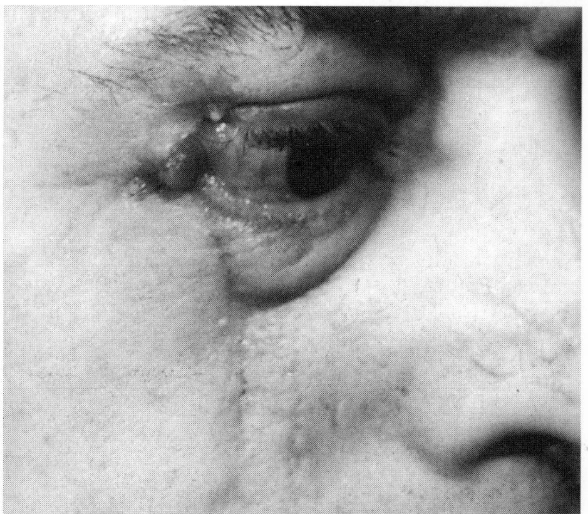

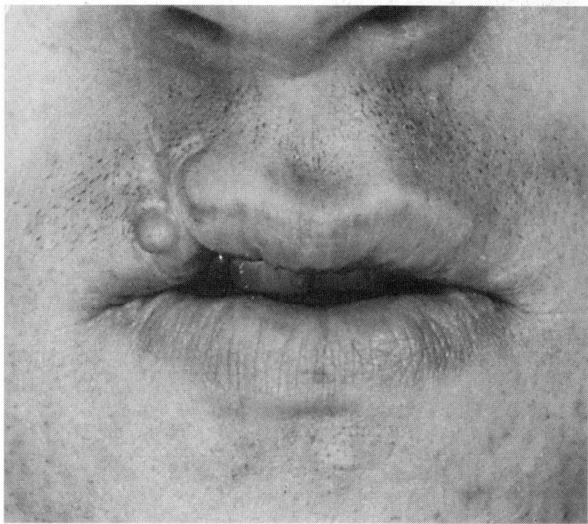

Fig. 1.6 Irregularities of the eyelid and the mouth, – the result of failure to suture matching points together accurately at the time of the initial treatment.

out and its safe extent vary in the different body sites (Fig. 1.7). In the face, the appropriate level is deep to the dermis, so that the plexus of subdermal vessels is included, while leaving undisturbed the branches of the facial nerve. The potential for advancement of facial skin depends very much on the degree of redundancy which was present previously. In the child, there is an absence of skin redundancy, and the potential is virtually nil; in the ageing wrinkled face, it is considerable. In the scalp, the plane is between the galea aponeurotica and the pericranium, and the vascular anatomy of the scalp is such that extensive undercutting can be carried out with safety. The galea rather than the skin is responsible for the inextensibility of the scalp, and it is multiple galeal 'relaxation' incisions which have been advocated to increase the amount of advancement. Experience indicates that the effectiveness of this manoeuvre has been greatly exaggerated. In the limbs and trunk, if undercutting is to be more than minimal, the plane between the superficial and deep fascia should be used.

Surgeons vary greatly in the extent to which they make use of undercutting in this way, but if more than minimal advancement is required to allow a wound to be closed, it is probably wiser to close the defect with a split skin graft.

STITCHCRAFT

When the surgeon is aiming to make his scar as inconspicuous as possible suturing of the wound

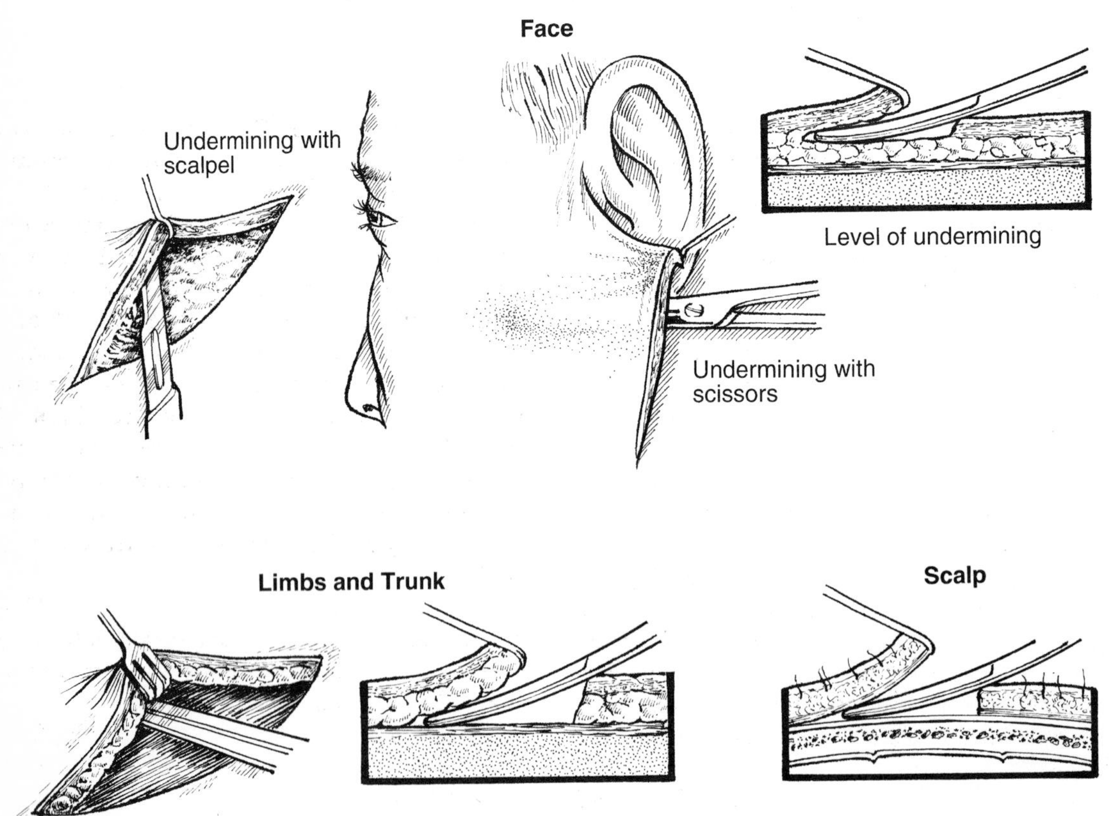

Fig. 1.7 The levels, and the methods used, in undermining in the face, limbs and trunk, and scalp.

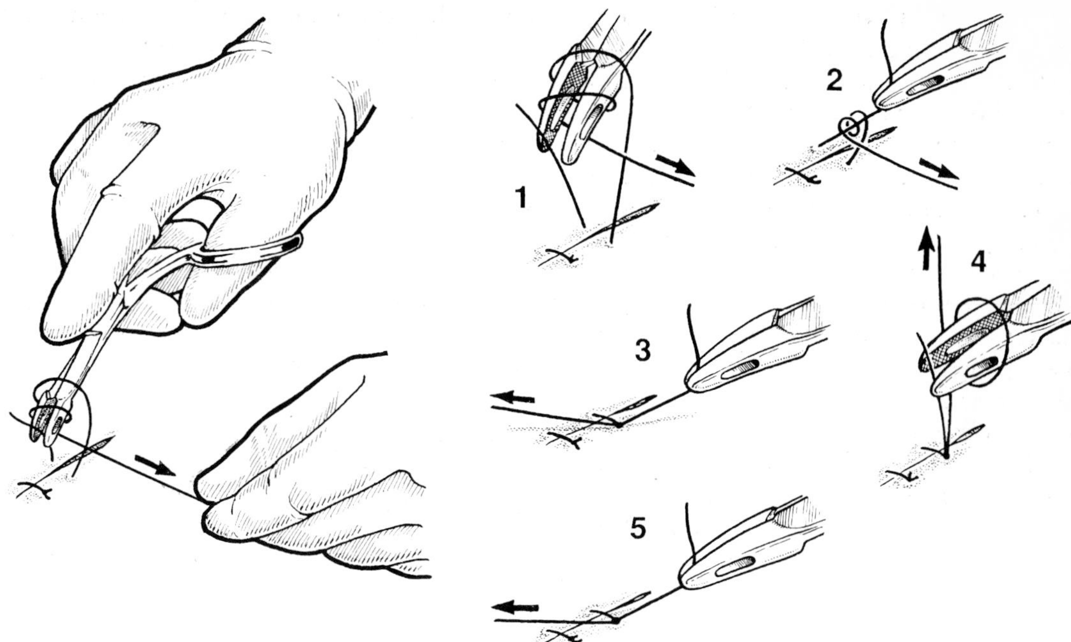

Fig. 1.8 Instrumental tying of a suture.

becomes an extremely precise procedure, preferably using the instrumental method of suture tying (Fig. 1.8). The necessarily small needles and fine suture materials make tying by hand clumsy and difficult. Instrumental tying allows the tension of the suture to be regulated, and knot placement to be carried out with much greater finesse, precision and expedition.

The more a wound is traumatised in the process of suturing the less good is the cosmetic result likely to be and the implements used for holding wound margins steady for suturing should be as atraumatic as possible. The skin hook may cause minimal trauma to the wound margins, but it is difficult to use with elegance and speed, and dissecting forceps are more routinely used. Individual preference will decide whether the toothed or non-toothed variety is used. The decision is immaterial as long as both are used with due regard to the trauma they are causing.

The aim is to produce an accurately and atraumatically coapted wound, and the technique of handling and suturing is merely a means to this end. First time accurate placing of the suture is a habit to acquire. The second attempt is all too often worse than the first, and only results in a moth-eaten wound edge and poor scar.

The needles used are curved and move most readily in a circle. The wrist must therefore be rotated as part of the movement involved so that insertion of the needle and its pull-through are in the line of its curve (Fig. 1.9). Slight oedema of the wound tends to develop for a short time after a wound is sutured and allowance should be made for it in tying the suture. The correct suture tension just avoids blanching the skin held by the suture. Tied too tightly, the suture cuts in more rapidly and is more likely to leave a suture mark.

Sutures may be *interrupted* or *continuous*. When the cosmetic result is all-important interrupted sutures are used, but continuous sutures are often adequate in other circumstances.

Interrupted sutures

The standard suture is the *simple loop suture* (Fig. 1.10). It consists of a simple loop knotted at one or other side of the wound, and aims to bring the

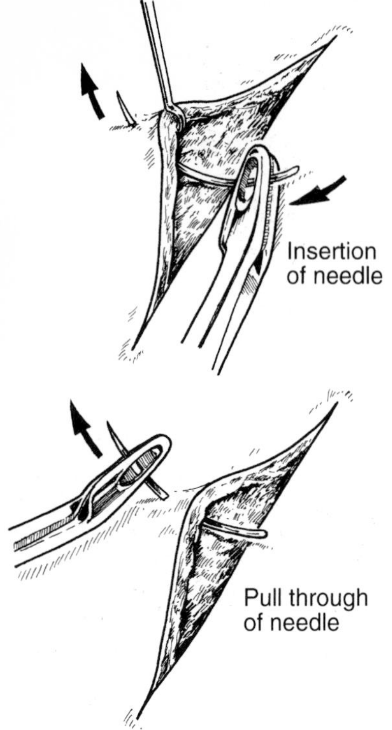

Fig. 1.9 Insertion and pull-through of a needle in the line of the curve of the needle.

skin edges together accurately with no overlapping of one margin. A general tendency towards slight eversion of the suture line helps to ensure complete dermal apposition. It also makes sure that inversion of the wound edges, which generally results in a poorer scar, is avoided.

The suture should include at least the entire thickness of the dermis, and the needle should take an equal bite of each side. The taking of an equal bite can be viewed as the 'coarse adjustment' of getting the wound edges level. One or other edge may remain a little lower than its fellow, and it can be raised to match the levels of the two edges by manipulating the knot in tying to that side of the wound. *Each suture has an optimal side for its knot, and its manipulation is the 'fine adjustment'.*

The desired degree of wound eversion is achieved in several ways. The taking of a slightly greater bite by the needle of its deeper part, dermis or fat, has the effect of approximating the entire face of the wound edge and creates a degree of eversion. The wound edges are also sometimes undermined for 2–4 mm and held everted as the needle is inserted, allowing its path to take the desirable greater deep bite. As already

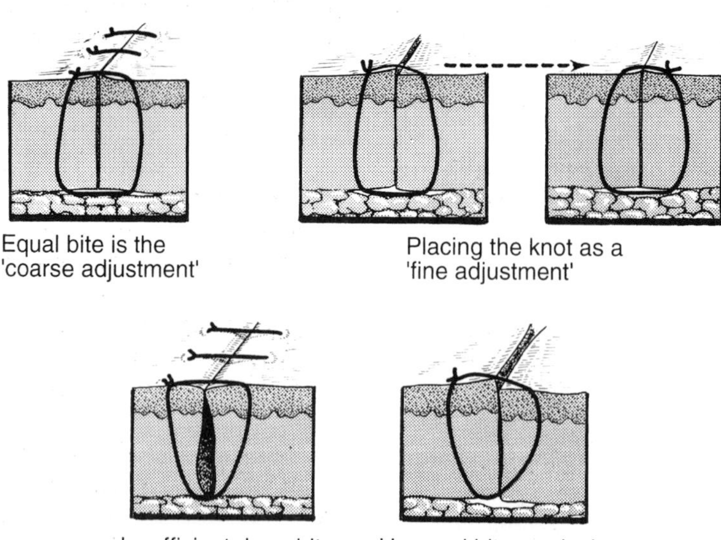

Fig. 1.10 The simple loop suture.

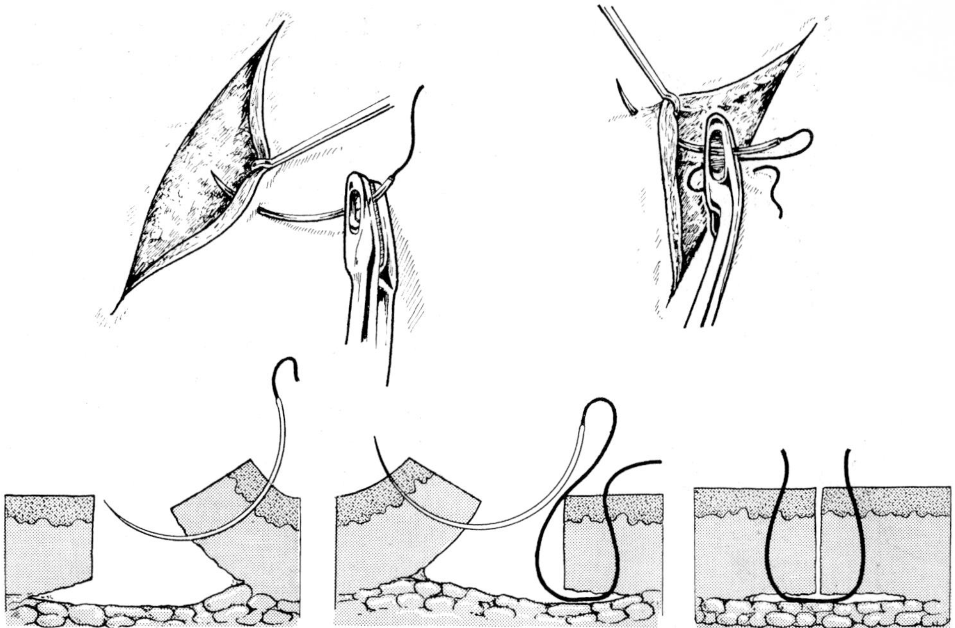

Fig. 1.11 Everting the wound edge with a skin hook before inserting the needle, and the path of the curved needle through the skin.

indicated a skin hook can be used to hold the wound edge everted (Fig. 1.11), though dissecting forceps are more usual. The side of the thumb can also be used effectively to evert the skin during the insertion of the needle (Fig. 1.12). As a rule it is technically easier to suture from the more mobile side of the wound to the more fixed side.

Where the skin is thin and poorly supported, or mobile on its deep surface, e.g. around the eyelids, it is particularly difficult to avoid inversion, and a solution may be to use the *vertical mattress suture* (Fig. 1.13). This suture has no greater tendency to leave suture marks than any other if it is not tied too tightly and is removed early, and if the superficial bite is minimal the tendency to invert is corrected.

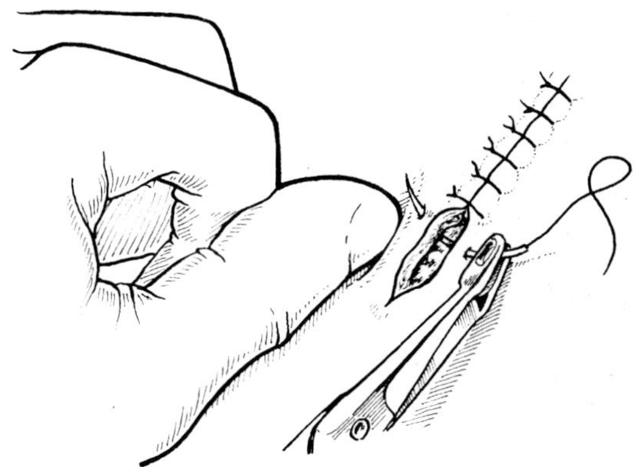

Fig. 1.12 The use of the thumb to evert the skin during the insertion of a suture.

When there is no tension of the wound interrupted sutures alone are adequate. When there is an element of tension the use of *buried absorbable sutures* (Fig. 1.13), or a *continuous intradermal suture* (Fig. 1.13), are described with the aim of allowing early removal of skin sutures without wound disruption or stretching.

Surgeons vary in the extent to which they use buried absorbable sutures to close the skin in layers, as opposed to relying on a single layer of skin sutures. The similarity in the results obtained by surgeons using both techniques would indicate that the routine use of layered closure is not strictly necessary. The method probably has its real value when it is used to eliminate dead space, and prevent haematoma.

The use of a continuous intradermal suture to diffuse wound tension has the merit that the suture can be left in for 10–12 days without

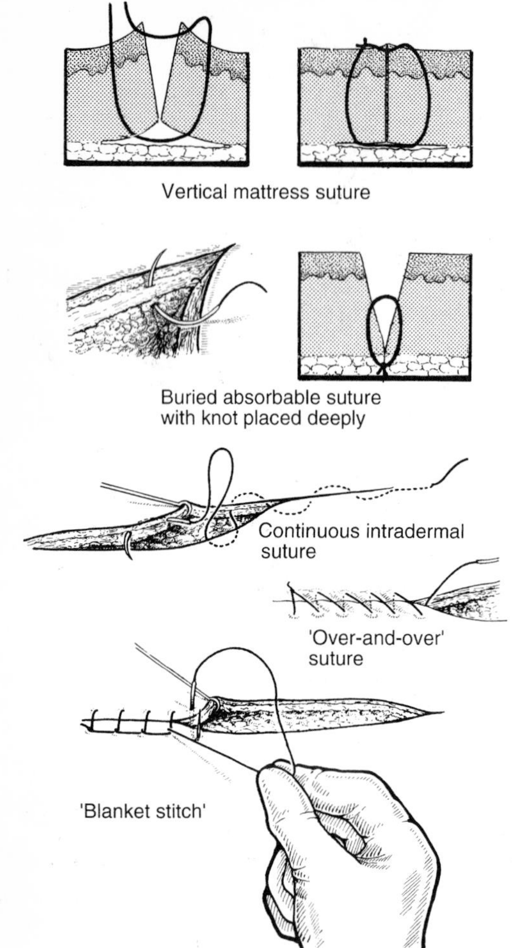

Fig. 1.13 Commonly used types of skin suture.

leaving suture marks. Although it may be used by itself, it will be found that really accurate skin edge apposition is only possible if additional interrupted skin sutures are used. Its role then is to reduce tension on the interrupted sutures, and the smooth surface of monofilament materials used in this capacity makes for easier removal.

Continuous sutures

The most useful continuous sutures are the *'blanket' stitch* and the *continuous 'over-and-over'* (Fig. 1.13). The blanket stitch has the advantage of not 'bunching up' the wound and a double turn at each stitch converts it into a locked suture. The 'over-and-over' suture unfortunately does tend to bunch the wound. Such sutures cannot be placed as accurately as the interrupted suture, but where an impeccable scar is not essential they certainly save time. It is sometimes stated that the continuous suture tends to strangulate the wound edge, but this is the result of unduly tight insertion rather than any inherent defect of the method.

Suture materials

Suture materials are now routinely swaged to an atraumatic needle, and the characteristics which separate one from another concern whether the material is non-absorbable and needs to be removed, or absorbable and can be left *in situ*, the extent to which it causes tissue reaction, and how it handles in clinical practice.

In its handling characteristics, silk remains the bench mark against which other non-absorbable suture materials are measured, but for many surgeons synthetic materials such as nylon and prolene have largely replaced it, because the tissue reaction to their presence is less marked. Their handling characteristics have also improved, though they still do not match those of silk. Using silk, the appropriate degree of eversion of the wound, the correct tension in tying the suture, and the placing of the knot to ensure that the wound edges are accurately apposed, are all easier to achieve than with the synthetics. Local reaction to the silk may be greater, but it lasts only until the suture is removed, when it immediately subsides. The multifilament silk is easier to remove atraumatically than the more rigid monofilament synthetic. In short, the technical aspects of suture insertion and removal are easier with silk than synthetics. The extent to which these virtues might legitimately be considered to offset the temporary adverse tissue reaction which it causes is debatable. There is no objective evidence to suggest that the results achieved with the synthetics are any better than those achieved with silk, but there is also no doubt that to use silk is currently viewed as old fashioned.

The absorbable materials produce a much more severe tissue reaction, and one which continues until they are completely resorbed. The reaction to buried catgut is generally considered to be greater than with the newer synthetic materials, such as Vicryl, Dexon and PDS. This generalisation requires to be analysed in a little more depth, since the amount of the reaction also depends on the volume of the buried material. Even the slower absorption of the newer materials is recognised to be accompanied by the presence of a granuloma at the site of each buried suture, even on occasion an abscess, and these persist as long as the material remains. The minimal reaction when 6-0 catgut is used in closing the skin in the primary repair of a cleft lip in a baby clearly reflects the small amount of catgut in the tissues, and it appears to be more than offset by the absence of the trauma involved in suture removal. Clearly a good deal depends on the circumstances in which the sutures are used.

There is an increasing trend towards the use of inverted absorbable sutures to hold the edges of the dermis together, used with the aim of taking up any tension in the wound, and used along with or without cutaneous non-absorbables or a continuous subcuticular suture. The rationale is that the incidence and severity of cross-hatching is reduced, and that the persistence of the buried sutures will allow formation of the scar to proceed with minimal tension, reducing the degree to which the scar will stretch. Here again, the evidence for this is derived from clinical impression.

DISTRIBUTION OF WOUND TENSION

When a wound is tending to distort, and it is difficult to distribute the tension evenly on both sides for suturing, it often helps to make the wound taut with a skin hook in each end so that a few key sutures can be placed accurately before inserting the intervening sutures. When distortion is to be expected, and especially in a curved incision, trouble will be saved by tattooing matching points (Fig. 1.14) with Bonney's Blue (Pig. Tinctorium, BPC) *(gentian violet, 10 g; brilliant green, 10 g; alcohol 95%, 950 ml; water to 2000 ml)* on either side of the projected incision before any cut is made.

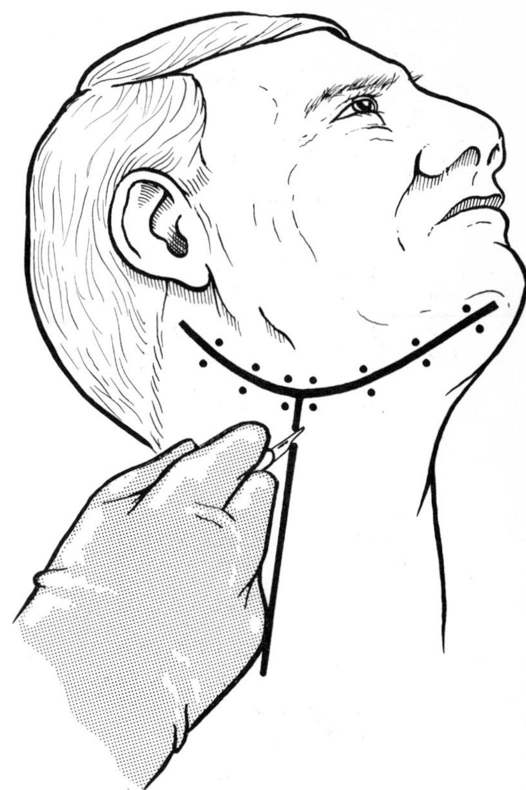

Fig. 1.14 Tattooing matching points with Bonney's Blue before making the skin incision to facilitate matching of corresponding points when the wound is being sutured.

THE THREE-POINT SUTURE

Where a triangular flap has to be inset, it is often difficult to get the tip of the flap to lie in position, yet multiple sutures placed through the full thickness of the dermis are apt to strangulate the tissue at the tip and produce necrosis. In such a situation the three-point suture (Fig. 1.15) helps to avoid necrosis while holding the tip in place. As frequently illustrated the suture tends to bunch the tip of the flap, and a minor variation is recommended which is theoretically sound and effective in practice in holding the tip without bunching. The points to be noted in inserting the suture are *to make sure that the suture leaves and enters the reception side of the wound at the same level in the dermis as its placement in the tip of the V flap* and *make the suture emerge well back on the reception side of the wound.*

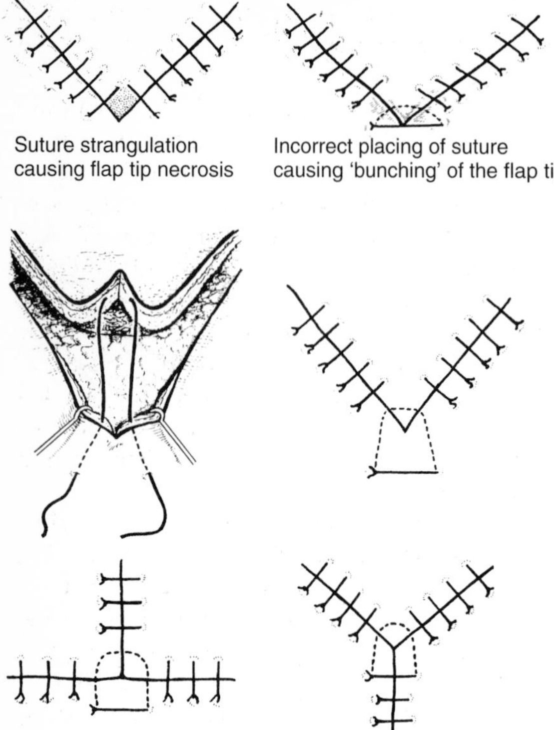

Fig. 1.15 The three-point suture.

The principle of the three-point suture can be extended for use where two flaps are being approximated to the third side of a wound.

LENGTH OF SCAR AND THE 'DOG-EAR'

When an oval or circular lesion is excised and the defect is closed directly the resulting scar is always considerably longer than the original lesion, a fact which it is always wise to explain to the patient.

When the curved lines, ellipse up to circle, resulting from the excision are brought together in a straight line the effect is to lengthen the scar. In addition, closure of the ellipse almost invariably leaves a 'dog-ear' at each end of the suture line, and the correction of this lengthens the scar still further.

To remove a dog-ear (Fig. 1.16) the wound should be sutured until the elevation becomes pronounced. A hook placed in the end of the wound and raised defines the extent of the dog-ear. The elevation is then excised by incising around the base on one or other side, finishing in the line of the wound. The resulting flap is brought across the wound so that the excess skin can be defined and removed. The resulting line has a slight curve and its direction, which depends on the side of the dog-ear cut initially, can be chosen to fit the best line cosmetically.

Failure to remove the dog-ear leaves a rather unsightly swelling (Fig. 1.17), and although it flattens somewhat with the passage of time, it does tend to remain prominent enough to mar an otherwise satisfactory result.

HAEMATOMA

The most important single factor causing complications and bad results where surgery, whether it be incision or flap transfer, has otherwise been soundly planned and adequately carried out is **haematoma**. It provides a culture medium for

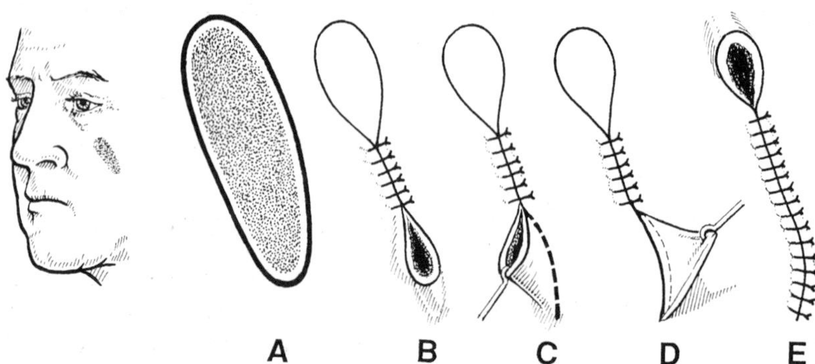

Fig. 1.16 Removal of a 'dog-ear'. Following excision of the lesion (**A**), the margins of the defect are closed directly (**B**) until the 'dog-ear' becomes apparent. The 'dog-ear' is defined with a skin hook, and the skin is incised (**C**) around the base. The excess skin is defined and removed (**D**), and suturing of the wound is completed (**E**).

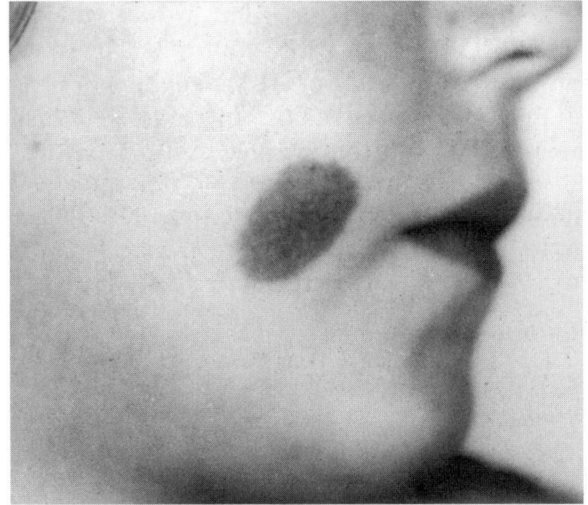

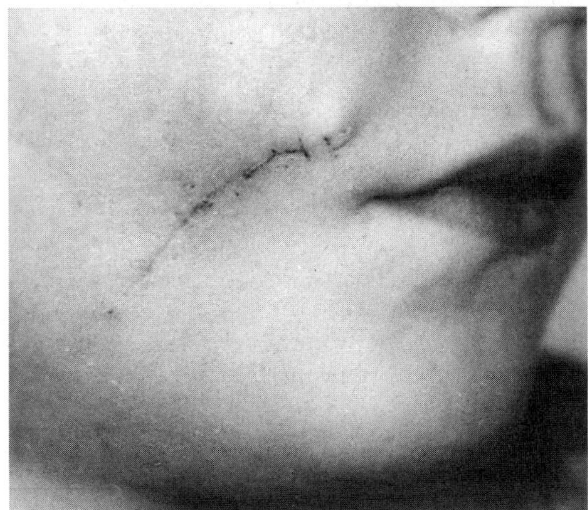

Fig. 1.17 The result of failure to excise a 'dog-ear'.

organisms which in its absence would merely be commensals, and is readily converted into a collection of pus. Even in the absence of infection its presence adds to the general tension of the wound. It acts as a foreign body which, unless evacuated, becomes organised, producing fibrosis and adding to scar tissue formation.

It is generally true that in a wound with an adequate blood supply and no obvious source of contamination, the occurrence of infection can nearly always be traced to haematoma. Indeed it is remarkable just how much contamination a wound can tolerate without clinical sepsis where there is no haematoma.

The aspects of haematoma specific to its occurrence in flap transfer are discussed in Chapter 4. Present discussion is concerned with the more general considerations of its prevention and management.

Even with the greatest care it is not always possible to avoid haematoma, and the problem of treatment then arises. One's natural instinct is to evacuate the clot as soon as it is diagnosed, but while early evacuation is sometimes effective the bleeding which gave rise to the original haematoma is apt to begin again and cause recurrence. In addition the suture line has to be opened enough to allow extrusion of the haematoma and the handling, pressure, etc., needed to squeeze out the fairly solid clot has an unfortunate habit of causing further wound dehiscence.

An alternative method of managing the situation is to await natural liquefaction of the clot, and aspirate it through a polythene intravenous cannula inserted obliquely at a distance from the suture line. At this stage there is no tendency to fresh bleeding and recurrence of the condition. The problem is that liquefaction can take up to 10 days, and in the interval it may become infected. Once infection develops, evacuation by opening the suture line, or even incision and drainage, may be needed although spontaneous discharge may occur. With a low-grade infection, aspiration may suffice if the clot *cum* pus has become sufficiently fluid.

Haematoma is very much a condition where prevention is better than cure, and the main measures used to prevent its occurrence are meticulous haemostasis and the avoidance of dead space. Where a potential dead space is unavoidable, the use of suction drainage is the most effective prophylactic. Apart from its effectiveness, it has the virtue, in contrast to the use of pressure dressings which hide the situation until the haematoma is well established, of allowing the local state to be continuously monitored.

POSTOPERATIVE CARE

The aim of good postoperative treatment is to *prevent haematoma*, *provide rest for healing*, and *prevent suture marks*. In practice this is achieved by the dressing, care in suture removal, and later support of the wound.

The dressing

In the past, the use of pressure dressings was standard, with or without a drain. The pressure dressing, apart from preventing haematoma, created the immobility and splinting which were considered to provide the best conditions for rapid, uneventful healing. With the increased use of suction drainage there has been a marked reduction in the use of dressings generally, with exposure of the wound site increasingly standard practice in combination with suction drainage if necessary.

When a dressing is used, the wide mesh of a single layer of tulle gras — *tulle fabric impregnated with petroleum jelly* — allows the passage of any discharge, and this combined with the petroleum jelly base make it a particularly good dressing, permitting its removal with the minimum of trauma from sticking. Over the tulle gras, gauze and wool followed by a crepe bandage will give adequate, cushioned pressure and immobility. Elastoplast may replace the crepe bandage in suitable circumstances, and the adhesive properties of the Elastoplast can be considerably enhanced by preliminary painting of the skin with Mastisol.

An alternative dressing which can be applied directly to the suture line is 'micropore' skin tape. It does not macerate the skin, supports the wound well and yet, peeled off slowly, sticks neither to suture or hair. Applied directly over the wound, its adhesiveness encourages the wound edges to lie flush, a useful attribute when flap tips are tending to lie a little proud of the wound as a whole. If no undermining has been used, such tape can provide the sole dressing. Apart from its role in the sutured wound, it can also on occasion be used to coapt wound edges and obviate the need for sutures at all, a considerable virtue when the young child with a laceration is being treated.

When the wound is exposed it is desirable to keep the suture line free of blood until the fibrin clot covering the line of the wound is firm and dry. A mild degree of reaction at the site of the sutures is not uncommon, settling when they are removed and seeming not to affect the final result adversely. The severity of the reaction seems to parallel the degree of sebaceous activity in the particular area of the face and in the individual patient. The use of Chloramphenicol ointment, conveniently applied from the small tube designed for ophthalmic use, has been found to eliminate this reaction to a considerable extent, and it has the incidental virtue of softening any minor discharge around the individual sutures and facilitating their removal.

Suture removal

Set days are apt to be laid down for the removal of sutures in various sites and under varying

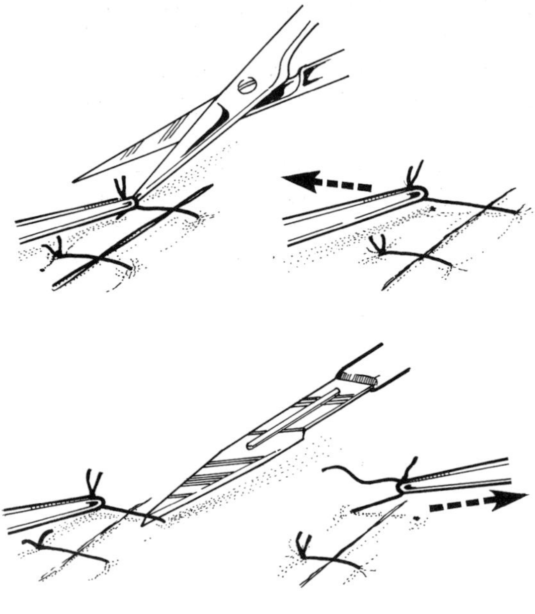

Correct methods

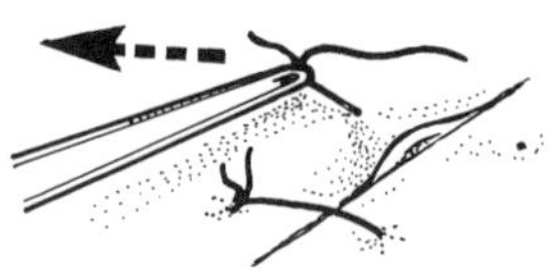

Incorrect method

Fig. 1.18 The technique of suture removal, showing the use of iris scissors and a No. 11 scalpel blade.

Correctly removed, the suture is pulled towards the wound. Incorrect removal, pulling the suture away from the wound, causes added tension across the wound, and is liable to result in dehiscence.

circumstances, but this approach is quite wrong. The principle is to remove at the earliest time judged safe, and this depends on so many factors, degree of tension, site, line of wound, etc., that it is quite impossible to lay down hard and fast rules. In any case clinical experience soon tells the surgeon when a suture may be removed safely.

In removing the suture (Fig. 1.18) it must be remembered that the tensile strength of the wound is minimal, and dehiscence is liable to occur on the slightest provocation. Where most care is needed, the sutures are usually smallest, and prerequisites for safe removal are a good light, fine, sharp scissors which cut to the point, and fine dissecting forceps which grip properly. The technique of removal is not radically different from suture removal in other surgical contexts, except for the degree of gentleness which is necessary and the fact that the suture, once cut, must be pulled out *towards* the wound, not away from it. In removal, as in insertion of the suture, the surgeon should have his elbows well supported, and work from wrist and fingers to give smooth movements without tremor. The patient should also be carefully supported so that the suture line stays absolutely still.

Scissors are not invariably sharp, nor do they always cut to the point, and a good alternative method is to use the triangular tip of a No. 11 scalpel blade (Fig. 1.18) to cut the suture. In a difficult situation its sharp point will often cut the suture with less disturbance of the wound than scissors.

Subsequent support of the wound

Early suture removal leaves the wound devoid of strength, and a sudden ill-judged tension strain may cause it to dehisce. For this reason the wound is best supported or at very least protected for up to a week after suture removal, and micropore skin tape works well in this role. It is seldom practicable to support the wound much beyond this, and indeed attempts to prevent later stretching of the wound by prolonged support are of little avail.

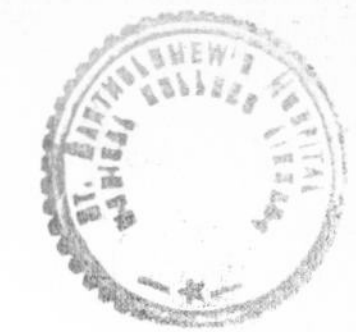

CHAPTER 2

The Z-plasty

The Z-plasty is a procedure which involves the transposition of two interdigitating triangular flaps. The name derives from the 'Z' shape seen when the three limbs of the flaps are drawn out on the skin. Transposition of the flaps has several effects (Fig. 2.1), of which two have special relevance:

1. There is a gain in length along the direction of the common limb of the Z.
2. The direction of the common limb of the Z is changed.

Exploitation of these effects has made the Z-plasty

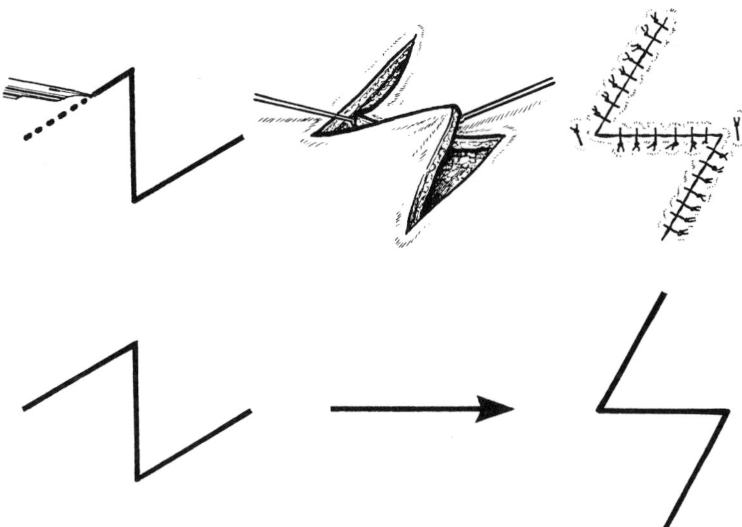

Fig. 2.1 The Z-plasty.

an extremely useful and widely used procedure. Its value has been most strikingly established in three sets of circumstances, in the **treatment of contracted scars**, when use is made of the gain in length, in the **management of facial scars**, when use is made of the change in direction of the common limb, and in the **prevention of scar contracture** in certain types of elective and emergency surgery, particularly in the hand. This latter usage is discussed in Chapter 11.

Lengthening and change of direction of the common limb occur together as a result of transposition, but it is usually only one of the two which concerns the surgeon at any particular time. The fact that the other is accomplished at the same time is usually a bonus, though it can be a nuisance.

THEORETICAL BASIS

The Z-plasty was originally used in releasing contracted scars, and its theoretical basis can be more easily understood if it is considered with that as the background.

The basic manoeuvre

When the Z-plasty is used to release a contracture, the common limb, i.e. the central limb of the Z, is positioned along the line of the contracture. The size of each of the angles of the Z is 60°, a compromise figure which has been reached as a result of experience. The reasons for selecting this angle size and the effects of altering it are discussed later, but 60° will be the size used in the present discussion.

Constructed in this way the two triangles together have the shape of a parallelogram with its shorter diagonal in the line of the contracture, its longer diagonal perpendicular to it. The two diagonals can conveniently be referred to as the **contractural diagonal** and the **transverse diagonal** (Fig. 2.2).

In order to understand the sequence of events when a Z-plasty is used in releasing a contracture it is essential to bear in mind that the common limb of the Z, being along the line of the contracture, is under tension. Its ends spring apart when the interdigitating flaps are raised and the fibrous tissue band responsible for the contracture is divided. The springing apart of the divided contracture results in a change in the shape of the parallelogram, and the triangular flaps become transposed, the contractural diagonal lengthens and the transverse diagonal shortens (Fig. 2.3).

It is important to appreciate that when a Z-plasty is used properly to correct a linear contracture the surgeon does not actively transpose the Z flaps. Flap transposition follows naturally from the change in shape of the parallelogram, as do the lengthening and the shortening.

The changes in length are such that the length of the contractural diagonal after transposition equals that of the transverse diagonal before transposition. The contractural diagonal has lengthened at the expense of the transverse diagonal, which

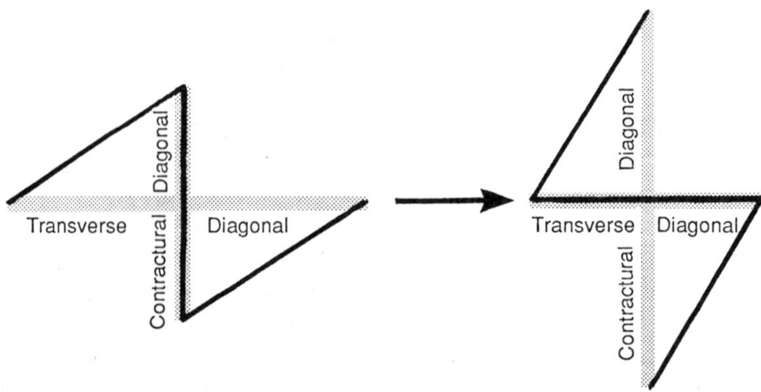

Fig. 2.2 The diagonals of the Z-plasty, showing how, with transposition of the Z-plasty flaps, the contractural diagonal is lengthened and the transverse diagonal is shortened.

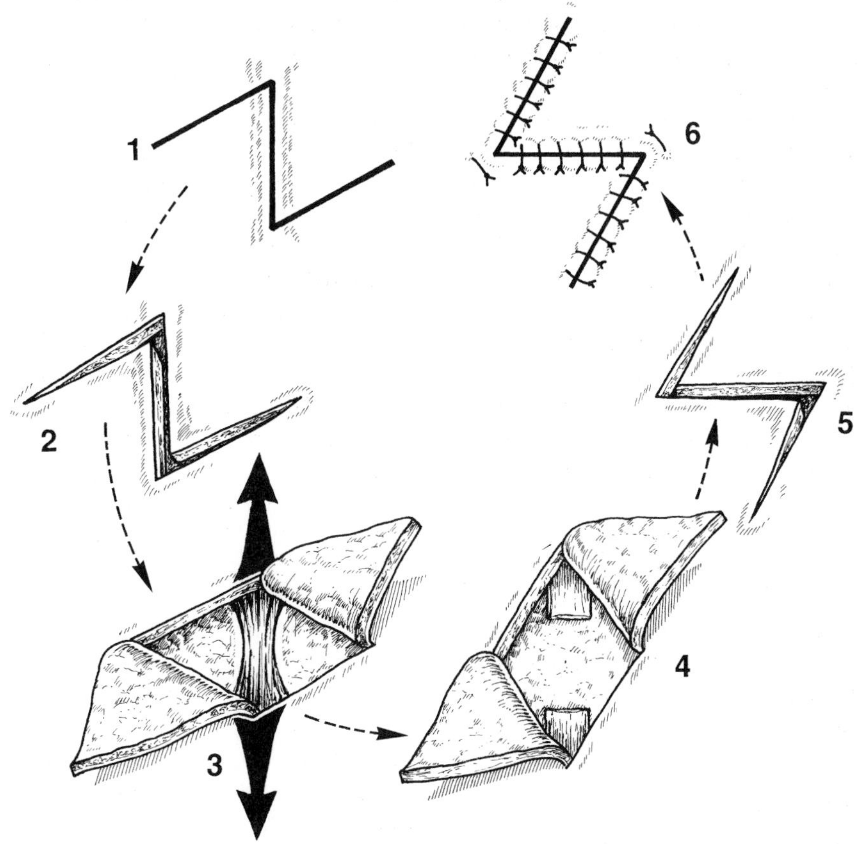

Fig. 2.3 The several stages of the Z-plasty, demonstrating how division of the contracture, shown diagrammatically as a single band, has the effect of changing the shape of the Z, lengthening the contractural diagonal and shortening the transverse diagonal.

has shortened as much as the contractural diagonal has lengthened.

Translated into practical terms this means that skin has been brought in from the sides with a tightening effect, as shown by the shortening of the transverse diagonal, to allow the lengthening of the contractural diagonal. The difference in length of the two diagonals indicates the actual amount of lengthening and shortening.

The surgeon's interest is in the lengthening rather than the shortening, but it is crucial to successful Z-plasty practice to realise that lengthening cannot take place without the transverse shortening. Translated into practical terms, this means that unless there is transverse skin slack available, equal in quantity to the length difference between the axes of the Z, the method will not work.

Variables in construction

Since the skin flaps must fit together in their transposed position the limbs of the Z are constructed equal in length. The angles of the Z are also usually made equal in size. The factors which do vary are **angle size** and **limb length**, and the ways in which variation in these factors affects the result provide an explanation of why specific constructions are used in particular sets of circumstances.

Angle size. Once the lengths of the limbs of the Z have been fixed the amount of lengthening to be expected is determined by the size of the angle, its amount increasing with increase in the size of the angle. With an angle of 30° there is theoretically a 25% increase in the original length, with 45° a 50% increase, and with an angle of

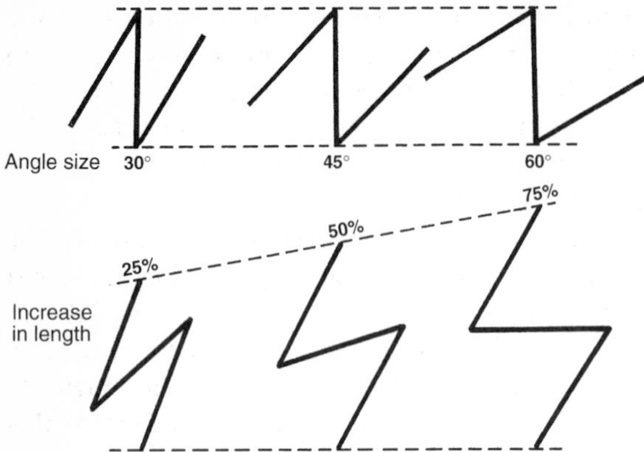

Fig. 2.4 The changes in the percentage increase of length which results from the use of different angle sizes.

60° the increase rises to 75% (Fig. 2.4). These increases are theoretical and they cannot be applied with strict accuracy to the clinical situation, though when account is taken of variations in skin extensibility, pre-existing scarring, etc., it is surprising how well they do apply. The theoretical lengthening usually exceeds slightly what can be achieved in practice.

In releasing a contracture the object of the Z-plasty is to maximise the amount of lengthening. Narrowing the angle much below 60° would defeat this object, since the smaller angle would reduce the gain in length, and adversely influence the blood supply of the flaps.

Increase in angle size much beyond 60° would increase the amount of lengthening, but it would also entail an equal increase in the amount of transverse shortening. Tissue for transverse shortening is seldom available in unlimited quantity, and it is found in practice that when the angle increases beyond 60° the tension produced in the surrounding tissues tends to be so great that the flaps cannot readily be brought into their transposed position. For this reason 60° is the compromise figure used for angle size.

Limb length. With the use of 60° as the routine Z-plasty angle, it is length of limb which provides the major variable in practice. The amount of tissue available on either side determines the practicable limb length — a large amount permits a large Z, a small amount correspondingly limits the size of the Z.

Single and multiple Z-plasty

The search for ways of reducing the amount of transverse shortening without significantly affecting the amount of lengthening has led to the development of the multiple Z-plasty, and its advantages are such that it has replaced the single Z-plasty in many clinical situations.

In the single Z-plasty one large Z extends along virtually the entire length of the contracture; in the multiple Z-plasty the contracture is viewed as having a number of segments, on each of which a small Z-plasty is constructed.

The contrast between the two types of Z-plasty can best be appreciated by using a concrete example. If we construct a single Z-plasty which is going to achieve 2 cm of lengthening, and at the same time construct a series of four small Z-plasties, each equal in size to a quarter of the single Z-plasty, they can be compared from the point of view of lengthening and shortening (Fig. 2.5).

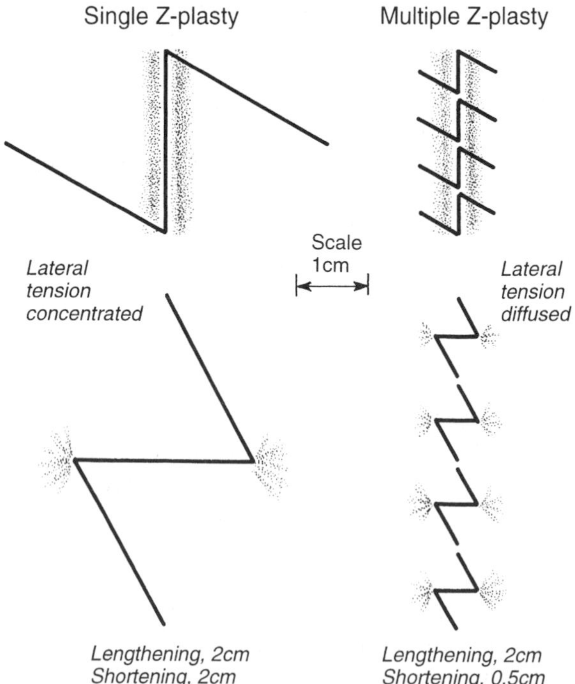

Fig. 2.5 Comparison of the lengthening and shortening produced by a single and a multiple Z-plasty. Note also how lateral tension is concentrated by the single Z-plasty and diffused by the multiple Z-plasty.

The single Z-plasty achieves 2 cm of lengthening and at the same time there is 2 cm of shortening in the transverse axis.

In the multiple Z-plasty, each of the four Z-plasties achieves 0.5 cm of lengthening with a corresponding 0.5 cm of shortening at each transverse axis. The lengthening which occurs is in series and consequently is additive, giving an overall lengthening of 2 cm, while the shortening is in parallel, and remains 0.5 cm at each Z. The amount of lengthening achieved by each is thus the same, but the shortening has been greatly reduced by the use of the multiple Z-plasty. Many clinical situations exist where a Z-plasty could be used to advantage, but the tissues cannot stand 2 cm of shortening, though they could tolerate 0.5 cm with ease, and for these the multiple Z-plasty is a possible solution.

The change from single to multiple Z-plasty also alters the form of the lateral tension. From being concentrated in the line of the transverse limb of the single Z, it is spread over the several transverse limbs of the multiple Z-plasty in addition to being reduced. These differences have obvious advantages from a vascular point of view.

In the multiple Z-plasty, as in the single Z-plasty, the theoretical lengthening is probably unattainable. Quite apart from the effect of scarring, etc., there tends to be some loss of lengthening in passage from one Z to the next. Nevertheless the comparison between the two, and the advantages of the multiple over the single, are still valid.

Blood supply of the flaps

The most frequent complication of a Z-plasty is necrosis of the tip of a flap and it is a particular hazard when there is scarring of the skin or, more commonly, when the skin flap raised has to be excessively thin, e.g. in Dupuytren's contracture involving the finger, a problem discussed in greater detail on p. 194. Precautions to avoid necrosis can be taken at all stages of the procedure — by providing the flaps with the maximum of vascular capacity, and by avoiding tension.

Provision of maximum vascular capacity. This is achieved by designing the flaps broad at the tip, by cutting the flaps as thick as possible, and by avoiding scarring across the base. The tip of the flap can be broadened by modifying its shape slightly without affecting its angle size (Fig. 2.6). The thickest flap practicable should always be cut, making use of the levels of undermining described on p. 10.

Avoidance of undue tension. Tension in the transposed flaps can be very difficult to avoid particularly when the contracture is a dubious candidate for a Z-plasty. Indeed its presence is usually an indication of this fact. The single Z-plasty, with its large flaps, is more prone to this problem, since it concentrates transverse tension; the smaller flaps of the multiple Z-plasty are less liable, since their effect is to reduce and diffuse the transverse tension, thereby minimising circulatory embarrassment.

CLINICAL USAGE

The Z-plasty is used in different clinical situations, in some of which the theoretical basis of the procedure is not immediately obvious, but in each one analysis of the changes which take place with transposition of the flaps is capable of explaining the effect of the change in terms of lengthening and shortening, or of a change in the direction of the common limb.

Use in contractures

From the theoretical discussion it follows that the Z-plasty is most effective where the contracture is narrow and the surrounding tissues are reasonably lax. Scarred and contracted tissue on either side can yield no 'slack' to allow lengthening, which explains why the postburn contracture is

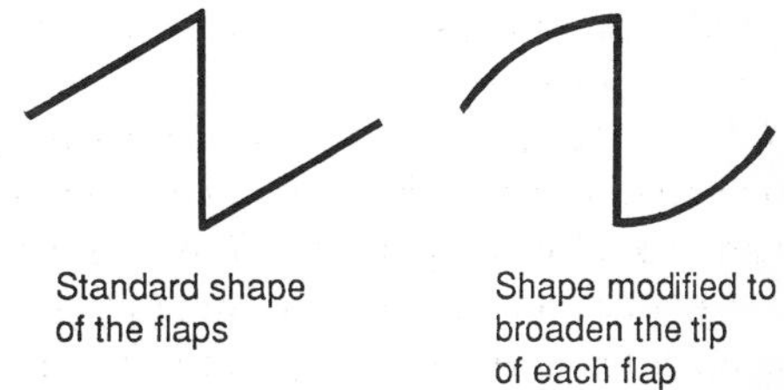

Fig. 2.6 The modified shape of the Z-plasty flaps which gives maximum vascular capacity.

so seldom totally correctable by a Z-plasty, single or multiple. In contracting, the burn scar contracts in all directions simultaneously, and although a contracture may be present clinically, skin has actually been lost in every axis. The contractural axis is only the most obviously tight. The transverse axis is just as short and it is unable to shorten any further in the way that would be needed for a successful Z-plasty.

Ideally, the central limb of the Z should extend the full length of the contracture but this requires a correspondingly large quantity of tissue to be brought in from the sides, tissue which is not always available. The problem arises in the limbs particularly, for such tissue as is available tends to be spread out along the length of the limb rather than being concentrated at one point. As has been discussed above, the solution in such circumstances is likely to lie in constructing a multiple Z-plasty rather than a single Z-plasty, bringing in from the sides smaller quantities of tissue along the entire length of the contracture (Fig. 2.5).

A good measure of the planning and execution of a Z-plasty is the behaviour of the flaps when the contracture is released. If the manoeuvre has been well planned and carried out the flaps should literally fall into their transposed position. Indeed it should be difficult to return them to their old relationship.

The Z-plasty, single or multiple, is most effective when the contracture is of the bowstring type. When the contracture is more diffuse it is less satisfactory, and a stage is eventually reached where the decision has to be made whether a Z-plasty is appropriate at all, or whether fresh skin should be imported from elsewhere in the form of a free skin graft or flap. The answer is usually to be found in the surrounding skin; transverse slack must be present if the contracture is to be released and if it is not obviously available there (Fig. 2.7) the Z-plasty will fail.

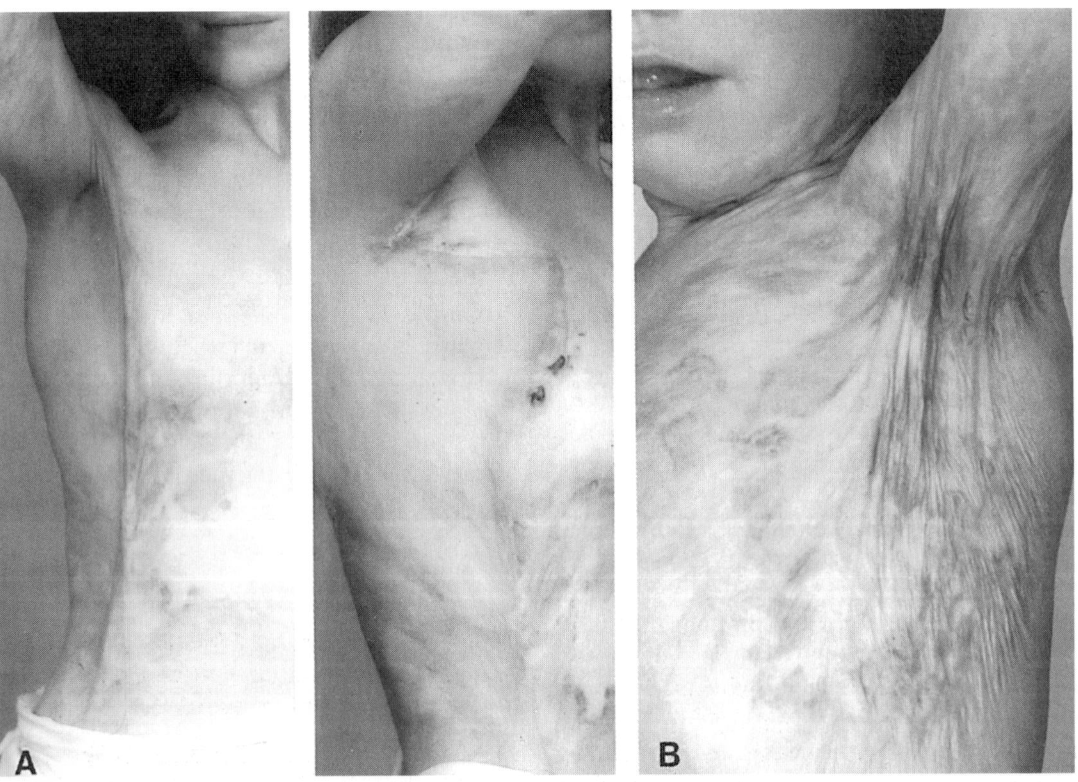

Fig. 2.7 A narrow axillary contracture (**A**), suitable for correction by a Z-plasty, and a diffuse axillary contracture (**B**), unsuitable for a Z-plasty, and requiring for its correction the insertion of a split skin graft.

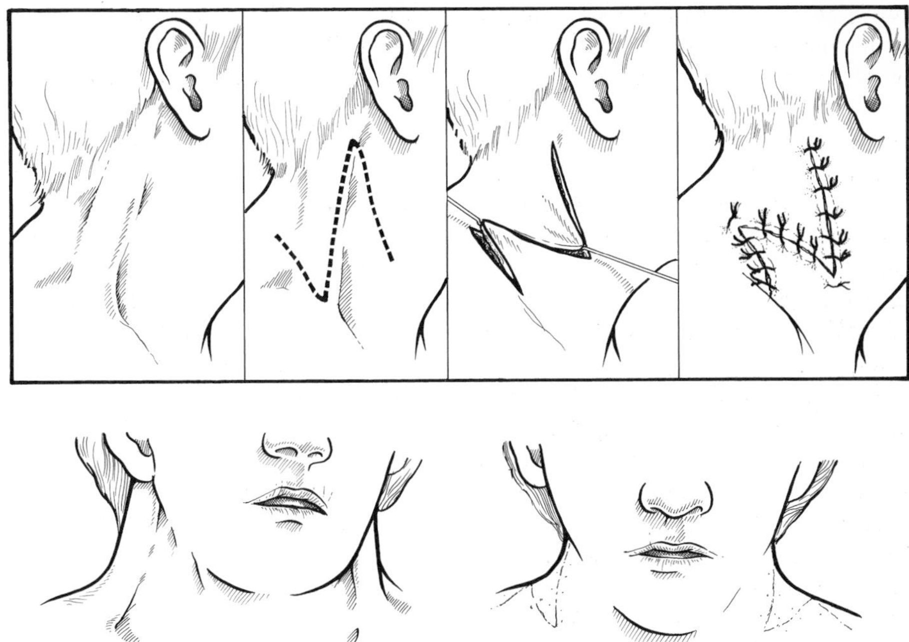

Figure 2.8 The use of a single Z-plasty to correct the neck webbing component of Turner's syndrome.

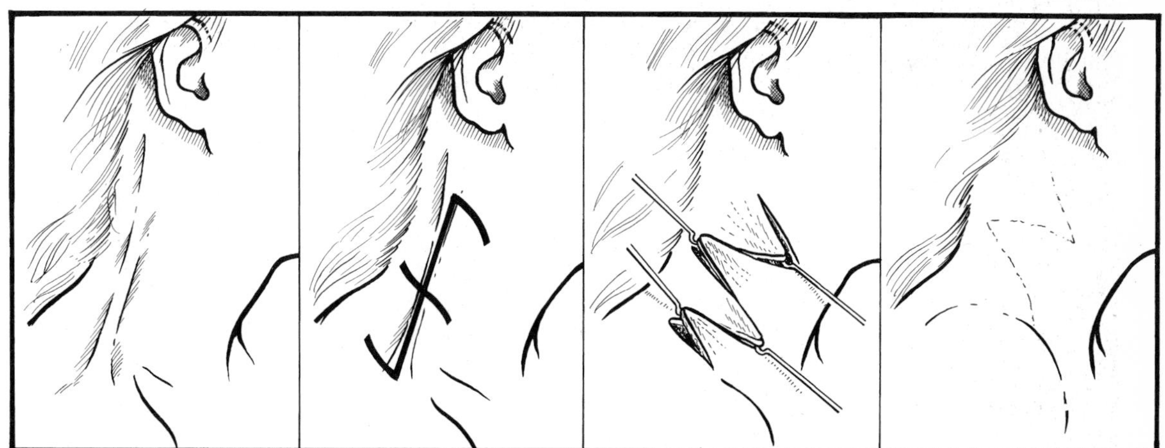

Fig. 2.9 The use of a multiple Z-plasty in correcting a localised postburn contracture of the neck.

Planning the Z-plasty (Figs 2.8, 2.9)

It may be difficult in planning the procedure to decide where the flaps should be. A good method is to draw an equilateral triangle on each side of the contracture (see Fig. 11.6), and to select the more suitable of the two sets of limbs from the resulting parallelogram. If neither has any demonstrable advantage either may be used.

Factors which might favour one set are:

1. The flap with the better blood supply is preferable. In particular a potential flap with scarring across the base should be avoided.

2. One flap may result in a scar which will fall into a better line cosmetically. The factors which would influence the choice in such circumstances have already been discussed in Chapter 1.
3. The lie of the flaps and the surrounding skin may permit one set of flaps to rotate more readily into their new position.

Skin which shows scarring has lost some of its normal elasticity and this may affect the planning of the flaps. A flap of scarred skin should be designed a little longer initially than its fellow of normal skin, otherwise the scarred flap will be found to be too short when it is sutured to the unscarred flap.

It is usual, although not essential, to have the two angles of equal size. On occasion a line of scarring can limit the angle of one flap and dissimilar angles may then have to be used. Lengthening and shortening then become the average of the amount to be expected from each angle alone. Indeed, if the full quadrilateral of any Z-plasty is drawn, complete with contractural and transverse diagonals, the transverse diagonal will provide an indication of the actual length to be expected when the flaps are transposed.

The multiple Z-plasty

In designing a multiple Z-plasty the line of the contracture can be viewed as a series of contracted segments, on each of which a small Z-plasty is constructed, creating a line of individual Z-plasties, but in practice it is more usual to construct them in the form of a **continuous multiple Z-plasty** (Fig. 2.10). In this, the Zs, instead of being individual, are designed as a continuous series with a single line along the length of the contracture and multiple Z side limbs (Fig. 11.7). In theory such a multiple Z-plasty can be constructed with the side limbs parallel or skew. The presence of scarring in a particular line may influence the construction and make skew flaps preferable, but the use of parallel limbs allows the flaps to rotate uniformly. It also avoids the construction of a broad-tipped flap with a narrow base, undesirable from a vascular point of view, and unavoidable with the skew construction.

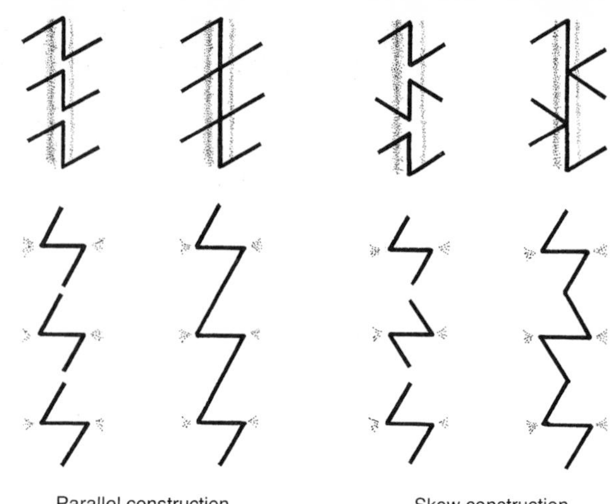

Fig. 2.10 The evolution of the parallel and skew types of the continuous multiple Z-plasty from a series of interrupted small Z-plasties.

Whether a multiple Z-plasty has to be used largely depends on the depth of the bowstring. It is unwise to take the side limbs much beyond the base of the bowstring, and if the making of a large Z would encroach on the surrounding flat skin to any extent, especially if the skin tends to be taut, a multiple Z-plasty (Fig. 2.9) is safer and on the whole just as effective.

Use in facial scars

Scars in the face tend to be more cosmetically acceptable the more nearly they lie in a line of election, and a problem of acceptability can arise when an otherwise satisfactory scar is more than 30° off the line of election. When a Z-plasty is used to improve the appearance of a scar, its effect as a rule is to break the line of the scar and change its direction. This change in direction involves the common limb of the Z-plasty, and the object is to place it postoperatively as nearly as possible in a line of election.

The success of the method used to place the common limb of the completed Z-plasty accurately in terms of size, site, and direction depends on two facts. First, if the Z-plasty incisions are made to end on the selected transverse line, transposition of the flaps will leave the common limb lying along the line as planned (Fig. 2.11).

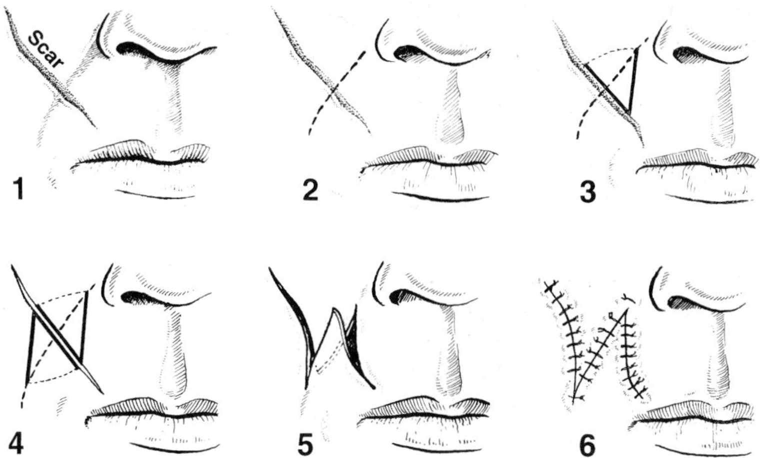

Fig. 2.11 The steps in planning a Z-plasty so that the transverse limb of the completed Z-plasty lies in a predetermined line, in this instance the line of the nasolabial fold.

Second, the limbs of the Z-plasty are equal in length.

The planning of the Z-plasty used for this purpose must be regarded as a formal procedure, marked out carefully on the skin with Bonney's Blue before any actual incision is made. The steps themselves are more easily illustrated than described (Figs 2.11, 2.12).

With the scar outlined (1), the line, preferably in a line of election, is selected for the postoperative common limb, and drawn out on the skin (2). The length of the intended common limb, which determines the size of the Z-plasty, is measured out on the line of the scar, proportioned approximately evenly on each side of the line already selected and drawn out as the postoperative common limb (3). From each extremity of this measured length, a line of equal length is marked out to meet the line drawn out to represent the postoperative common limb (4). These steps outline the Z-plasty flaps (5). The fact that the two oblique lines have been made to end on the selected transverse line means that transposition of the flaps will bring the common limb into the desired line as planned regardless of its direction (6).

Altering the obliquity of the line selected for the postoperative common limb has the effect of altering the size of the Z-plasty angle. Increase of obliquity reduces the angle and decrease of obliquity increases the angle, to a maximum of 60°, at which point the common limb becomes perpendicular to the line of the scar.

As the common limb departs from the perpendicular the flap becomes narrower and the blood supply to its tip increasingly tenuous. Facial skin with its excellent blood supply is more tolerant of narrow flaps than skin elsewhere on the body surface, but even in the face there is a limit to permissible narrowness. A tip angle of 35° is as narrow as can be used with safety. Even then care in suturing near the tip of each flap is necessary (Fig. 2.13). Fortunately the angle size can be gauged at the planning stage before any incision is made.

In the long facial scar it may be desirable to break the line with more than a single Z-plasty. Scars are not invariably straight and lines of election usually run in different directions in different parts of the scar. Each Z-plasty has generally to be planned strictly on its own, with its individual and quite distinct obliquity. The effect is to convert the single linear scar into a series of smaller scars joined by transverse limbs in lines of election, ideally in actual wrinkle lines. Even at worst, several small scars tend to be less conspicuous than a single long scar. It is also found that a large Z-plasty does not give as good a result as the smaller Z-plasty. In planning therefore, the estimated length of the transverse limb should be kept fairly small (Fig. 2.13).

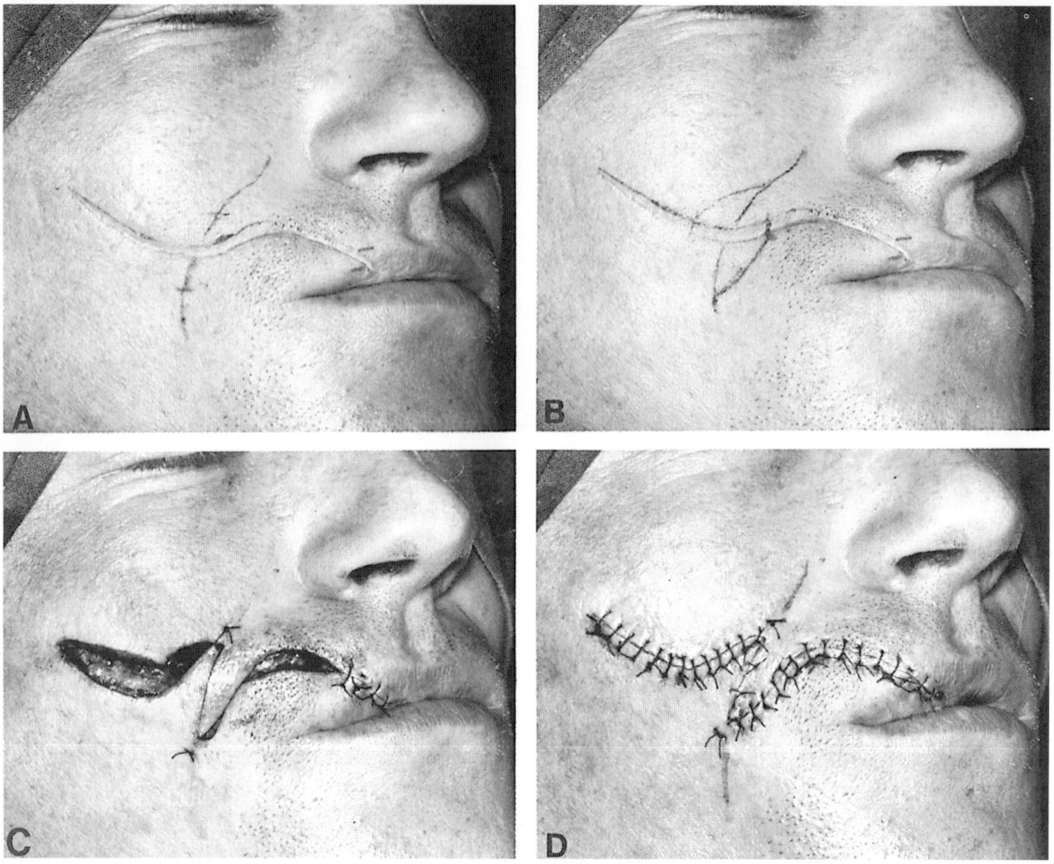

Fig. 2.12 The use of the method shown in Figure 2.11 in revising a scar crossing the nasolabial fold.

A The scar outlined, and the line of election – the nasolabial fold.
B The lines of the Z, all equal in length, and with each oblique line ending on the line of election.
C The scar excised, and the Z flaps transposed.
D The procedure completed with the transverse limb of the Z lying along the line of election as planned.

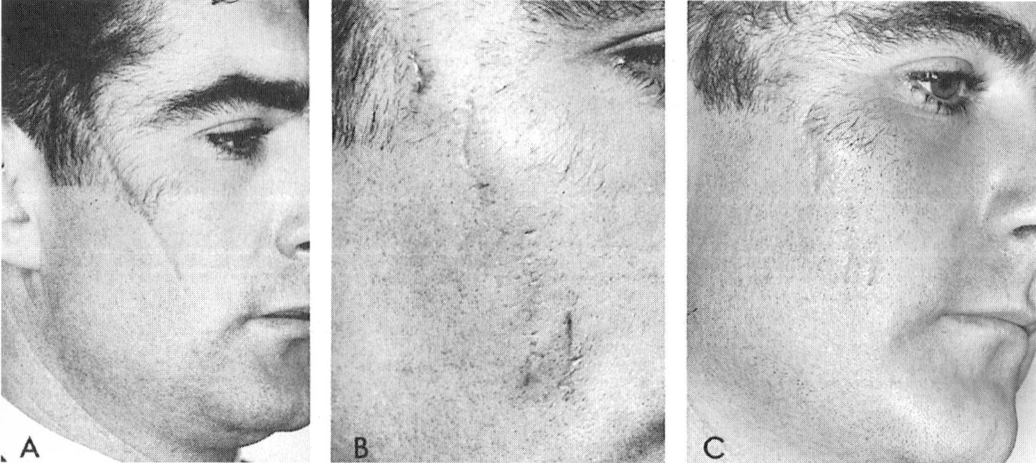

Fig. 2.13 Scar excision with three Z-plasty inserts. Each insert has been individually planned to place its transverse limb in the direction of the local line of election.

When a multiple Z-plasty is used to break up a facial scar simultaneous lengthening takes place, and this shows as an overlapping of the flaps as they pass from one Z to the next. Trimming of the overlap is usually required in order to reduce the overall lengthening.

Patient selection

Whether or not to incorporate a Z-plasty in revising a particular facial scar can be an extremely difficult decision. Revision, with or without a Z-plasty, is generally postponed until the scar has largely settled, and the improvement in its appearance is near maximal. Revision, incorporating one or more Z-plasties, involves increasing the length of the wound significantly, and the early result all too often appears disappointing both to surgeon and patient. Only once the reaction has slowly settled, and the scars soften once again, does the benefit become apparent.

Consideration of how the original scar has behaved may be of help in deciding. Any suggestion of hypertrophy of the original scar should be seen as a warning against any revision, let alone one which incorporates a Z-plasty. The patient who already has a marked wrinkle pattern tends to be a better than average candidate, particularly if the scar has become pale and matches the surrounding skin well. The smooth, uncreased adult skin should be viewed with caution.

The completely settled scar which has remained conspicuous because it continues to be redder than the surrounding skin, as some scars do even though they have become quite soft, is a bad candidate. The end result is likely merely to be a longer red scar, for each transverse limb stays as red as the rest of the scar and its line fails to merge into the background despite being in a line of election. The problem is seen most often in the patient with the so-called Celtic skin.

A conservative approach to the use of the Z-plasty in facial scars has much to be said for it, confining its use to the patient in whom revision will allow an obvious line of election, such as the nasolabial fold, to be used in breaking the line.

The use of the Z-plasty in the revision of facial scars in children is generally contraindicated. Scars as a whole are not considered to behave well in children in any case, but an added reason is the smoothness of their skin, and the absence of wrinkles in which a scar can be concealed.

Use in bridle scars

When a scar crosses a hollow, contraction along its length tends to give rise to a ridged or bridle scar bridging the hollow. Such a scar has similarities to a straightforward contracture and the solution is equally the use of a Z-plasty (Fig. 2.14).

Correction of the bridle element requires an increase in the length of the scar to allow it to sit into the hollow which it is bridging, but it is also necessary to shorten the distance from the skin in the hollow on one side of the scar as it rises to the line of the scar and drops to the hollow on its other side. These two axes are at right angles to each other, and if they are viewed as the axes of a Z-plasty constructed around them, transposition of the flaps will result in lengthening of the axis along the line of the scar allowing it to sit into the hollow, while shortening of the other axis will pull the line of the scar down into the hollow (Fig. 2.15).

When the scar is short and the hollow is deep the lengthening of the scar which follows transposition of the flaps of a single Z-plasty may be matched by the reduction in length of the transverse axis crossing the line of the scar, and a single Z-plasty (Fig. 2.15(1)) extending along the greater part of the length of the scar is then likely to be effective.

Where the bridle scar is longer and relatively shallow the amount of shortening of the axis crossing the line of the scar may be quite small compared with the amount of lengthening required to allow the scar to lie in the hollow, but the shortening may need to be repeated along the line of the scar. In such a situation a multiple Z-plasty would be the version to use (Fig. 2.15(2)). Depending on the site of the bridle scar, the detailed planning of such a multiple Z-plasty may involve the added complication of trying to fit the transverse limbs into a line of election. As long as it is remembered that each transverse limb can be positioned independently using the method shown in Fig. 2.12, this does not pose insuperable difficulties.

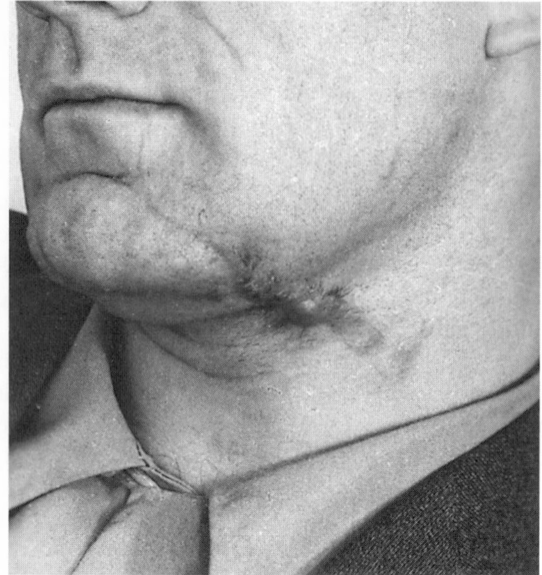

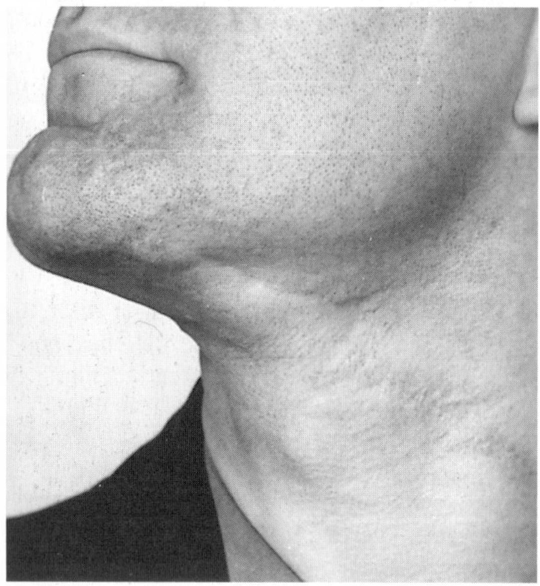

Fig. 2.14 The use of Z-plasties in revising a bridle scar crossing the submandibular concavity.

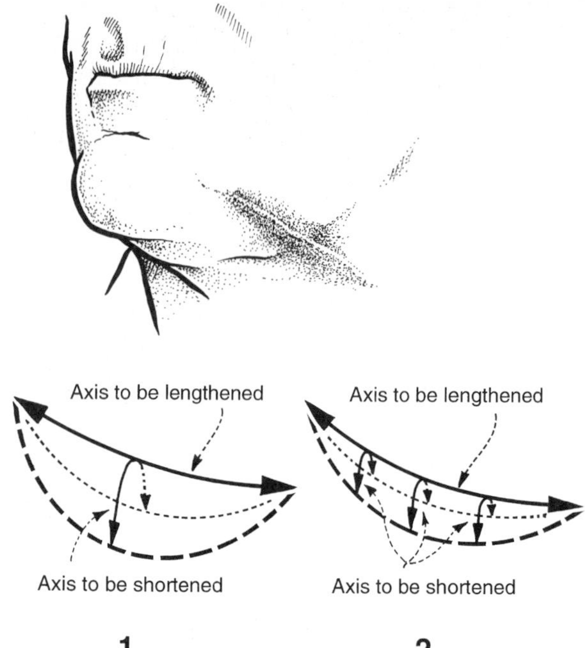

Fig. 2.15 The use of the Z-plasty in bridle scars, showing (**1**) the rationale of the use of a single Z-plasty in the scar bridging a deep hollow, and (**2**) a multiple Z-plasty in the scar bridging a shallow hollow.

Use in curving scars

This problem is seen in its worst form when a trap-door of skin which has been uplifted, usually as a result of trauma, is sutured back in place. Contraction of the margin of the resulting scar causes elevation of the tissue within its concavity. Seen later the result may be assumed, not unreasonably, to be due to bad suturing, but excision of the scar, trimming of the flap quite flat, and resuture with the greatest care only results in recurrence of the original state of affairs within a matter of weeks (Fig. 2.16).

Lengthening of the scar by judicious use of the Z-plasty is necessary to prevent recurrence. Here, as in correcting the bridle scar, an effort should be made to place any Z-plasty in a line of election, although with the curving scar the planning of the Z-plasty to give the best result from every point of view can be an extremely difficult exercise and one in which facility comes only with experience (Fig. 2.17).

On occasion the problem of the curving scar takes a slightly different form, as when the two sides of a wound to be sutured are unequal in length, as in the excision of a ‘comma-shaped’ scar. The taking of unequal bites in suturing can partially equate the lengths but this has limited effectiveness. The Z-plasty can then sometimes help further to reduce the discrepancy in lengths (Fig. 2.18).

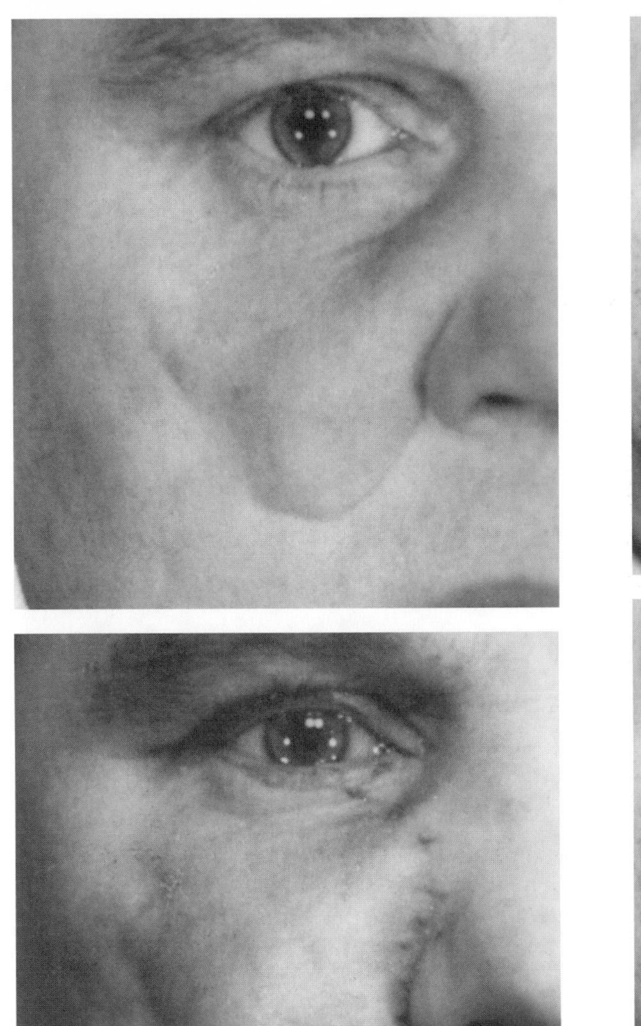

Fig. 2.16 The recurrence of trap-door scarring of the cheek following simple excision and suture of the scar.

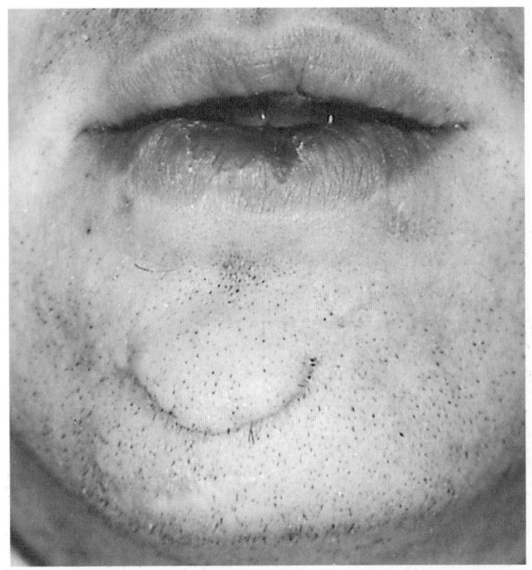

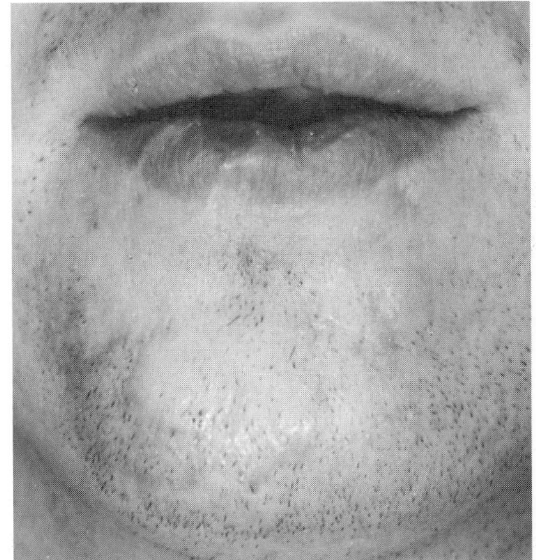

Fig. 2.17 The correction of a trap-door scar of the chin following excision of the scar with the insertion of Z-plasties.

Use in overriding scars

Where there is a tendency to overriding of the tissue on one side of a scar the junction between the two sides can usually be smoothed by incorporating one or more Z-plasties when the scar is being excised (Fig. 2.19), and here again the use of lines of election should be remembered.

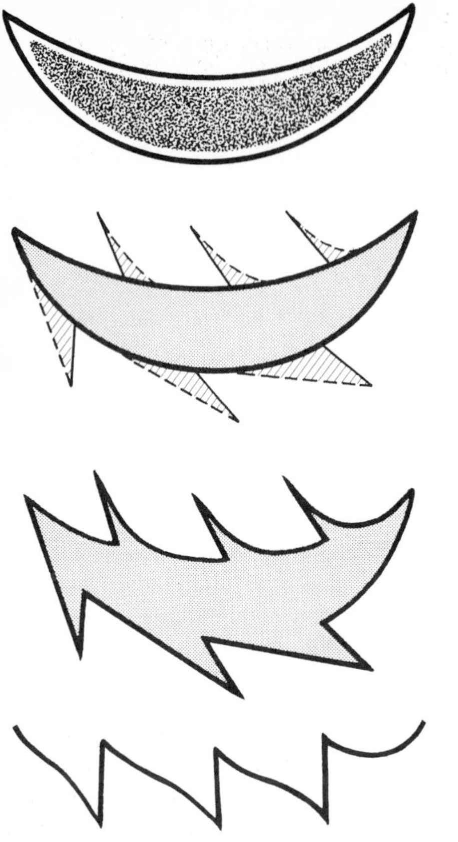

Fig. 2.18 The use of Z-plasties in equalising the lengths of the two sides of a wound which were previously unequal.

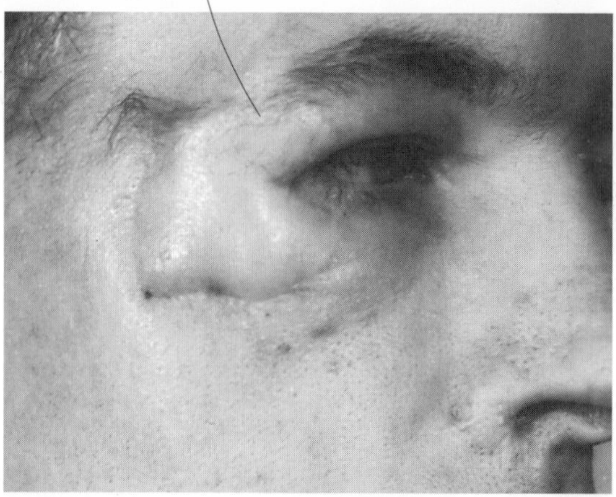

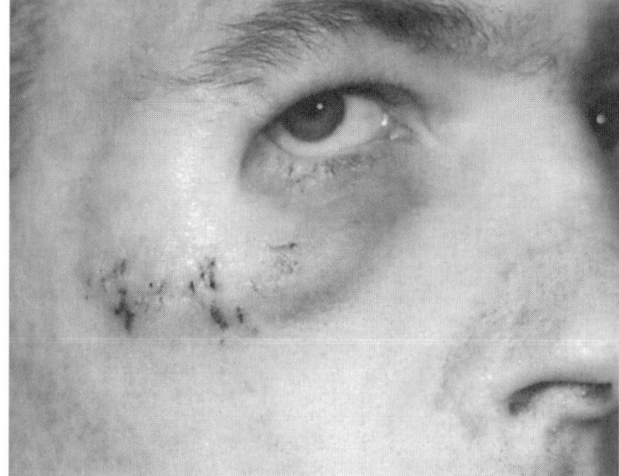

Fig. 2.19 The incorporation of Z-plasties during revision of a scar at the margin of a flap, used in conjunction with thinning of the flap, to give a smooth junction between the flap and its surroundings.

CHAPTER 3

Free skin grafts

Free skin grafts (Fig. 3.1) are of two kinds:

1. **Full thickness skin graft** consisting of epidermis and the full thickness of dermis.
2. **Split skin graft** consisting of epidermis and a variable proportion of dermis. Split skin grafts are described as **thin**, **intermediate** or **thick** according to the thickness of dermis included.

These various categories of graft are not really completely distinct from each other. They merely represent convenient reference points on a continuous scale of decreasing thickness from the full thickness skin graft to the graft consisting of little more than epidermis. The real difference in practice is between the full thickness skin graft and the split skin graft. The full thickness skin graft is cut with a scalpel while the split skin graft, of whatever thickness, is usually cut with a special instrument.

The full thickness skin graft, once cut, leaves behind no epidermal elements in the donor area from which resurfacing can take place; the split skin graft leaves adnexal remnants, pilosebaceous follicles and/or sweat gland apparatus, as foci from which the donor site can resurface. As a result the donor area of a split skin graft heals spontaneously, and requires no care other than that usually accorded any raw surface; the donor area of a full thickness skin graft has to be closed by direct suture or, if it is too large for this, covered with a split skin graft. This limits the size of the full thickness skin graft which can usefully be cut in practice. Extensive defects are split skin grafted; the full thickness skin graft is restricted to small defects.

While the properties of the full thickness skin graft are relatively constant, those of the split skin graft depend in some degree on the thickness of its dermal component, the thicker split skin graft approximating to the full thickness skin graft in its characteristics.

The full thickness skin graft takes less readily than the split skin graft, and before it can be used successfully conditions have to be optimal.

The full thickness skin graft remains virtually at its original size; the split skin graft tends to contract subsequently if circumstances permit, e.g. across a flexure. Within broad limits, the thinner a graft the more it contracts secondarily. The stability of a graft depends on dermis, and the thicker graft stands late trauma better than the thin graft.

During its transfer from donor to recipient site a free skin graft is completely, even if only

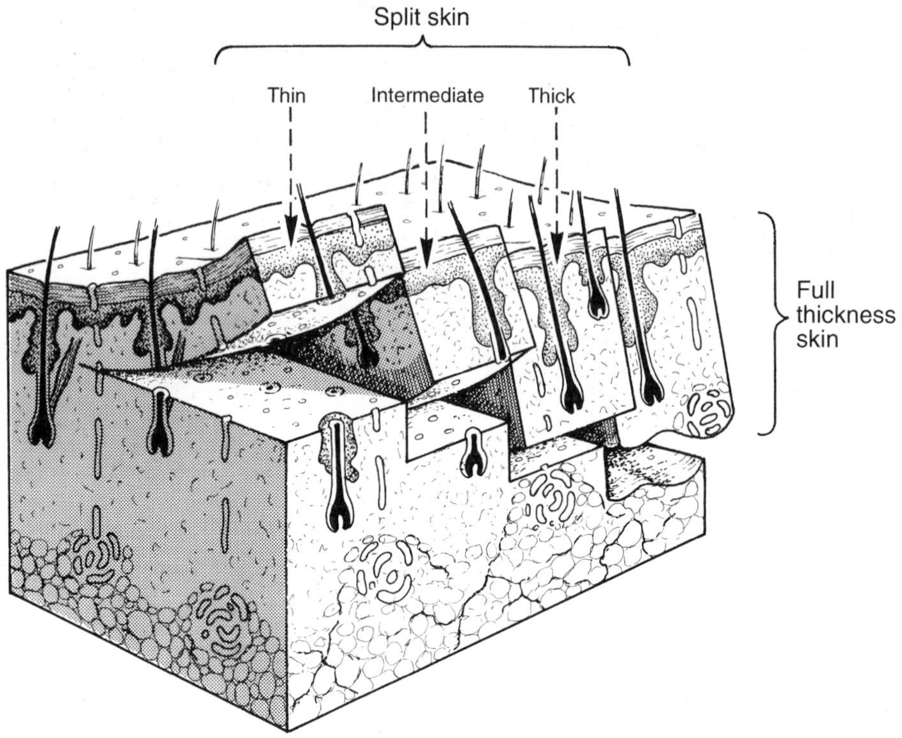

Fig. 3.1 The thicknesses of the various types of free skin grafts, showing the constituents of each.

temporarily, detached from the body. While so detached such a graft remains viable for a limited period whose precise limit depends on the ambient temperature at which the graft is maintained (see p. 47). In order to survive permanently it has to become reattached, and obtain a fresh blood supply from its new habitat. The processes which result in its reattachment and revascularisation are collectively referred to as **take**.

THE PROCESS OF TAKE

The graft initially adheres to its new bed by fibrin, and revascularisation is achieved by the outgrowth of capillary buds from the recipient area to unite with those on the deep surface of the graft (Fig. 3.2). This link-up is usually well advanced by the third day.

Coinciding with the vascular link-up, the fibrin is infiltrated by fibroblasts which gradually convert the initial tenuous adhesion provided by the fibrin clot into a definitive attachment by fibrous tissue. The strength of this attachment increases quickly, providing an anchorage within 4 days which allows the graft to be handled safely if reasonable care is taken. More slowly a lymphatic link-up is added and, even more slowly, nerve supply is re-established, although imperfectly and not invariably.

Of these various processes the ones most relevant in clinical practice are vascularisation and fibrous tissue fixation. The speed with which they are provided, and their effectiveness, are determined by the characteristics of the **bed** on which the graft is laid, the characteristics of the **graft** itself, and the **conditions under which the graft is applied to the bed**.

The graft bed

The bed on which the graft is laid must be capable of providing the necessary initial fibrin anchorage, and also have a rich enough blood supply to vascularise the graft. Vascularisation is achieved by the outgrowth of capillary buds, and the more rapid the process and profuse the out-

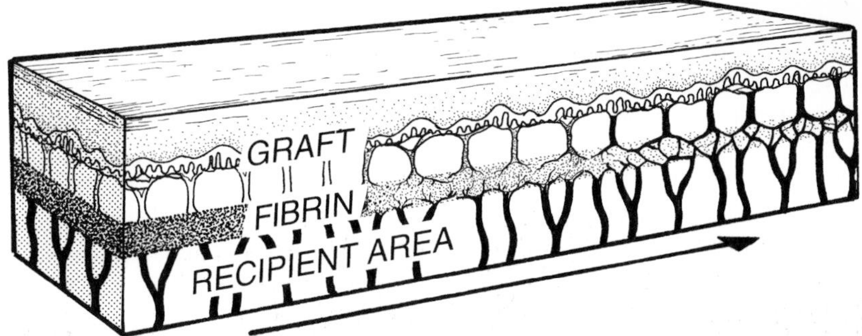

Fig. 3.2 A diagrammatic representation of the process of 'take' of a free skin graft – the initial adhesion of the graft to the bed by fibrin, the growth of capillaries from the bed into the fibrin layer to link up with the capillaries in the graft, and the growth of fibroblasts into the fibrin clot to convert the initial fibrin adhesion into a fibrous tissue attachment.

growth the more suitable the surface is for grafting. Capillary outgrowth is also the key factor in the production of granulation tissue, and here too, speed and profusion of outgrowth determines the effectiveness of the process. The fact that capillary outgrowth is common to both processes makes it possible for the surgeon to assess the suitability of a surface for grafting by considering the speed with which it would be expected to granulate, if left ungrafted. In the extreme clinical situation, *the potential recipient area which is not capable of producing granulations will not take a free skin graft* (Fig. 3.3). *The surface which granulates rapidly and well will take a graft readily; one which granulates only slowly takes a graft less readily.*

Muscle and fascia accept grafts readily, but the ease with which fat can be grafted varies with the site. On the face, fat is extremely vascular and grafts take easily; elsewhere its relatively poor vascularity makes it a less satisfactory surface to graft. Cartilage which is covered with perichondrium, bone covered with periosteum, and tendon covered with paratenon, whether parietal or visceral, all accept grafts readily. Bare cartilage and bare tendon cannot be relied on to take a

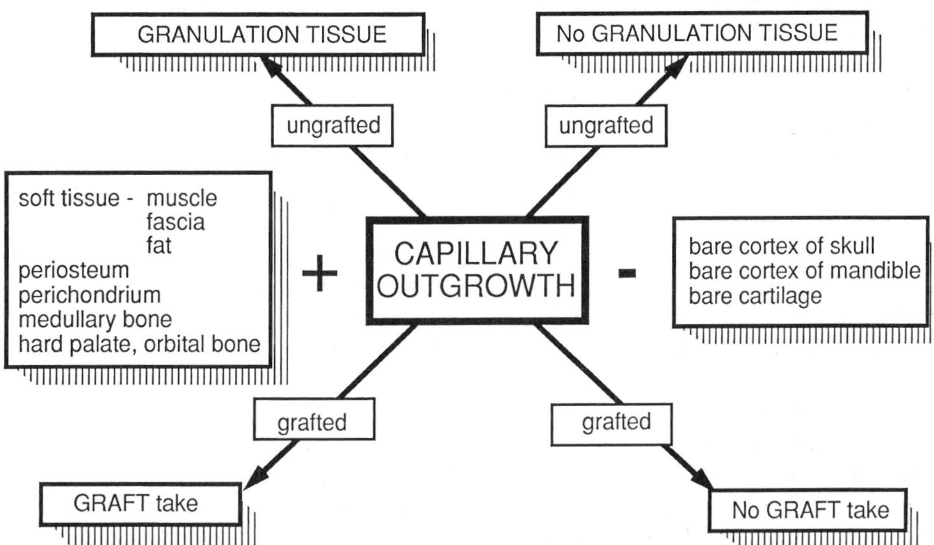

Fig. 3.3 Capillary outgrowth as the common factor in determining the ability of a tissue surface to produce granulation tissue and its capacity to accept a free skin graft. A surface which, left ungrafted, will granulate quickly and effectively, is capable of accepting a graft. A surface which, left ungrafted, will not granulate quickly and effectively, will not accept a graft.

graft, although if the area is small enough, the blood supply of the surrounding tissue may be sufficiently profuse to allow the graft in its vascularisation to bridge the defect and cover it successfully (Fig. 3.5).

Bone requires more detailed consideration because its behaviour varies in different sites. Bare cortical bone as typified by outer table of skull or subcutaneous border of tibia lacks sufficient vascularity to take a graft successfully. The hard palate and the bony orbit are both capable of taking grafts. The bone of the diploë, exposed when the outer table of the skull has been removed, and medullary bone generally, will also take a graft successfully. In each instance the ease of graft take parallels the speed and effectiveness with which each would granulate left ungrafted.

Any surface suitable for grafting on the basis of its vascular characteristics has fibrinogen and the enzymes which convert it into fibrin in sufficient quantities to provide the necessary adhesion unless the surface is harbouring organisms which destroy fibrin. The organism *par excellence* which does this is *Streptococcus pyogenes*, probably by virtue of its potent fibrinolysin. This problem arises mainly when granulating surfaces are being grafted, and is discussed on p. 50.

A striking example of how the ease with which a graft takes parallels the vascularity of the bed is shown by the effect of radiation on vascularity. A site which shows radiation injury is rarely capable of being successfully grafted, despite the fact that in the absence of such injury it is grafted routinely without difficulty.

The graft

Skin grafts can vary both in their thickness and the vascularity of the skin from which they are taken. Each of these variables affects their speed of vascularisation and consequently the ease with which they take.

Variations in graft thickness relate to the thickness of their dermal component and this influences their vascularity, dermis in general being less vascular in its deeper part. The number of cut capillary ends exposed when a thick skin graft is cut is smaller than with a thin graft (Fig. 3.14) and the full thickness graft has even fewer. With vascularisation slower the thicker the graft, thin grafts are generally easier to get to take than thick grafts. In order to get the thickest grafts to take, conditions have to be little short of ideal. These facts apply to grafts taken from sites other than the head and neck — the abdomen, thigh, arm, buttock, etc. The head and neck sites commonly used as donor areas have such a rich blood supply that full thickness grafts from one of these sites compare very favourably in their vascular characteristics with thin split skin grafts taken from elsewhere.

Conditions for take

Rapid vascularisation is all-important, and the distance to be travelled by the capillary buds in order to link-up clearly needs to be as short as possible. The graft has therefore to be in the closest possible contact with the bed. The most frequent cause of separation is bleeding from the bed, the resulting haematoma acting as a block to link-up of the outgrowing capillaries (Fig. 3.4).

The graft has also to lie immobile on the bed until it is firmly attached. In particular, shearing strains which tend to make the graft slide to and fro and prevent capillary link-up are to be avoided (Fig. 3.4) until the initial fibrin adhesion

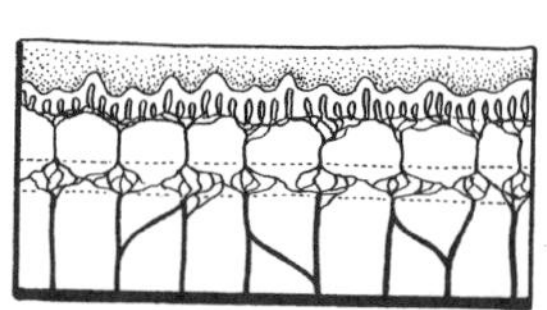

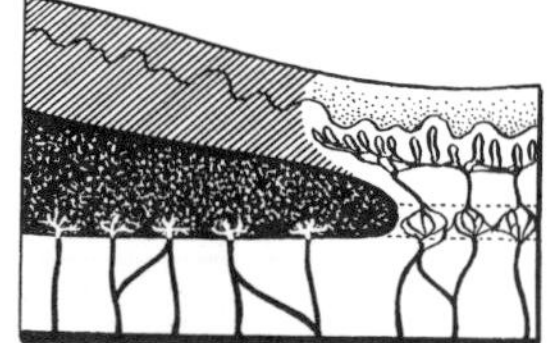

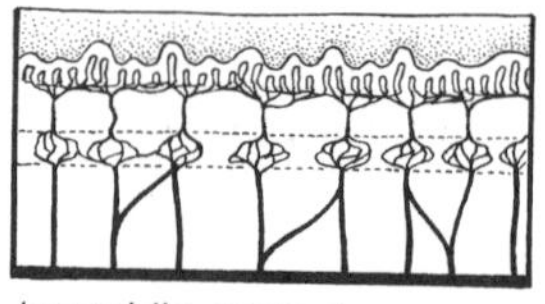

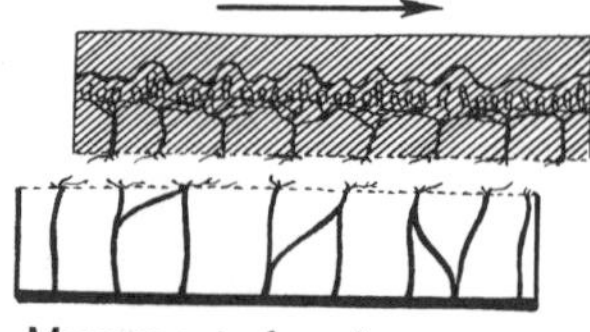

Fig. 3.4 The influence of *close immobile contact* on the vascularisation of a free skin graft.

has been converted into a strong fibrous tissue anchorage.

In summary, *given a bed capable of providing the necessary capillary outgrowth to vascularise a graft, and free of pathogens inimical to graft take, the conditions necessary for successful take are close, immobile contact between graft and bed.*

The most frequent cause of graft loss is the presence of a haematoma which separates the graft from its bed and/or shearing movements which prevent adhesion between graft and bed, each in its own way preventing capillary link-up and vascularisation. The methods used in clinical grafting practice vary according to the clinical situation, but in each instance the particular method adopted is used because it is considered to be the one most likely to prevent haematoma and avoid shearing movement.

The phenomenon of bridging

A graft may survive over bare cortical bone, tendon or cartilage, and even if separated from its graft bed by blood clot, provided the area is small enough. In such circumstances the graft survives by bridging (Fig. 3.5), a phenomenon of interest in view of the light which it throws on the process of vascularisation. It provides confirmatory evidence of a link-up with the existing vascular network of the graft since it could not occur if vascularisation took place solely by capillary invasion from the graft bed. In most circumstances bridging is strictly limited in area and beyond this the graft will not survive. It cannot be relied on to cover significant areas of bone, tendon or cartilage successfully.

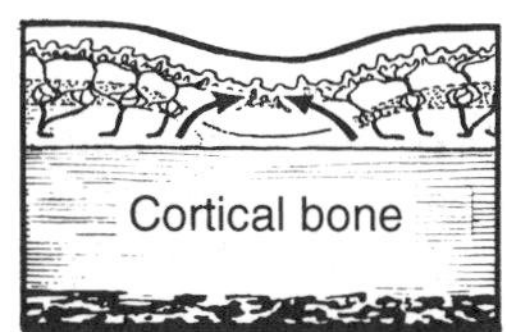

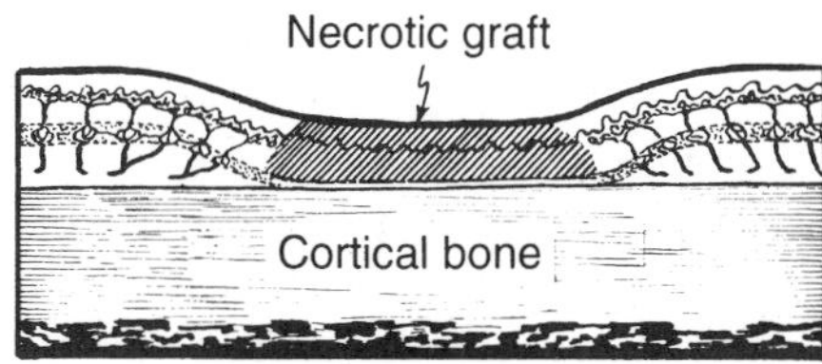

Fig. 3.5 The phenomenon of bridging.

Where a particularly rich vascular network is present both in a graft and its bed, bridging may be possible over a much larger area, and the use of a composite free graft of ear skin and cartilage to reconstruct alar defects succeeds or fails largely on the extent to which bridging is successful.

THE FULL THICKNESS GRAFT

The thickness, appearance, texture and vascularity of skin vary greatly in different parts of the body and have a strong influence on the donor site appropriate to a particular surgical situation.

Postauricular skin

The posterior surface of the ear extending on to the adjoining postauricular hairless mastoid skin (Fig. 3.6) makes the best donor site when the face is being grafted. It gives a most excellent skin colour and texture match, and when replacing eyelid skin is often virtually undetectable. The vascularity both of the graft and the sites to which it is usually applied make it the easiest of full-thickness skin grafts to get to take. It is the smallness of the area of skin available which limits the size of the defect which it can be used to cover. The donor site is closed by direct suture.

Upper eyelid skin

In the adult, skin is nearly always available on the upper eyelid (Fig. 3.6), and this can be useful particularly when the defect is of another eyelid. The match of colour and texture is outstandingly good. The area available is obviously limited, though the redundancy of the upper eyelid skin usually present in the older age group, the group in which such grafts are most often needed, allows more skin to be harvested than one might expect.

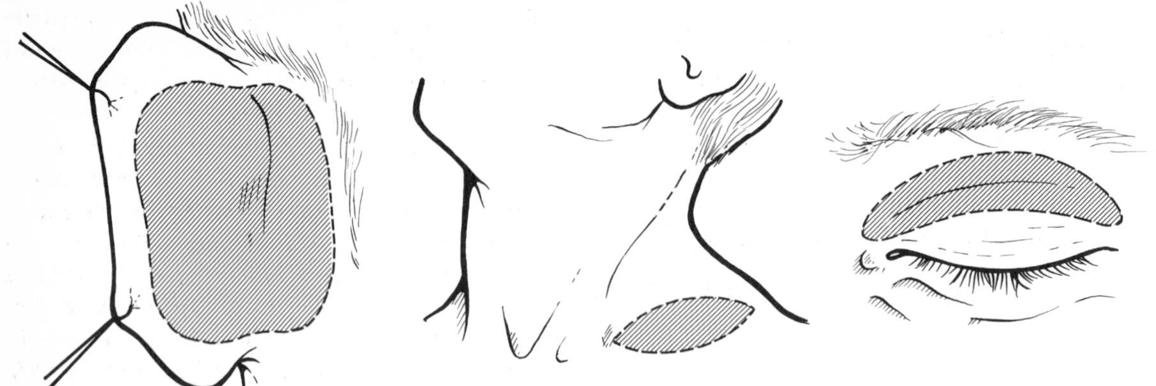

Fig. 3.6 The areas in the postauricular, supraclavicular, and upper eyelid sites, within which full thickness skin grafts can be harvested.

Supraclavicular skin

The skin of the lower posterior triangle of the neck (Fig. 3.6) gives a reasonable colour and texture match used on the face although one distinctly inferior to postauricular skin. A larger area of skin is available but, unless the neck defect is grafted the increase is not sufficient to make it more obviously useful. Grafting the neck defect creates a cosmetic defect of its own and one which is likely to be particularly undesirable in the female where the donor area is often exposed. These adverse factors restrict its usefulness considerably and it is not often needed.

Flexural skin

The antecubital fossa and the groin are both described as possible donor sites. The dermis is thinner than average, and the skin is mobile on the deeper tissues, but only a limited width is available unless a graft is used to cover the donor site. On the face the cosmetic result is comparable to that using supraclavicular skin.

In the antecubital fossa, even if the donor site defect can be closed directly, the resulting scar is very obvious, and if closure is under much tension, hypertrophy of the scar is a hazard. Its use as a donor site is not recommended. The groin area is useful if a long narrow graft is needed, closure in such circumstances being relatively simple. Its main use is in hand surgery, particularly in managing flexion contractures.

Thigh and abdominal skin

The texture and colour match of thigh and abdominal skin grafted to the face is usually poor. The skin either stays extremely pale or becomes hyperpigmented relative to the rest of the face. An added deficiency is a loss of the constantly varying fine play of normal facial expression, the grafted area taking on a rather mask-like appearance, due possibly to its thicker dermis.

Both sites provide a source of skin for the palm of the hand. The thickness of the dermis in both sites, where there is no ageing skin atrophy, provides a good pad to take the necessary pressure when used on the sole of the foot. If a graft of any size is used the donor site must in its turn be grafted and even when the donor site can be directly sutured the scar usually stretches badly.

METHOD OF USE

The full thickness skin graft is accurately fitted to the defect, and a pattern of the defect to be grafted is made to ensure that the graft is at normal skin tension in its new site (Fig. 3.7). Aluminium foil and polythene sheet are materials most often used for making patterns.

The pattern of the area to be grafted is made before excision or after excision, whichever is more convenient. If the defect is irregular, matching points can be tattooed with Bonney's Blue on the defect, and on the graft before it is cut. When the pattern can only be made once the

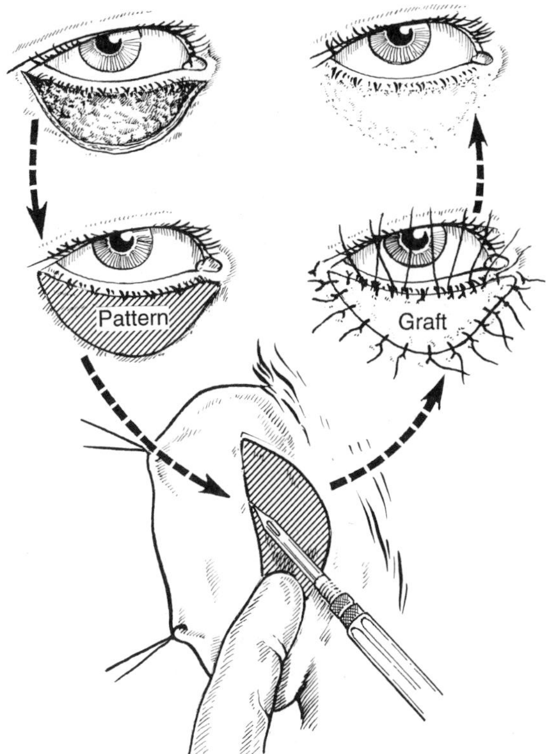

Fig. 3.7 The use of a pattern in cutting a postauricular full thickness skin graft which will accurately fit the defect. The same principle applies in harvesting full thickness skin grafts from other sites in other clinical situations.

defect is surgically created, the defect should be displayed to the full before making the pattern. This applies with particular force when the defect is of the eyelid, when failure to make the pattern and consequently the graft of a size to fill the defect in full results in residual ectropion.

It is generally considered that the full thickness skin graft should be carefully cleared of fat on its deep surface. Time and care can be spent in the cutting of the graft so that no fat is left on its deep surface (Fig. 3.8). Alternatively, the graft may be cut without special regard to the inclusion of fat, the fat being subsequently removed with scissors.

Excision of the fat after the graft has been cut is a tedious business, but to cut the graft without fat requires both skill and care. It is probably easier for the surgeon who seldom uses the method not to attempt it lest the graft be button-holed in the process. Most surgeons gradually acquire a feel for the correct plane at the time of cutting the graft and, by cutting parallel to the skin surface, stay in that plane.

The graft is easier to cut if the area is ballooned with fluid, usually 1 in 200 000 noradrenalin. Using the pattern already made, the outline is marked on the skin with Bonney's Blue, incised and undercut. It often helps to pull the skin of the graft taut over the knife with hooks so that the knife is cutting blindly, largely by touch. Alternatively, the graft can be held turned back so that cutting is done under vision. This method is less precise and usually results in more fat being left on the graft.

In the case of donor sites other than postauricular and upper eyelid, the relative avascularity of fat makes the caveat regarding its removal almost certainly valid, but in the case of the postauricular and upper eyelid sites its validity is more dubious. The skin of the upper eyelid in the average patient where the source is used virtually peels off, and there is little if any fat to remove. In the postauricular site, having been taught scrupulous trimming of fat, a gradual change to increasingly less scrupulous removal has not been attended by poorer take of the graft.

Behind the ear and in the upper eyelid, closure by direct suture is usually straightforward. Elsewhere, direct suture should be used where possible, but if the defect is too large it has to be split skin grafted.

THE SPLIT SKIN GRAFT

This graft has a much wider usage than the full thickness graft, and within limits the surgeon is able to control its thickness and make use of that variable in its characteristics and clinical behaviour.

DONOR SITES

The donor site is chosen in any set instance by such factors as the amount skin required; whether a good colour and texture match is needed; local convenience, as in grafting from forearm to hand with need for only one dressing; the necessity of having no hair on the graft; the cutting instrument

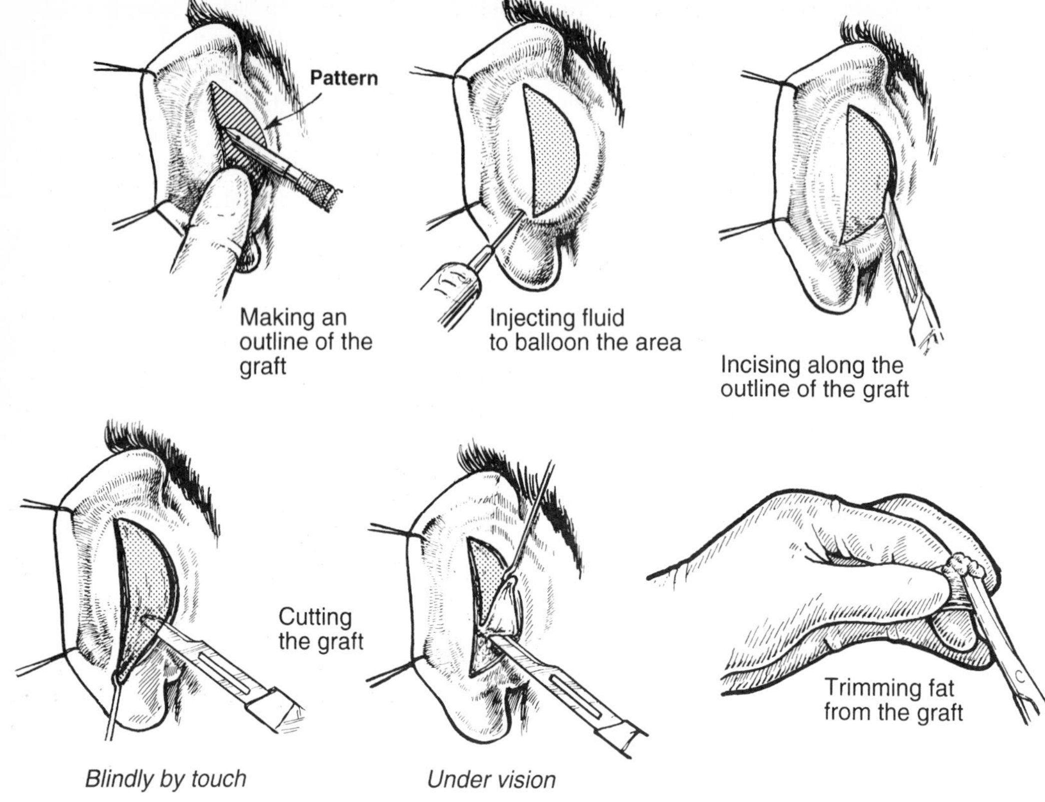

Fig. 3.8 The method of harvesting a postauricular full thickness skin graft. A similar technique is used in harvesting full thickness skin grafts from other sites.

available; the desirability where possible of avoiding the leg in the aged or outpatient.

The sites usually used as donor sites are:

1. The thigh and upper arm.
2. The flexor aspect of forearm.
3. Virtually the whole of the reasonably plane surface of the torso.

When these sites are not available or all possible sites are needed skin can also be cut from:

1. The other aspects of forearm.
2. The lower leg.

LOCAL ANAESTHESIA FOR GRAFT CUTTING

Local anaesthesia can be used for harvesting split skin grafts by injection of the local anaesthetic agent or by the topical application of the local anaesthetic to the skin area being harvested.

When the anaesthetic agent is being injected, the addition of hyaluronidase to the solution makes it possible to cut a reasonable size of graft readily. The exact amount of hyaluronidase which has to be used is not critical; 1500 IU added to 100 ml of anaesthetic solution works satisfactorily. The mixture diffuses rapidly and leaves a uniformly flat skin surface. The diffuse increase in tissue turgor also increases the dermal thickness and makes the area slightly more rigid, valuable when a thin graft is required.

The topical anaesthetic agent used is the commercial preparation EMLA (Astra Pharmaceutical), a mixture of lignocaine and prilocaine. Both agents are very slowly absorbed into the superficial layers of the skin, with negligible absorption into the blood stream, and this allows larger areas to be anaesthetised, though the anaesthesia may not extend to the deeper part of the dermis. Since its deep effectiveness cannot be assessed preoperatively, it is wise to restrict the grafts cut to those of medium thickness.

The area of anaesthesia required should be marked out on the skin, and the area covered liberally with the anaesthetic cream, preparatory to the application of an occlusive dressing to enhance its absorption. As a rule, at least an hour should be allowed for sufficient absorption to permit the cutting of a graft. Although pallor of the skin area is often seen, it is not a reliable indicator either of the presence of the anaesthesia or its surface extent. The patient has to be tested for both. Tissue turgor is not noticeably increased, though the skin often has a slightly 'corrugated' appearance. This is probably due more to the occlusive dressing used to enhance absorption rather than to any property of the cream itself.

GRAFT-CUTTING INSTRUMENTS

The instruments commonly used for cutting grafts are:

1. The Humby knife.
2. The power-driven dermatome.

The Humby knife (Fig. 3.9)

The instrument originally used to cut split skin grafts freehand was a knife with a blade approximately 25 cm long, referred to as a Blair knife after the American plastic surgeon who developed it. To cut a graft of any size with a uniform thickness using the Blair knife was something of a virtuoso performance, and it was only when Humby, an English plastic surgeon, added a roller mechanism, that consistency of graft thickness became a reality. Modified versions of the Humby knife, of which the Watson modification is currently the best, have since been produced. There is also a scaled-down version, the Silver knife, with a razor blade to provide the cutting edge, useful when only a small graft is required.

The Humby knife can only be used on convex surfaces, but despite this its convenience makes it the most frequently used instrument for routine graft cutting.

The donor site most often used is the thigh, and the positioning of the leg for this purpose will be described in detail, but the principles outlined can be applied to any other donor site.

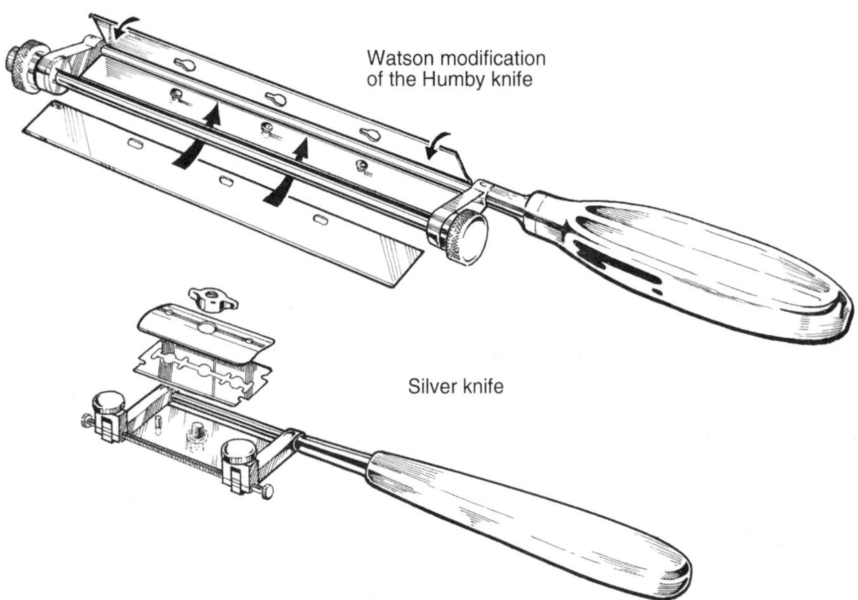

Fig. 3.9 The Watson modification of the Humby knife, and the Silver knife. The Silver knife is essentially a miniature version of the Humby knife, used when a small graft is required.

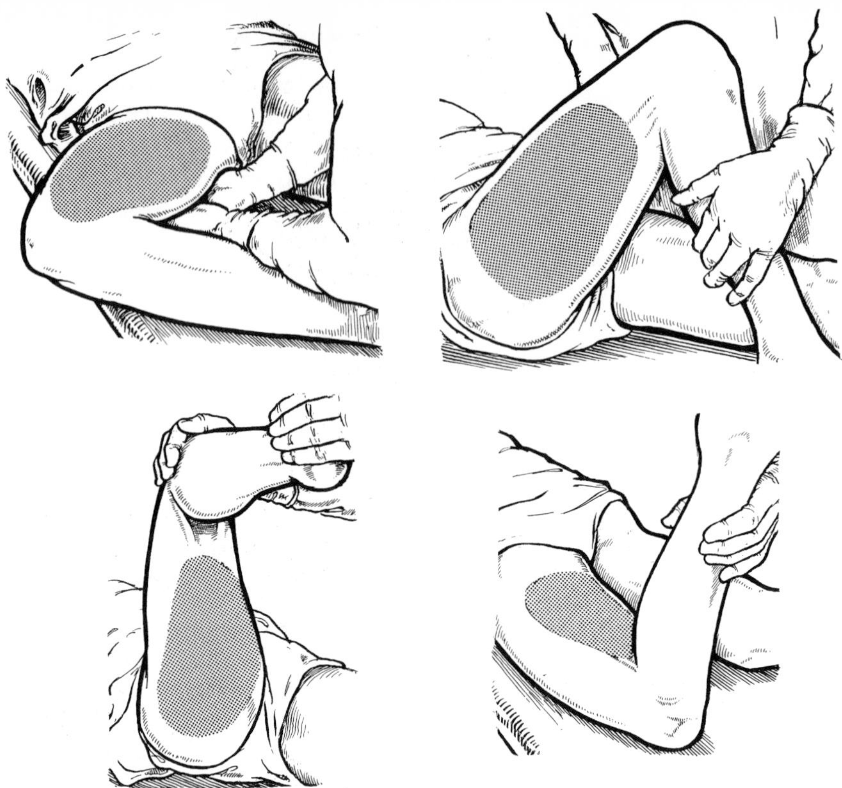

Fig. 3.10 The positioning of the thigh for cutting a split skin graft from its various surfaces, and the way the surface is presented to provide the maximum area of flat skin.

The leg is placed with the appropriate group of muscles relaxed (Fig. 3.10) so that by pressing the muscle group either medially or laterally the maximum of plane surface is presented to the knife.

For the **medial side of the thigh**, the hip is slightly flexed and externally rotated. The assistant presses from below with the flat of both hands pushing round the hamstrings and adductors to give the necessary wide flat surface for cutting a broad graft.

When the **lateral aspect** is used, the surface presented when the assistant presses laterally is less satisfactorily flat in its lower part because of the depression which the iliotibial tract creates between vastus lateralis and biceps femoris. The depression becomes less noticeable proximally, and the overall surface is flatter.

For the **posterior aspect**, flexion of both hip and knee are needed to get at the surface unless the subject is prone. The ridges produced by the diverging hamstrings make a good graft difficult to obtain in the distal part, but passing proximally the flat surface broadens and a good graft can be cut readily.

Because of the prominence of the femoral shaft the **anterior aspect** does not give a broad plane surface and the site tends not to be used unless all donor sites are needed or a narrow graft is specifically desired.

In the **arm** (Fig. 3.11) positioning and pressure are used as in the thigh to create the broadest plane surface.

Cutting the graft

Graft thickness is controlled by adjusting the distance between the roller and the blade. Despite the presence of a gauge on the instrument most surgeons assess thickness by holding the knife up to the light to see the clearance between blade and roller. Clearance of a little less than 0.5 mm

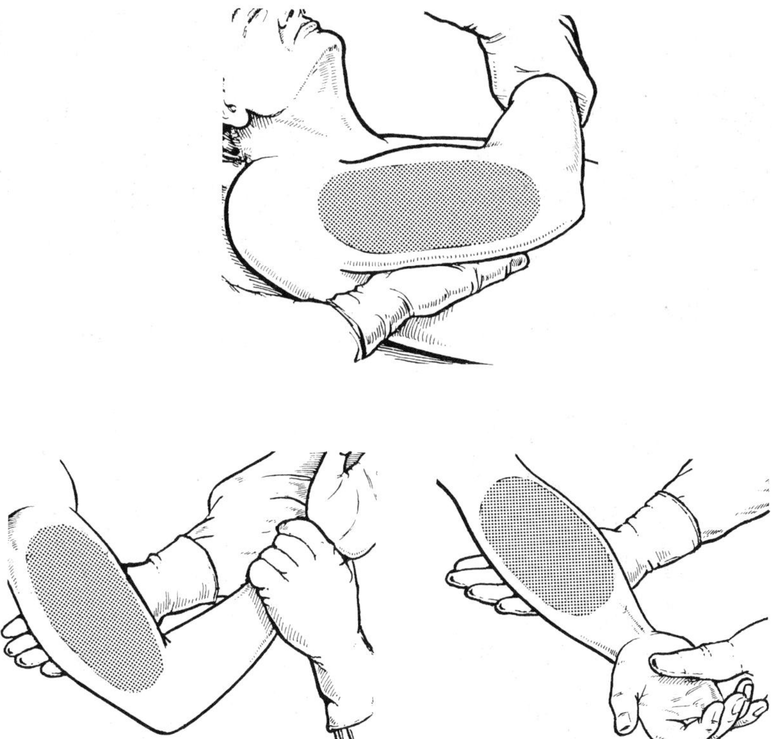

Fig. 3.11 Positioning the arm for cutting a split skin graft.

will be found as a rule to give a graft of average thickness, but this initial assessment is controlled, and an adjustment made if necessary, by watching both the graft as it is cut and the bed from which it is being cut. The guiding characters of graft thickness are described below.

Ideally, the blade when cutting moves to and fro smoothly over the skin surface which does not move at all with the knife. Drag, the result of friction between the blade and the skin, causes the skin to oscillate to and fro with the knife, making the graft more difficult to cut. It cannot be completely eliminated, but lubrication with liquid paraffin of the skin surface and the surface of the blade next to the skin does reduce it considerably.

In cutting the graft the surgeon should work from the more convenient side of the patient, cutting down the limb or up according to his position. A little in front of the knife and moving smoothly a fixed distance from it, a wooden board is held pressed down on the skin (Fig. 3.12). The board serves the double purpose of steadying the skin and flattening it as the blade reaches it. The edge of the board which is pressing on the skin is lubricated also with liquid paraffin so that the forward movement of the knife is in unison with

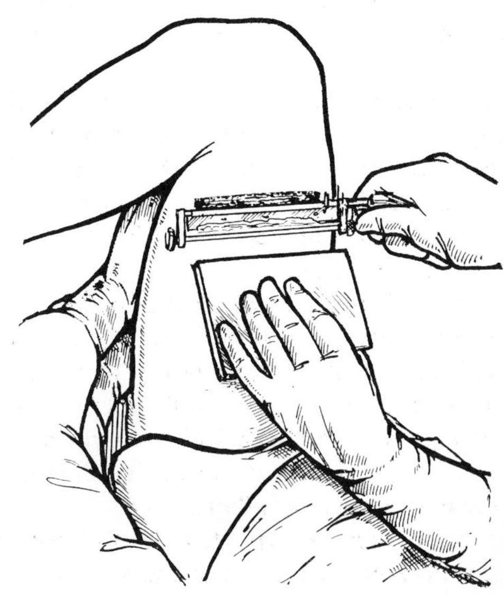

Fig. 3.12 Cutting a split skin graft with the Watson modification of the Humby knife.

the movement of the board, the distance between the two remaining constant. To get knife and board moving smoothly together takes practice. It is best achieved by concentrating on an even to and fro motion rather than on the forward moving of the knife as it cuts the graft.

The presence of a further assistant holding the skin with a wooden board just behind the knife before it starts to cut may help to keep the area steady and taut. The board is kept still as the knife moves forward in cutting the graft. This manoeuvre is mainly of use when the skin is atrophic, lax and mobile, as in the aged or emaciated subject, helping to eliminate drag which is otherwise liable to be a problem.

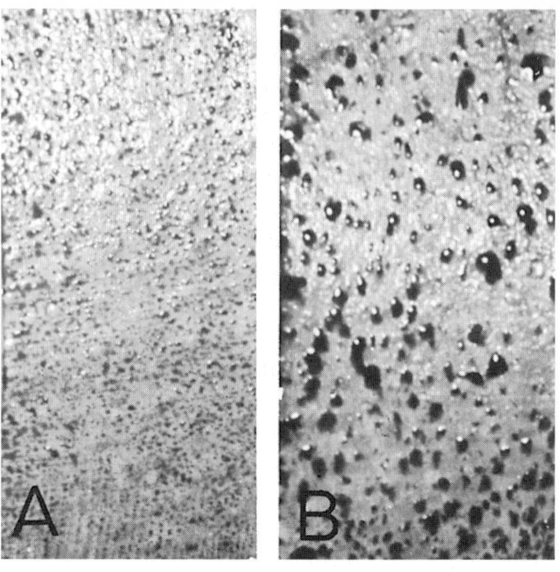

Fig. 3.14 The pattern of bleeding from the donor site of a thin split skin graft (**A**), and a thick split skin graft (**B**).

Assessment of graft thickness

Although a setting of the roller has been suggested, the surgeon must be prepared to modify it if necessary. The first 6 mm or so of the graft cut provides an initial indication of its thickness and the setting can be adjusted accordingly.

The **translucency of the graft** is the main index of thickness (Fig. 3.13). The very thin graft is translucent and not unlike tissue paper; the grey of the knife blade shows through. Opacity of the graft increases with increasing thickness until the full-thickness skin graft has the colour and appearance of cadaver skin. A split skin graft of intermediate thickness is moderately translucent.

The **pattern of bleeding of the donor site** gives a further indication of thickness (Fig. 3.14).

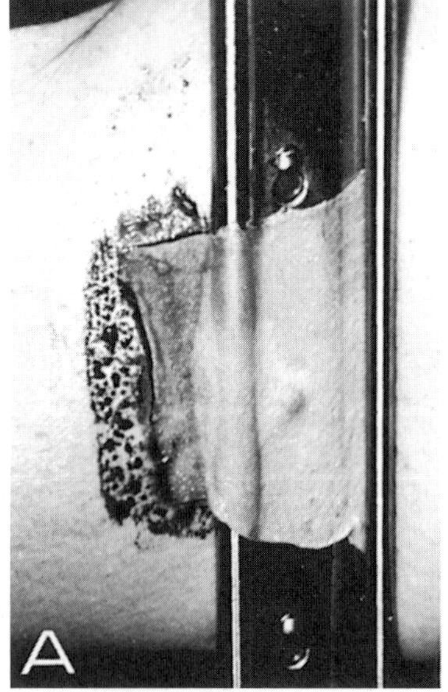

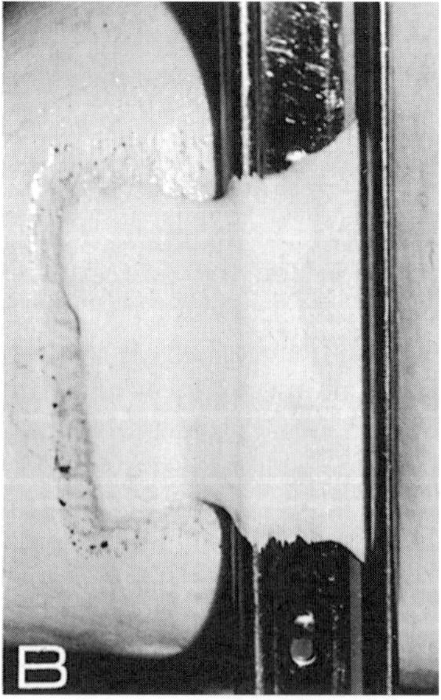

Fig. 3.13 The degree of translucency of a thin split skin graft (**A**), and of a thick split skin graft (**B**).

The thin graft produces a high density of tiny bleeding points; the thicker graft gives a lower density of larger bleeding points.

While these criteria are generally applicable, they should always be correlated with the clinical appearance of the skin in the individual patient, particularly as to signs of clinical atrophy. With the papery skin of the aged, the graft must be correspondingly thin and the distribution of bleeding points gives no help in such cases.

The thickness of the skin from the point of view of clinical atrophy and graft cutting, and the presence of remnants of the adnexa from which the site can heal, seems to vary in different parts of the limb. In general, lateral is thicker than medial, and distal thicker than proximal. In the thigh when atrophy is clinically obvious, the lateral aspect should be chosen if at all possible. The donor site is much more likely to heal without trouble.

The power-driven dermatome

The power-driven dermatome is a complex and fragile instrument. Its great merit lies in its ability to cut a graft of controlled width and accurately controllable thickness from almost any part of the trunk or limbs. It is also capable of cutting a thin graft — a thing that other instruments are less able to do with comparable consistency.

In appearance it is not unlike a large hair-cutting machine (Fig. 3.15), and the resemblance is maintained in action with the rapidly oscillating cutting blade which is driven electrically or by compressed air. With the skin held steady, and lubricated with liquid paraffin, the instrument is able to move forward smoothly.

It is in the grafting of the extensive deep burn that the power-driven dermatome has proved its worth. Its ability to cut skin from almost any part of the body surface has considerably extended the available donor areas. The straight margin, and the uniform thickness of the graft which it cuts, mean that a limb can be flayed with scarcely any wastage of skin between adjoining donor sites in the knowledge that the whole area will heal uniformly and quickly. This facility makes it a practical possibility to cut successive crops of skin from the same donor site, a most valuable property when skin is at a premium.

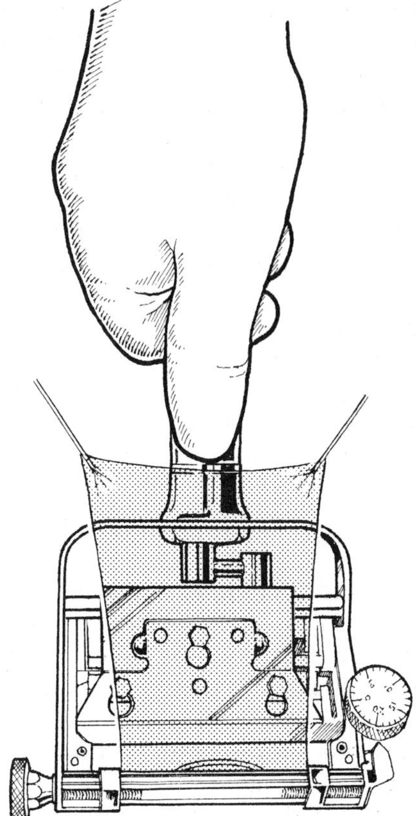

Fig. 3.15 Cutting a split skin graft with the Brown dermatome.

STORAGE OF SKIN

By storage at a low temperature, skin cut in excess of current requirements can be preserved viable for later use as needed. The increase in the use of delayed exposed grafting has greatly increased the need for storage. Within the temperature range 0–37°C the survival time of a stored graft is a function of its temperature, the lower the temperature the longer the survival time.

The graft is wrapped in gauze moistened with saline and placed in a sterile, sealed container. Unless specially long survival, e.g. up to 21 days, is needed, the storage temperature is not of paramount importance, but it seems probable that 4°C is likely to give the best results.

HEALING OF THE DONOR AREA

(Fig. 3.16)

The cutting of a split skin graft leaves greater or lesser portions of the pilosebaceous apparatus and the sweat glands in the donor area and, from these multiple foci, epithelium spreads until the area is resurfaced with skin. The remnants of the pilosebaceous apparatus are much more active as foci of epithelial regeneration than the sweat gland remnants, which react sluggishly. The sweat glands also extend more deeply than the hair follicles. These differences affect the healing patterns of sites from which thin and thick split skin grafts have been cut. It is difficult to give precise healing times of donor sites, because assessment depends on whether the way in which the site is managed leaves the area covered with a dry scab or keeps it more moist. The donor site of the thin graft, with its full complement of cut pilosebaceous follicles, heals in approximately 7–9 days, while the donor site of the thick graft, depending virtually entirely on sweat gland remnants, heals more slowly, taking 14 days or more. The quality of the healed donor site skin which is derived solely from sweat gland remnants is also poorer. Most grafts are of intermediate thickness and leave a percentage of pilosebaceous follicles so that healing takes 9–14 days.

If the thickness of the graft is such that no pilosebaceous follicle or sweat gland remnants are left in the donor area, or infection of the area destroys any remnants which were left, the area will granulate, and healing then takes place from its margin unless in the interval it is split skin grafted.

DONOR SITE MANAGEMENT

Management of the donor area has been, and to some extent still is, one of the less satisfactory aspects of skin grafting. The problems are pain, the provision of the optimal local environment for the healing process, and removal of the dressings.

Pain usually settles within 3–4 days, and is often followed by itching. Although itching is a useful clinical indicator of satisfactory progress, it is more difficult to treat, and can cause more discomfort to the patient than pain. Pain can be reduced by the perioperative application of topical local anaesthesia in the form of a jelly, or by impregnating the dressings with a liquid form of

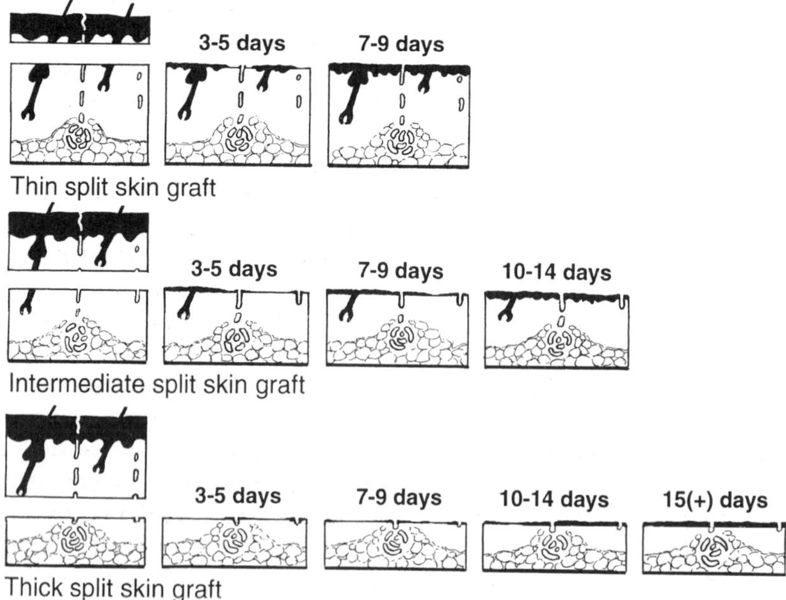

Fig 3.16 The healing patterns of the donor sites of the various thicknesses of split skin grafts.

the anaesthetic agent. Use of a long-acting agent often gets the patient over the most painful period without the need to use potent analgesics.

Traditionally, donor areas were dressed with tulle gras, over which was laid absorbent gauze, the whole held in position with a crepe bandage. The dressing became dry, hard and adherent to the healing skin. Its removal was not merely painful, but in the process regenerating epithelium was pulled off. Alternatively, the dressing was left *in situ* until it separated spontaneously, an approach which was only practical if it remained dry.

The ideal donor site dressing would remain non-adherent during the healing phase, be absorbent, maintain a moist environment, and minimise the potential for bacterial colonisation, these being factors considered to encourage epithelial migration. Such a dressing does not exist at present, but the materials now available have steadily improved. Alginate dressing materials (Kaltostat) produce more rapid haemostasis, and reduce the blood present in the dressings, in this way reducing management problems. Kaltostat has greatly improved the patient's lot, and should be largely standard management. It is claimed on its behalf that wound healing is also expedited, but experience is that waiting for 10–14 days before removing the dressing leaves a more robust wound, better able to cope with the trauma involved in its removal. The dressing which has failed to separate after 14 days is probably best soaked off, most effectively in a bath, a routine hallowed by long usage, and as valuable now as in the past.

Management of the donor site using dressings is standard practice in temperate climates, but in hotter climates, particularly where the humidity is high, infection is a very real hazard when dressings are used, with *Pseudomonas aeruginosa* a common pathogen. Treating the area by exposure once haemostasis has been achieved, which allows the area to become dry and prevents colonisation with *Ps. aeruginosa*, is a useful alternative.

Newly healed donor areas are often covered with a flaky keratinised layer, and the use of an emollient, non-irritant cream for 3–4 weeks is usually effective if it is creating a problem for the patient.

When part of the graft has been thicker, the corresponding segment of donor area heals less rapidly and may even granulate with resulting discharge, necessitating removal of the dressing if it is extensive, merely noticed to be present when the dressing is removed if the area is small. Such an area can be allowed to heal spontaneously if it is small, but if it is of any size it should be grafted without delay.

When the graft is being cut, and part or all of the donor area looks doubtful from the point of view of depth, particularly if fat is showing to any extent, a useful prophylactic is to cover it immediately with a thin split skin graft. The problem is most likely to arise in the older patient with atrophic skin. As already discussed (p. 47), the skin of the lateral aspect of the thigh is less prone to this problem, and can usefully be used as a graft source in these circumstances.

The colour of the recently healed donor site can vary from 'more deeply coloured than normal' to deep cyanosis, both colours slowly fading in time to leave the area paler than normal, often with areas of variation in pigmentation, indicative of local minor variations in the thickness of the graft cut.

A late problem which can arise in a donor area is the development of hypertrophic scarring. Most often this affects the abdomen and buttock, and the inner aspect of thigh and upper arm, though any donor site can be affected. One's impression, difficult to prove, is that the thicker the graft cut and the younger the patient the greater its proneness to occur. Warning of its probable development is a complaint of severe itching of the donor area. Left untreated, the condition does eventually settle, but at the expense of a white, atrophic-looking patch of scarred skin. A clinical impression, again difficult to prove, is that the use of one of the locally active steroids in ointment form reduces both the incidence and severity of the complication. Such treatment certainly relieves the itch consistently, and is probably best applied as soon as itch is reported by the patient, and continued until the area is showing signs of settling, as indicated by its clinical appearance.

THE RECIPIENT SITE

Free skin grafts are applied either to raw surfaces surgically created, or at least surgically clean, or to granulating wounds. The practice of grafting varies with the two types of surface as does preparation for grafting.

THE SURGICALLY CLEAN SURFACE

Preparing the recipient area

Although a full thickness skin graft or split skin graft may be used in different clinical situations the underlying principles of preparation do not vary. Failure of a graft where it might reasonably be expected to take well is most often due to **haematoma**, and a completely dry field is therefore essential before the graft is applied.

To achieve this several measures are used. Without doubt the use of time is the most important single factor in achieving haemostasis. The steps of the operation should be planned to give the area to be grafted the longest possible time for the normal haemostatic processes to become effective. While waiting for bleeding to cease, the area may be left covered with gauze soaked in saline.

In controlling obvious bleeding points only the actual bleeding point should be picked up by the mosquito forceps so that the necrosis caused by the short fine catgut tie is minimal. The precision of bipolar coagulation makes it a useful alternative. Graft take is not significantly reduced by either method provided the block of tissue killed is small enough.

During the excision the sucker can play a valuable part in allowing the surgeon to see precisely where he is cutting. The defect once created, however, suction applied to the raw area only keeps bleeding going. If a specific clot has to be sucked off, the sucker nozzle should not actually touch the tissue, otherwise the bleeding point will surely begin again.

Unless the graft bed is absolutely dry it is good practice once the graft is sutured in place to flush out under the graft with saline using a 20 ml syringe with blunt cannula, before the tie-over bolus is applied. Any small clot which remains can be removed by inserting a moistened Q-tip. As the Q-tip is twirled, the clot is caught by the cotton wool and can be removed with the stick.

THE GRANULATING AREA

In assessing a granulating area for grafting two factors are of importance — **clinical appearance** and **bacterial flora**.

Clinical appearance

Healthy granulations are flat, red and vascular, do not bleed unduly readily, and are free from a covering surface film. Good marginal healing is presumptive evidence that granulations will accept a graft, for it can be assumed that infection virulent enough to destroy a graft would be inimical to marginal epithelial growth.

Left ungrafted, granulations generally become more fibrous and less vascular, and grafting is liable to become more problematic. Infection tends to add to the difficulties of grafting in those circumstances. Subjected to inadequate pressure, granulations become oedematous and in this state are often misnamed exuberant. Such granulations need pressure rather than excision, and with successful application of a graft the oedema settles quickly.

Bacterial flora

Any of the common organisms may colonise a raw surface according to site and circumstance but, with the exception of *Str. pyogenes* and *Ps. aeruginosa*, such organisms are of little consequence as a general rule. Clinical appearance is a better guide than bacterial flora in assessing suitability for grafting.

Streptococcus pyogenes

The presence of *Str. pyogenes* is an absolute contraindication to any grafting procedure and, when the area involved is extensive, as for example following a burn, its possible presence makes routine bacteriological examination of exudate necessary before grafting is contemplated. Why a graft should fail when it is present is not exactly known, although interference with the normal fibrin attachment of the graft by the fibrinolysin which it produces may possibly be the cause.

Classically, granulations harbouring *Str. pyogenes* are glazed, gelatinous, and bleed readily at the slightest touch; the marginal epithelium is seldom healthy and growing. With the routine use of antibiotics this picture may not be seen and the granulations may look quite healthy, but this deceptively tranquil behaviour of *Str. pyogenes* does not mitigate its destructive effect on grafts. It must always be eliminated before grafting is attempted.

Pseudomonas aeruginosa

Infection with *Ps. aeruginosa* reduces graft take but not to an extent comparable with *Str. pyogenes*. Its presence is a nuisance rather than a disaster. When it infects the surface of an extensive burn the problem of preventing systemic spread as well as that of controlling the local infection exists, but systemic spread from less extensive raw surfaces is not a significant hazard. Attention is concerned more with reducing or eliminating it locally as a step in preparing the granulations for grafting. Infection may be a mixed one with *Proteus mirabilis*, and in many instances the general measures, discussed under preparation of granulations for grafting, for controlling local infection are adequate. In any case while *Ps. aeruginosa* may reduce graft take by 5–10% at most, grafting of the area does tend to end the infection. Grafting regardless of its presence and accepting any small reduction in take gives excellent results.

In short a positive culture of *Ps. aeruginosa* is not a contraindication to grafting if the granulations are clinically healthy.

Other pathogens

The other pathogens which commonly infect wounds are *Staphylococcus aureus*, *Escherichia coli*, and *Proteus mirabilis*. In this situation *Staph. aureus* is seldom more than a commensal. *E. coli* and *Pr. mirabilis* are especially common in the badly managed, heavily contaminated, granulating area. They are associated as a rule with a very typical, profuse, foul-smelling discharge and often occur as a mixed infection with *Ps. aeruginosa*. In the extensive deep burn they may be impossible to avoid, but all too often they are allowed to contaminate quite small granulating surfaces from which they could be excluded by ordinary care.

Preparing granulations for grafting

It is axiomatic that the granulating area is being treated, not its flora, and so antibiotics should not be used blindly on the basis of sensitivity reports. *Str. pyogenes* apart, the flora is largely immaterial provided the granulations look healthy, and the fastest way to eliminate the flora is to skin graft the area.

In deciding the appropriate steps to eliminate *Str. pyogenes* from a granulating area the organism cannot be considered in isolation. It might appear logical to use an appropriate systemic antibiotic, but experience is that systemic antibiotics to which organisms are sensitive are ineffective in eliminating them from a granulating surface. An antiseptic such as chlorhexidine (Hibitane) applied locally is likely to be more effective.

The presence of slough creates a suitable environment for continuing infection, and it is likely to continue as long as the slough remains. Surgical excision is a rapid and highly effective method of eliminating it. In removing the slough, excision to fascia is preferable to excision to fat. The Humby knife with the roller widely open has been used to excise both slough and heavily infected granulations and is most effective in the role.

Where a slough is being allowed to separate naturally, pus is inevitable, and if there are no signs of invasive infection it is not necessarily undesirable, for its enzymes play a valuable role in separating slough from viable tissue. In the absence of invasive infection the flora is to be regarded as innocuous. It can only be eliminated when the slough has gone.

Granulations, once clean and free of slough, should be grafted without delay. During such waiting as is unavoidable an innocuous dressing which will not damage the granulations when removed should be used, and tulle gras is usual. Unless *Str. pyogenes* is present an antibiotic is not essential. A meticulous dressings technique, adequate cover both in area and thickness of dressing, and infrequent dressings provide a better insurance against superadded infection than a blind reliance on antibiotics. The other factor which will keep granulations as healthy as possible for the longest time is pressure, and crepe bandages are usually necessary to provide this. Although the rationale is far from clear it is a common finding that hydrocortisone ointment sometimes improves unhealthy granulations or granulations showing little progress towards healing with or without grafts.

Despite all efforts the situation can arise where production of granulation tissue is either poor or non-existent. The common factor is generally ischaemia of the area. This can be the result of peripheral vascular disease reducing the local blood flow, and a similar situation can result from the effects of radiation. In both there is an indolent ulcer, poor granulations or none at all, and an absence of marginal healing. The aetiology is usually obvious, and generally nothing can be done to the area to improve the situation. Poor vascularity can also take the form of an inadequate throughflow of oxygenated blood, as seen in gravitational ulceration. This can be temporarily improved by supportive bandaging, and successful grafting achieved, but the success is likely to be only temporary until the venous problem is tackled effectively.

APPLICATION OF THE GRAFT

A skin graft can be applied to a defect in one of two ways, with **pressure** applied to the graft, or with the graft left **exposed**.

If full use is to be made of the virtues peculiar to each of these methods it is essential to see how in different clinical situations each provides close, immobile contact between the graft and the bed, the conditions necessary for graft take.

As already stressed, the factors which in practice are largely responsible for loss of a graft are separation of the graft from its bed by blood clot, and/or prevention of the graft from adhering to its bed because it is allowed to slide to and fro on its bed. Whether the pressure method or exposed grafting is used in the particular clinical situation it should be the one most likely to prevent **haematoma** and **shearing movements**.

PRESSURE METHODS

Pressure is usually applied in two ways. It is applied directly and very precisely to the graft by means of a bolus overlying the graft, the sutures used to fix the graft in position around the margin of the defect being left long and tied over the bolus to hold it in position. It is for this reason that the method is also referred to as **bolus grafting**. A further pressure dressing is then applied to the area generally, using crepe bandaging and/or Elastoplast. This provides additional pressure but, just as significantly, it adds to the immobilisation of the area.

For technical reasons, discussed on p. 57, the use of a tie-over bolus is not feasible when a granulating area is being grafted using the pressure method, and a pressure-immobilising dressing applied to the area generally is relied on.

Applying the graft (Fig. 3.17)

The **full thickness skin graft**, cut to its prescribed pattern, fits the defect accurately and is sutured edge to edge along its margin. Sufficient sutures are inserted to give as accurate edge apposition as would be demanded in the suture of a wound and, as in suturing a wound, care should be taken to avoid inversion of the edges. Sufficient sutures are left long to provide a snug tie-over; the remainder are cut short.

The **split skin graft** is cut large enough to cover the defect with an overlap, and the sutures used to hold it in its overlapped position are left long to provide for the tie-over. The graft takes to the margin of the defect and the overlap is trimmed off when the graft is dressed.

Dressing the graft (Fig. 3.17)

Care in packing of the graft area with the bolus material is essential to ensure that the graft as a whole is subjected to uniform pressure. The bolus should be bulky and extend to the margin of the

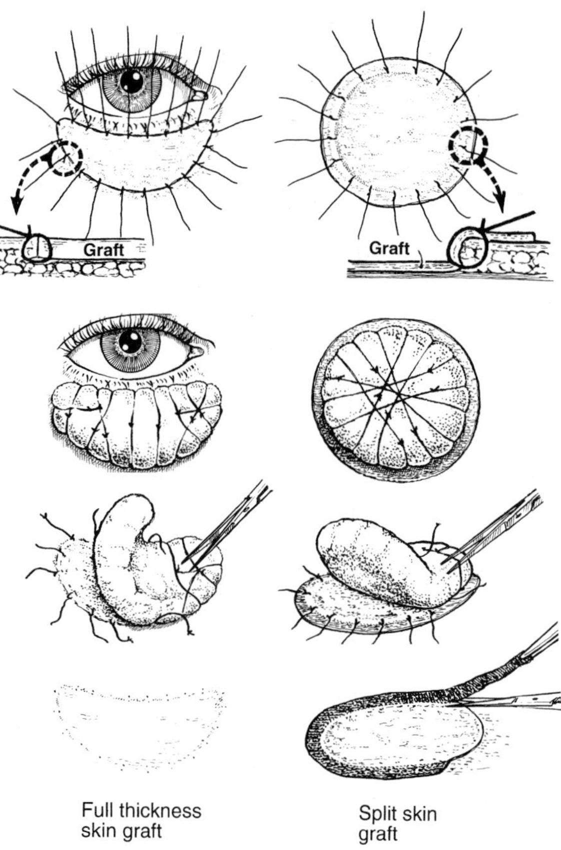

Fig 3.17 The use of the tie-over bolus dressing technique in the pressure method of skin grafting. The full thickness skin graft is sutured edge to edge with the margins of the defect. The split skin graft overlaps the defect, the overlap being trimmed away at the first dressing.

graft, the long tie-over sutures being then tied tightly over the bolus, anchoring graft and bolus in a single mass. A layer of tulle gras laid over the graft before the bolus is applied tends to ease the first postoperative dressing, but is not essential.

The bolus material classically used in the United Kingdom is cotton wool prepared with flavine emulsion.* Possible alternatives are cotton waste, cotton wool moistened with saline or tightly wrung out with liquid paraffin, and polyurethane foam. Of these materials flavine wool has the considerable virtue of being water-repellent and has desirable fluffing properties.

Over further cotton wool padding to diffuse the pressure, crepe bandages are applied. If the site lends itself better to immobilisation by Elastoplast this should be used instead. The objective is as complete immobility as can be achieved, and both the Elastoplast and crepe bandages are used to this end. Plaster of Paris should be used in addition if it is felt that it will add significantly to the overall immobility of the grafted area.

Bolus grafting is the standard method used when a graft is being applied primarily, and is routine with full thickness skin grafts, these being virtually always used primarily. The pressure acts as a haemostatic factor preventing the haematoma which might otherwise separate the graft from the bed. It is most effective in those areas which are easy to immobilise, for example the limbs and face. The face is admittedly mobile, but the tie-over bolus, coupled in the early stages with the addition of an overall immobilising crepe bandage and Elastoplast, is effective in preventing movements of the facial muscles.

In areas such as the trunk and the groin the problems of bolus grafting become more obvious, because pressure is extremely difficult to apply and effective immobilisation is virtually impossible to achieve. In these areas it has been found wanting, despite the use of increasingly elaborate methods of immobilisation, and it is in these areas that exposed grafting has provided the solution.

EXPOSED GRAFTING

The exposed grafting technique was initially developed as a solution to the ineffectiveness of bolus grafting in areas which cannot easily be immobilised. Even with the most elaborate methods of fixation and immobilisation the bolus

---

*PREPARATION OF FLAVINE WOOL. The materials used are flavine emulsion and best quality cotton wool or Gamgee. A sheet of cotton wool is soaked in the emulsion, previously warmed to reduce its viscosity, until it is completely impregnated. The excess of emulsion is then removed from the cotton wool. It is at this point that the usefulness of Gamgee becomes apparent, for the covering gauze adds to the strength of the material which can be rolled up and wrung out by hand. This must be done thoroughly until the cotton wool appears virtually dry and no more emulsion can be extracted. The sheet of cotton wool is left to dry off on a warm surface and when autoclaved is ready for use. For ease of handling it can be wrapped in cellophane or packed in a tin.

dressing with the underlying graft tended to slide to and fro, setting up shearing movements between graft and bed which prevented vascular link-up (Fig. 3.4). The pressure dressing, instead of being the means of providing immobile contact, became the means of preventing it.

Removal of the dressing had the effect of eliminating these shearing strains. With the graft laid in position and protected from being rubbed off, the natural fibrin adhesion between graft and bed allowed the graft to tolerate minor movements of the patient without interfering with the sequence of vascularisation and fibrous tissue fixation (Fig. 3.18).

Exposure solved the problem of shearing movements, but not the problem of haematoma, and the method which has been developed to solve it governs many of the practical details of current technique. Problems of haematoma did not arise when a granulating area was grafted using exposed grafting, and this fact provided the key to success in the post-resection defect — by the use of **delayed exposed grafting**.

It is theoretically possible to use exposed grafting primarily, but pressure cannot be employed effectively once the graft has been applied and this means that haemostasis must be most rigorous. By watching the graft carefully in the immediate postoperative period it is possible to evacuate any little haematoma by carefully snipping the overlying graft, but the method is nonetheless not at its best used primarily.

In delayed exposed grafting application of the graft is held over until haemostasis is assured. The gap in time between creation of the defect and application of the graft is not critical, 24–48 hours being an average time. In practice, the graft can be applied as soon as the surface has been cleared of clot.

Exposed grafting demands a degree of co-

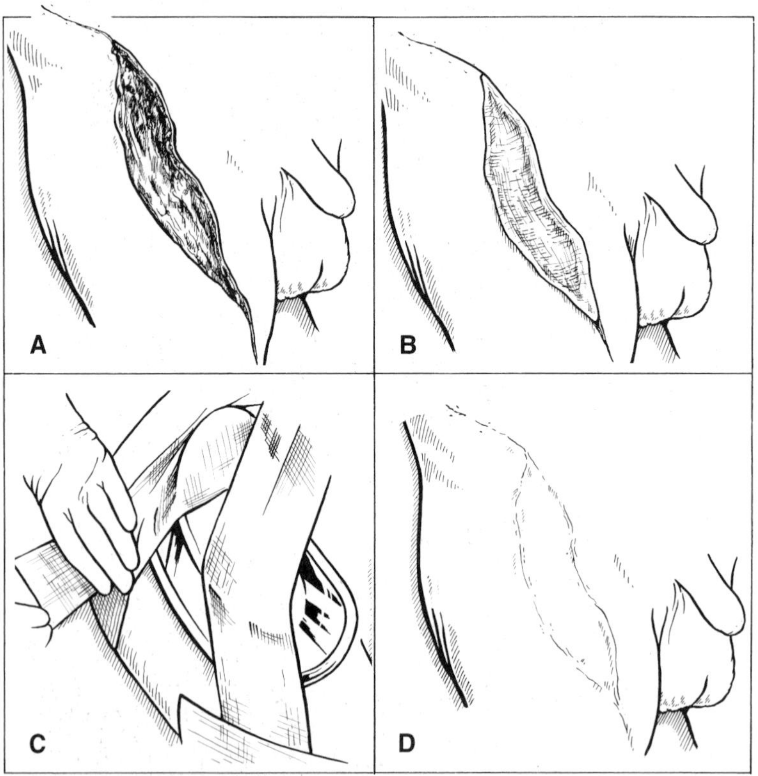

Fig. 3.18 The use of delayed exposed grafting in the management of a granulating area in the groin which followed skin necrosis complicating an inguinopelvic lymph node clearance for metastatic squamous carcinoma. The granulating surface (**A**) was covered with the split skin graft (**B**), and protected by the inverted kidney dish (**C**). **D** shows the end result.

operation from the patient, and it has to be used with discretion in children. Even in adults co-operation cannot be expected during recovery from the anaesthetic and transfer from operating theatre to bed, an added reason for postponing the application of the graft. Instead a temporary dressing is applied to the defect.

The graft is usually cut at the time of the excisional procedure and stored in the refrigerator (see p. 47) until it is required. It is then applied with the patient in bed, awake and co-operative.

Experience of using the technique over a prolonged period has demonstrated that the responsibility of applying the graft can safely be given to the nursing staff once they have been shown the steps involved. The graft should be allowed to overlap the margin of the defect and any air bubbles under it can be massaged out using a Q-tip. It adheres firmly to its bed remarkably quickly.

Protection of the graft has to be improvised, but it need not be elaborate, since it is possible to discard it in a day or two if the patient is reasonably cooperative. When the area is small an inverted stainless steel bowl or kidney dish strapped over the defect is adequate. Kramer wire is also a useful and versatile material used in this context.

The success of the technique in difficult sites has led to its use in previously undisputed pressure-grafting territory. This extension of its

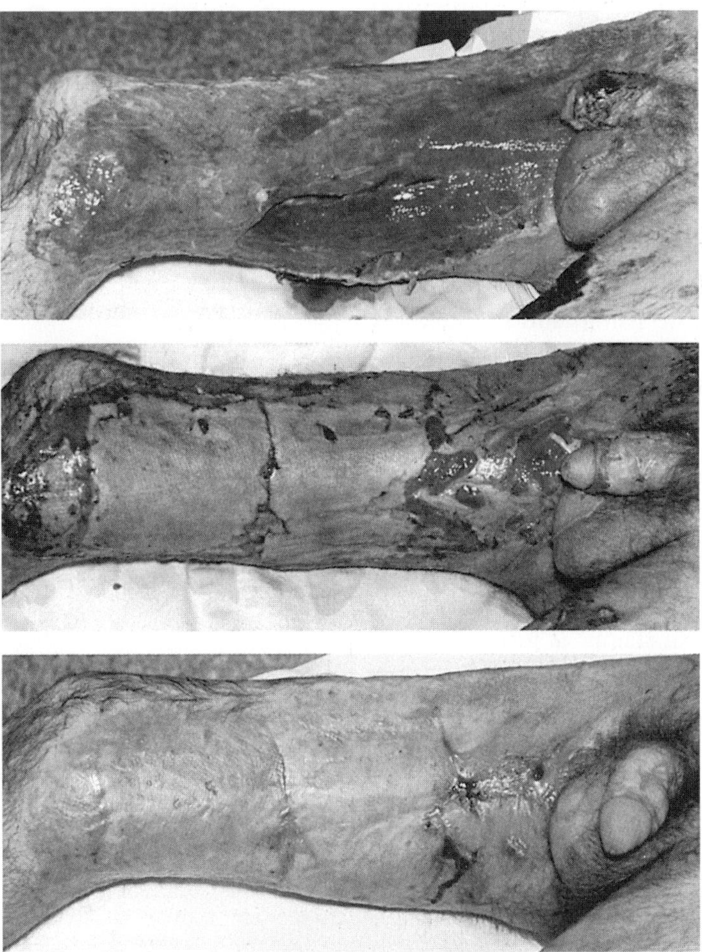

Fig 3.19 The use of sheet split skin grafts in covering a granulating area of the thigh.

role has demonstrated that many areas can be grafted successfully using either pressure or exposure. Choice tends to be a matter of personal preference, but the saving of operative time, and the ease and convenience of exposed grafting have made it increasingly popular when a single surface is being grafted. It is clearly not possible to use it if the site cannot be kept clear of the bed clothes, and this makes it generally inappropriate when the raw surface is circumferential.

GRAFTING GRANULATING SURFACES

When the grafting of granulating surfaces was first widely introduced, it was used in the management of full thickness skin loss burns, and the grafts were applied in the form of stamp-sized grafts. Each stamp formed a focus from which epidermis spread to cover the intervening areas, the healed site ending as a mosaic of graft alternating with spread epidermis. The appearance showed wide and quite unpredictable variation. At one extreme the spread epidermis was smooth and not unlike the stamps; at the other it became hypertrophic. Initially redder, it gradually paled in most patients to a colour more nearly matching the stamp. The spread epidermis was also less stable than the stamp, and in the lower limb it was necessary to provide support with elastic or crepe bandaging for a considerable period. Gradually the area became more stable, stability and cosmetic improvement usually progressing together.

With increased confidence in grafting techniques the stamps gradually increased in area to become sheets, and today sheets are used in preference to stamps when ample skin is available (Fig. 3.19). The use of stamps is justifiable only where skin is in short supply or the site creates particular difficulties, as in the perineum or axilla, stamps then being considered less likely to be dislodged than a sheet of skin.

The mechanics of applying the graft are similar regardless of whether pressure or exposure is to be used. Spreading the graft on a sheet of tulle gras (Fig. 3.20) eases handling; tulle gras and graft can then be applied to the granulating area. It is not usual to suture the graft in place, although in a difficult situation a few tacking

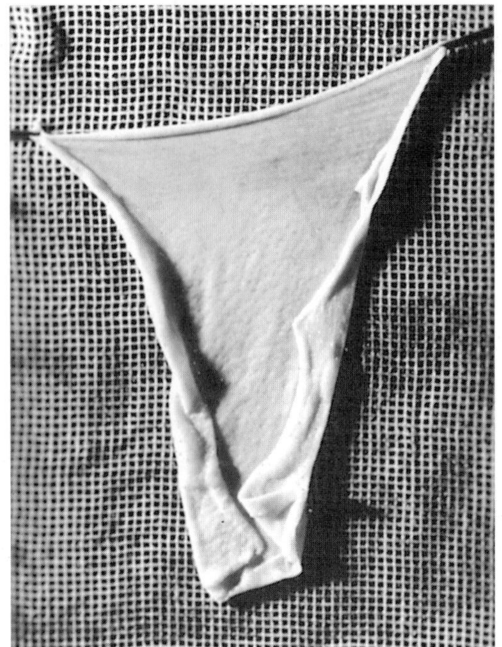

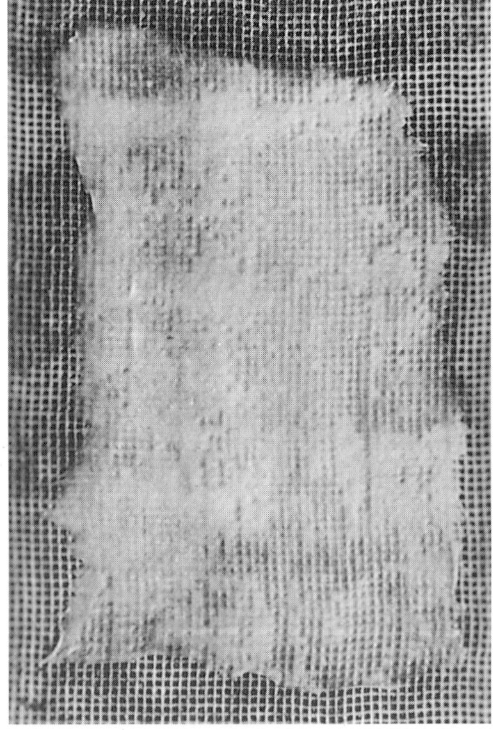

Fig. 3.20 The handling of a split skin graft on tulle gras, showing the graft laid on the tulle gras, which has been spread on a wooden board, and then spread on the tulle gras.

sutures may help prevent it from sliding off the granulations while the dressing is being applied. The sutures cannot be used for a tie-over dressing, for in the skin immediately adjoining a granulating area they are likely to cut out rapidly. The use of sutures to provide added fixation of the graft to the surrounding skin in this way has largely been replaced by micropore tape, though even it is not often considered necessary.

MESH GRAFTING

The meshing of grafts has given a considerable boost to the concept of expanding the area which an individual graft is able to cover, previously only possible by dividing it into stamps. The graft, cut in the usual way, is passed through an instrument from which it emerges shredded into a regular meshwork of skin. Traction applied to the four corners of the graft expands the mesh (Fig. 3.21) giving a considerable increase in area. The advantage of the meshed graft over the stamp graft lies in the regularity of the mesh and the uniform distribution of the graft as a source of spread epidermis (Fig. 3.22). The area between individual strips is reduced and the healing time becomes relatively short. As with stamps, the final cosmetic result varies greatly, and this is its main fault, but when cosmesis is a secondary consideration it does allow skin to be applied with success to surfaces where doubt might otherwise exist regarding the likelihood of take. In general, however, meshing is used in order to expand the extent of the area the graft is being used to cover. The possibly greater ease with which it may take is a bonus.

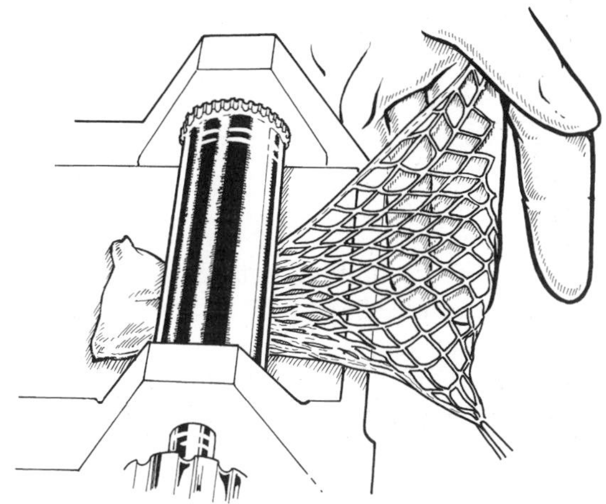

Fig. 3.21 Meshing a split skin graft. The graft, fed between the rollers, emerges meshed so that, stretched, it can be expanded to provide cover over a much greater area.

When pressure dressings are being used, the graft and the dressing can be applied in the operating theatre. The outer pressure dressing consists of the usual gauze, cotton wool, and crepe bandage or Elastoplast. Fixation is naturally less secure than that provided by a tie-over dressing, and when a crepe bandage is being used care is needed during the first few turns of the bandage to make sure that the graft does not slide off the granulating area. Bulk of dressing may be enough to produce immobility but plaster of Paris should always be used if necessary to reinforce the dressings.

When the exposed method is being used, application of the skin should wait until the patient is awake and back in bed. The graft is then protected until it is well fixed.

QUILTED GRAFTING

In addition to the conventional methods of applying a graft, whether using pressure or exposure techniques, it is the practice of some surgeons to routinely 'fenestrate' the graft. By this is meant the making of multiple slits in the graft with the object of 'allowing the escape of any fluid which might otherwise separate the graft from its bed'. The fact that the skin grafts of surgeons who do not habitually fenestrate them take equally well demonstrates that, except in specific instances, fenestration is unnecessary.

The sole useful niche of fenestration is as an element of the **quilted grafting** technique. Quilted grafting is used when the site involved is for practical purposes impossible to immobilise, and it finds its main application in grafting defects of the mobile parts of the oral cavity, most frequently the side of the tongue (Fig. 3.23).

The graft is sutured with catgut to the margins of the defect and multiple additional sutures are inserted through the graft and the underlying tongue muscle, anchoring the two together, and giving the overall appearance of a 'quilt'. The

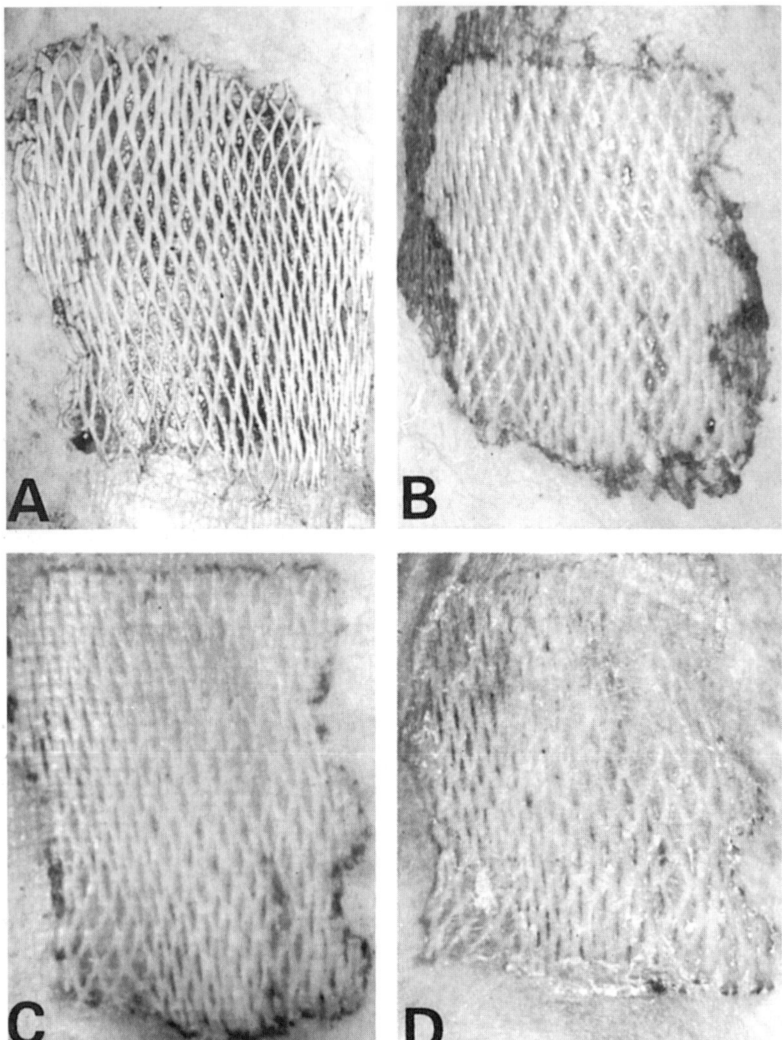

Fig. 3.22 The clinical use of meshed graft.

A The graft applied to a granulating area.
B, C The intermediate stages of healing by epidermal spread from the graft, seen by the increased blurring of the margins of the graft.
D The healed result, with the pattern of the original mesh still visible.

effect of the sutures is to convert the single large area of the defect into a mosaic of small areas, in each of which, despite the background of continuing mobility of the tongue, there is sufficient immobility to allow the graft to become attached and vascularised.

Effective haemostasis of the bed is obviously a prerequisite to successful use of the technique, but even with complete control of bleeding prior to application of the graft the inevitably blind insertion of the quilting sutures generally gives rise to some bleeding. It is in coping with this bleeding that fenestration of the graft has the beneficial effect of allowing any blood clots to escape, massaged out by the continuing movement of the tongue.

THE SEROMA

When a graft has been applied to a concave

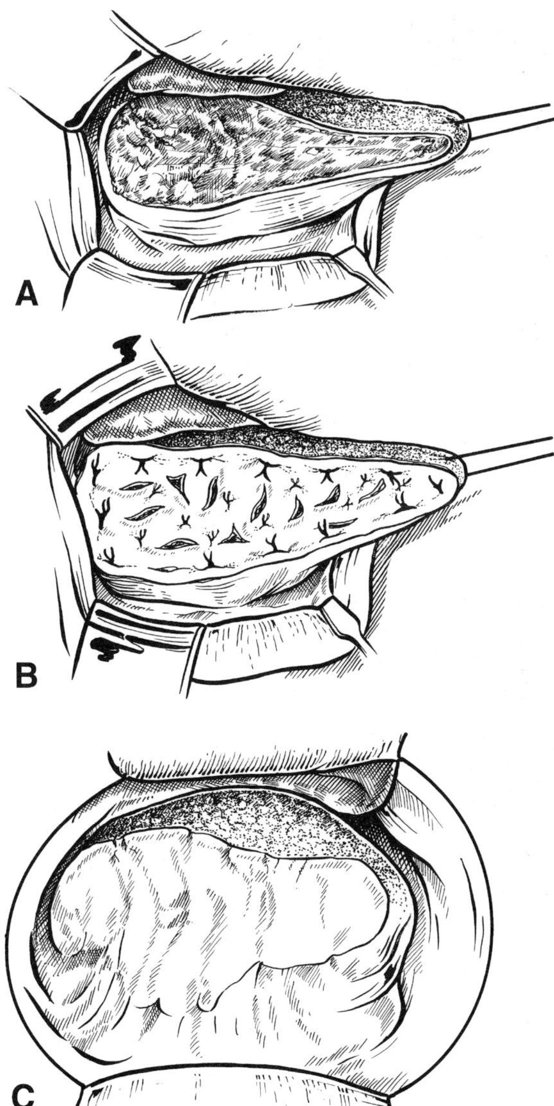

Fig. 3.23 Quilted grafting, used in resurfacing a defect of the side of the tongue.
A shows the tongue defect, and **B** the split skin graft, sutured to the margins of the defect in the standard manner, with the quilting sutures to provide foci of immobile contact between the graft and the bed, and intervening fenestrating slits in the graft to allow extrusion of any blood clots resulting from bleeding from the unavoidably blind insertion of the quilting sutures. **C** shows the final result.

surface it sometimes, after it has become vascularised but before it has become firmly anchored to its bed, becomes detached from this bed over part of its area and tents across the concavity. This leaves a space underneath which fills with serum, creating a **seroma**. It tends to occur following the use of a pressure dressing, and detachment takes place when pressure is removed a week after grafting. Aspiration of the serum is ineffective; the seroma rapidly reforms. While it is detached the graft remains surprisingly well vascularised from the surrounding attached graft.

Untreated, the graft proceeds to epithelialise on its deep surface from the cut ends of the pilosebaceous apparatus and eventually 'heals' completely. Since the graft cannot become re-attached once 'healing' has taken place, treatment is a matter of some urgency.

Once it is recognised that the condition is due to contraction of the graft with resulting detachment and that the seroma is secondary to this, treatment is obvious. The graft must be cut open over the area of detachment in such a way that it can lie completely and demonstrably quite freely on its bed. A cruciform cut may be needed before all tendency to tenting is corrected, for the graft has contracted in all axes. If the condition is treated without delay these measures suffice, but if several days have elapsed it must be assumed that some 'healing' has occurred and it is advisable to remove this epithelium by gently curetting the deep surface of the graft so that it can re-adhere. Alternatively the detached area of skin can be removed completely and a fresh graft applied.

With the increase in the use of delayed exposed grafting, the incidence of seroma has dropped markedly.

CHAPTER

4

Flaps

A flap, in contradistinction to a skin graft, contains within its substance a network of blood vessels, arterial, capillary and venous, and it is the effectiveness of the circulation through this network in perfusing the tissues of the flap at each stage of its transfer from donor to recipient site which determines its survival. The anatomical basis of the vascular network varies considerably in different sites of the body, and flaps with a striking diversity of tissue content and vascular patterns have been developed to exploit these variations.

The major flap types are largely named according to the tissue transferred. A flap which consists of skin and superficial fascia is referred to as a **skin flap**. When the investing layer of deep fascia is included, the flap becomes **fasciocutaneous**. A flap may also consist of a muscle, usually detached at one end, and moved to cover a surface which is unsuitable for grafting, for example bare cortical bone. When covered by such a **muscle flap**, the surface which results accepts a graft readily. The principle of the muscle flap has been extended to include the skin overlying the muscle, on occasion also bone to which the muscle is attached, the composite flap being **myocutaneous** or **osteomyocutaneous** depending on the constituents.

Prior to the development of the technique of joining small blood vessels together, flaps had to retain a vascular attachment to the body throughout their transfer, but it is now possible to transfer a flap *en bloc* to a distant site in a single stage, as a **free flap**, anastomosing its vascular system to suitable vessels in the recipient area.

Much of the jargon used in flap description derives from the vocabulary developed to describe skin flap practice. It will be discussed in that context, but it can be freely transferred to describe other flap types.

A flap is transferred to reconstruct a **primary defect**, and is **inset** into this defect. The transfer usually leaves a **secondary defect** which in most instances is closed by direct suture, or covered with a free skin graft.

The flap may be raised as a **local flap** from the tissues in the immediate vicinity of the primary defect, its movement usually taking the form of **transposition** or **rotation**, the term applied to the flap. Alternatively, the transfer may involve the movement of tissue at a distance from the primary defect, and is then called a **distant flap**.

The entire flap, or its greater part, may be inset into the defect at the initial transfer, and the proximal segment is then referred to as its **base**.

Alternatively, only the **distal segment** of the flap may be inset into the defect, its central segment and base remaining unattached. The base is then often referred to as the **pedicle** of the flap and the central segment as its **bridge segment**. These two, pedicle and bridge segment, act as the carrier of the flap and provide the channel of blood supply to its distal segment. It is desirable to eliminate unnecessary raw surface in such a flap, and so reduce the likelihood of infection, and this explains the practice of either tubing the bridge segment of a flap, or lining it with a split skin graft depending on the local circumstances. It is seldom technically possible to tube or line the local flaps commonly used in the face, but infection is rarely a problem because of the excellence of the local blood supply.

Once the distal segment of the flap is established in its new site, which usually takes 3 weeks, the bridge segment is divided, and either returned to its original site or discarded depending on the local situation. Insetting of the distal segment is then completed.

The pedicle of a skin flap usually consists, like the rest of the flap, of skin and subcutaneous tissue, but it is occasionally reduced to its subcutaneous component. In such circumstances it is the distal segment, with a full complement of skin and subcutaneous tissue, which is transferred as an **island flap**.

A distant flap can be transferred to its destination in several ways. It can be **directly applied** to the primary defect, it can be **waltzed**, pivoted on its pedicle, or it may be attached to a **carrier**, usually the wrist, on which it is conveyed to its destination. The wrist is selected as a carrier because its reach makes it possible for the flap to leap-frog a considerable distance in a single step. Waltzing of a flap tends to be used only when the distance between the flap and the primary defect is not great, and the transfer can be completed in a single movement. Transfer using a wrist carrier is an extreme rarity today.

It is sometimes felt that the blood supply of a flap would not be adequate for its survival if it were raised and transferred straightaway. Its vascular efficiency can be enhanced by surgically outlining the flap prior to its actual transfer, the procedure and its effect both being referred to as a **delay**. The term has also come to be applied to any surgical procedure used to improve the blood supply of a flap during transfer.

Most local flaps have a centre around which they rotate or are transposed, and this is referred to as the **pivot point**. When the flap is being designed, it is from this point that measurements are made to ensure that its geometry will allow it to achieve its transfer safely. When a flap is leap-frogging over intact tissue an alternative technique, **planning in reverse**, is used.

A difficulty which arises in describing in a systematic manner the flaps which are used most frequently today is that some belong to more than one category. Among the group of muscle and myocutaneous flaps some are used solely as muscle, and some only as myocutaneous flaps, while some are used in either form. To complicate the situation still further, some in each category are transferred as free flaps. A similarly confused situation exists in relation to certain of the skin and fasciocutaneous flaps.

With the development of free tissue transfer, problems of nomenclature have arisen in distinguishing between grafts and flaps, most obviously in discussing the transfer of vascularised bone. In such a transfer, the pre-existing vascular structure of the bone is maintained intact, its blood supply merely temporarily interrupted, rather than re-established through vascular link-up at a capillary level, as in a graft. To refer to such a transfer as a graft, admittedly a vascularised graft, may be regarded by the purist as a misnomer, but it has become standard usage, and as such has probably to be accepted.

VASCULAR ASPECTS OF FLAPS

Effective tissue perfusion determines the viability of all flaps, and dominates every aspect of their design and transfer. Skill in the design and use of flaps is very much a matter of balancing the demands of blood supply against those of flap geometry.

Flaps which lack a clear-cut directional orientation of blood flow, and have no focal point where arterial input and venous outflow are recognisably concentrated, tend to have inefficient perfusion characteristics and poor safety records. A well-defined directional orientation of blood flow, and anatomically recognisable vessels providing input and outflow, go with safety in transfer.

ANATOMICAL BACKGROUND

In the body sites which are considered to have major potential for use as skin and fasciocutaneous flaps, the skin is perfused from a vascular network running horizontally in relation to the investing layer of deep fascia. The network is fed from vessels which emerge at intervals from the deeper tissues, referred to as **perforators**, direct branches of the system of arteries and veins whose primary function is to perfuse the deeper structures, muscles and bones. A contribution to the skin circulation is also made by small vessels which reach it from the muscles which lie directly under the skin. *Such evidence as exists would suggest that under normal physiological conditions these vessels do not contribute significantly to perfusion of the skin*, but in some sites they are certainly capable of sustaining skin viability in the absence of other sources, since they form the vascular basis of myocutaneous flaps.

The pattern of sites at which these perforating vessels emerge shows a striking consistency, and following their emergence they run horizontally, giving off branches as they go. The great majority of these branches are not terminal, but instead link-up with vessels of a similar calibre. The richness of the resulting anastomoses and the calibre of the vessels involved vary in different sites, but the effect is to create a largely uniform and apparently random vascular network with little evidence of separate territories fed from individual perforators. It is this plexus (Fig. 4.1) which provides the background to the circulation from which the skin is perfused.

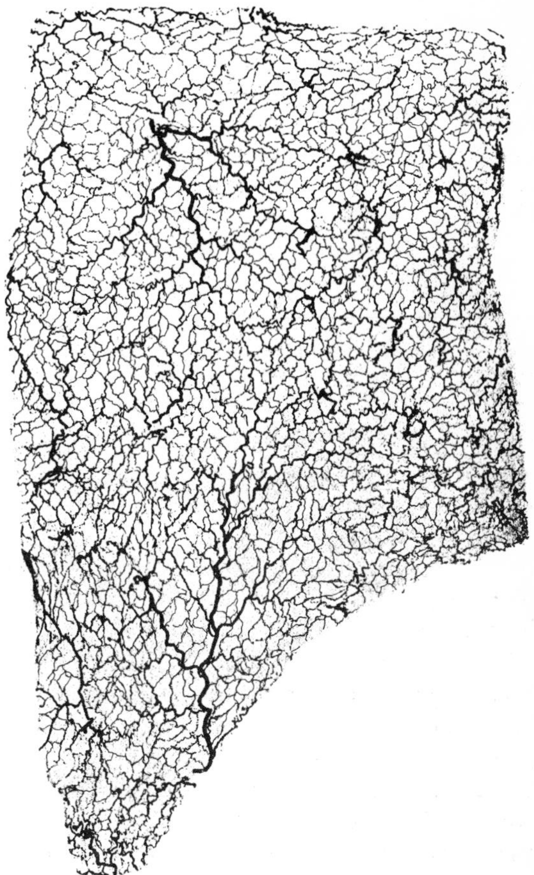

Fig. 4.1 The plexus of small arteries which provide the perfusion sources of the skin, in this instance of the anterolateral abdominal wall. Several perforating vessels providing arterial input are clearly visible, but the uniformity of the background plexus is very striking. (From *M. Salmon, Artères de la Peau, Masson, Paris, 1936*)

The **face and scalp** have in common an extremely rich skin blood supply, but the differences in their anatomical features have resulted in different vascular patterns above and below the level of the zygomatic arch (Fig. 4.2).

Below the zygomatic arch there is a rich dermal and subdermal plexus of small vessels fed mainly from branches of the facial artery, but also from the transverse facial artery and the vessels emerging from the bony foramina, infraorbital and mental. The branches of the facial artery emerge between the facial muscles which radiate from the angle of the mouth, the transverse facial artery emerges from the parotid gland, becoming subcutaneous a little above its duct, and the infraorbital and mental arteries emerge from the corresponding foramina. Multiple anastomoses unite the three systems, and from this background the subdermal and dermal circulation is fed.

Above the zygomatic arch a wealth of vessels of a sizeable calibre form an anastomotic pattern running horizontally between the skin and the galea. They are derived from vessels which reach the area from its periphery and they have no deep connections. This absence of deep connections means that delay of a scalp flap need never

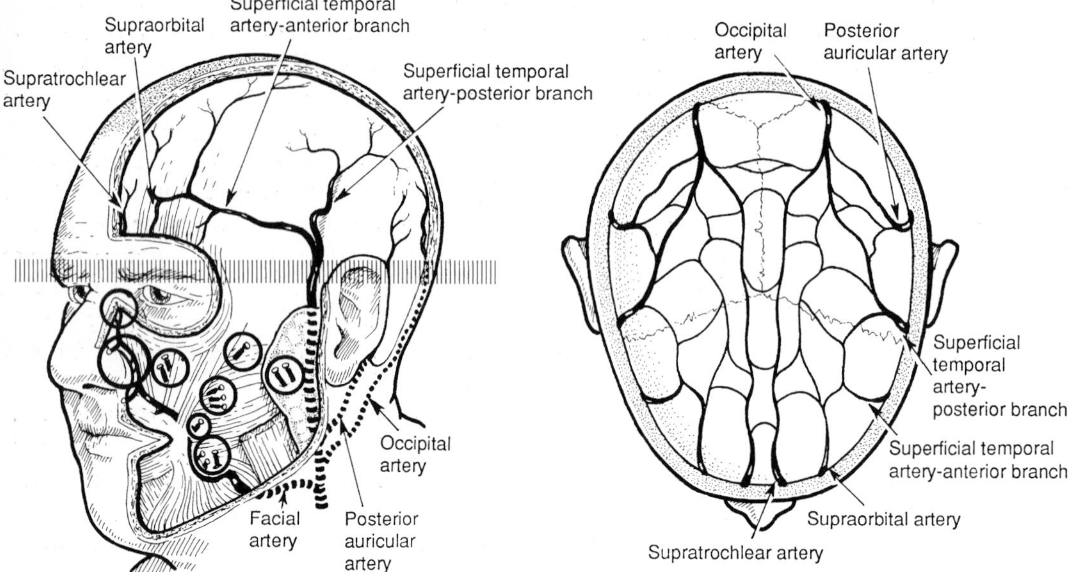

Fig. 4.2 Vascular patterns above and below the zygomatic arch.
Below the zygomatic arch there is a rich subdermal vascular plexus fed from perforator branches of the deeper pattern of anatomically named vessels. Above the arch a network of blood vessels runs horizontally in the fascial layer between the skin and galea with no significant deep connections, fed from the vessels around the margins of the scalp.

include elevation. Axial pattern flaps (see p. 70) are raised on the scalp and forehead, using the superficial temporal vessels and the supraorbital: supratrochlear system, but the number of vessels forming the anastomotic pattern, and their individual calibre, allows flaps with no overt axial pattern to be raised both in the scalp and forehead which behave in transfer as though they did have such a pattern.

The **neck skin**, together with platysma, receives the bulk of its blood supply from branches of the facial artery, mainly its submental branch, and branches of the transverse cervical artery. It has little in the way of deep vascular connections.

In the **trunk**, the deep fascial layer is not a very distinct entity, and flaps are raised in the plane of surgical cleavage rather than in conscious relation to the fascial layers. The surgical plane includes the layer in any case since, depending on the part of the trunk, it leaves the underlying muscle bare or the aponeurosis covered with a fine layer of areolar tissue.

Perforating vessels emerge into the superficial fascia from the underlying muscle or aponeurosis through which they have passed. In the super-

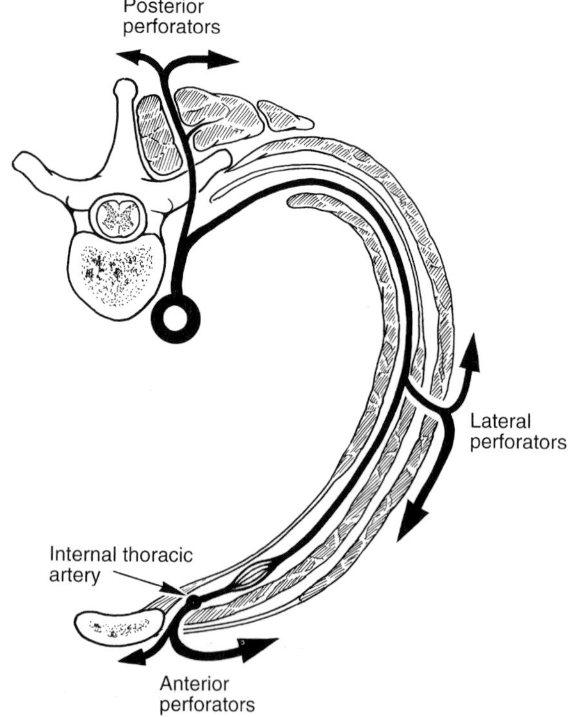

Fig. 4.3 The segmental intercostal vascular system with its pattern of anterior, lateral and posterior perforating branches.

ficial fascia they run in an essentially horizontal direction, branching, and becoming smaller in diameter. At their peripheral extent they have a diameter similar to their main branches, and link-up with corresponding branches of the adjoining perforating vessel systems, as seen in Fig. 4.1, to create the continuous vascular network from which the skin is perfused. The siting of the perforating vessels is consistent, as is also their direction once they have emerged into the superficial fascia.

The segmental intercostal neurovascular system (Fig. 4.3) has anterior, lateral, and posterior perforators. In the chest the lateral perforating vessels are in the line of the axilla and there is a corresponding increase in the lateral extent of the territory of the anterior perforating system. Branches also emerge from the pattern of vessels perfusing the large muscles of the shoulder girdle, particularly pectoralis major, latissimus dorsi, and trapezius. They contribute little to normal skin perfusion, and play no part in the design of skin and fasciocutaneous flaps, but they have a significant role in perfusing the myocutaneous flaps which involve the muscles from which they emerge.

In the **chest** (Fig. 4.4), perforators emerge from each intercostal space just lateral to the sternum, and pass laterally across the anterior chest wall, providing the basis of the *deltopectoral flap* (p. 91). In the scapular area, in addition to the segmental lateral and posterior perforating branches of the posterior intercostal vessels, cutaneous branches of the circumflex scapular vessels perfuse the skin area overlying the scapula (Fig. 4.5), allowing construction of the *scapular flaps* (p. 116).

Below the level of the 6th space the intercostal neurovascular bundles continue the initial downward direction of the ribs rather than pursuing the upward curve of the costal margin. This brings them on to the **anterior abdominal wall** (Fig. 4.6) where they run between the internal oblique

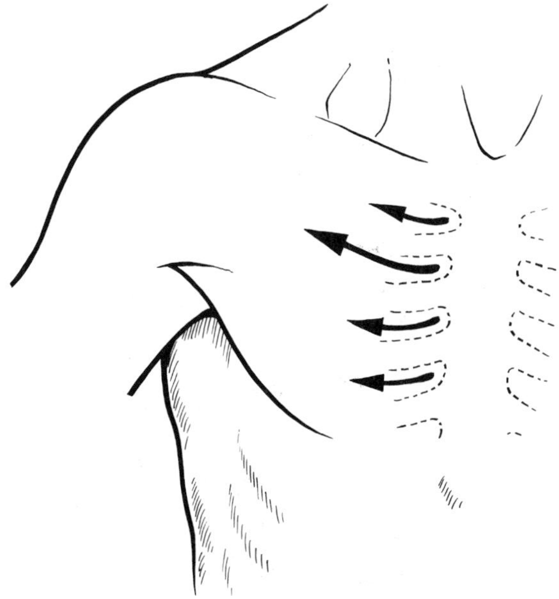

Fig. 4.4 The perfusing system of the skin of the anterior chest wall.
Anterior perforating vessels, derived from the intercostal segmental system, shown in Figure 4.3, emerge lateral to the sternum in the intercostal spaces and pass laterally over the chest wall.

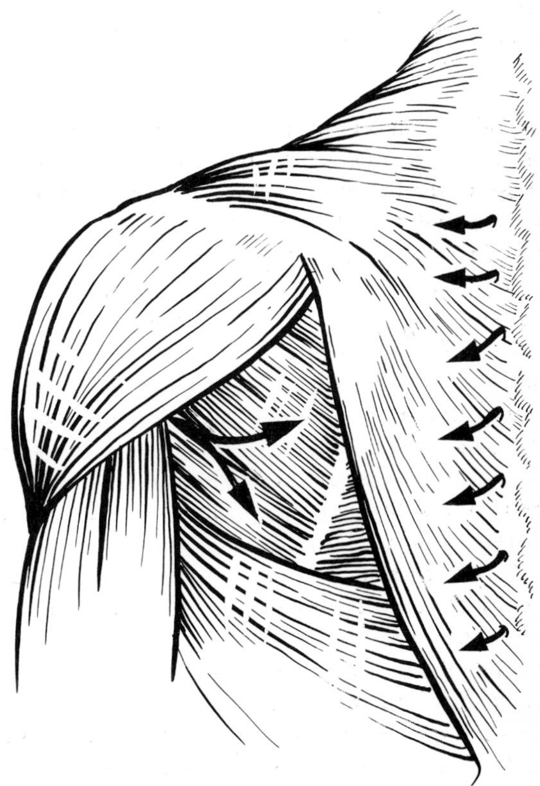

Fig. 4.5 The perfusing system of the scapular area.
The cutaneous branches of the circumflex scapular artery act as perforating vessels, and combine with the posterior perforating arteries of the segmental system.

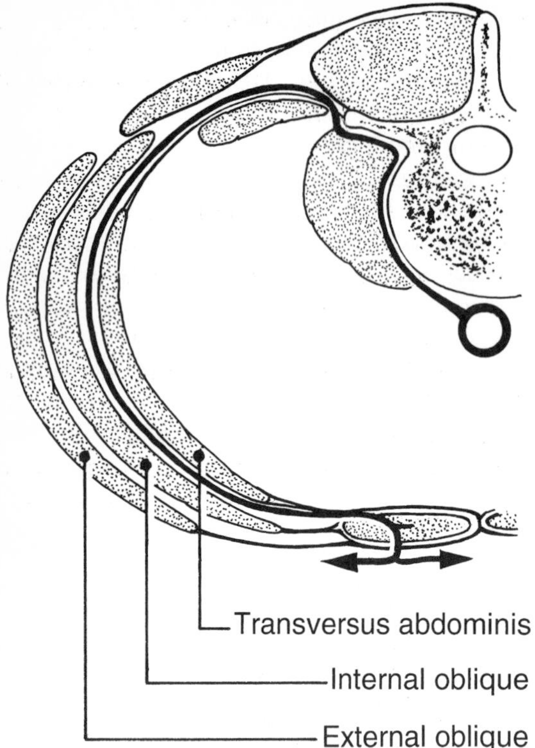

Fig. 4.6 The segmental system of vessels in the abdomen.
These vessels pass forward in the intermuscular plane between the internal oblique and transversus abdominis muscles, pierce the posterior layer of the rectus sheath and reach rectus abdominis, anastomosing with the superior and inferior epigastric vessels, and contributing to the system of perforating vessels emerging from the anterior layer of the rectus sheath.

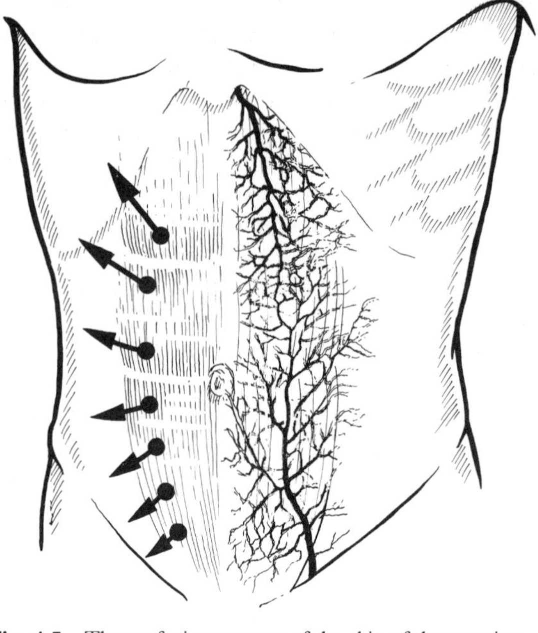

Fig. 4.7 The perfusion sources of the skin of the anterior abdomen.
This is provided by the perforating branches of the superior and inferior epigastric systems of vessels, anastomosing with one another within the rectus sheath, in combination with the abdominal segmental system of vessels (Fig. 4.6).

and transversus abdominis muscles, reaching the posterior layer of the rectus sheath which they penetrate. They continue through the rectus abdominis muscle and emerge as perforators from the anterior rectus sheath near the midline.

Within the rectus sheath a further vascular system is present deep to and within the substance of rectus abdominis, formed by the anastomotic junction of the superior and inferior epigastric vessels. This system intermingles with the segmental vessels and contributes to the system of perforators (Fig. 4.7). In the hypogastrium there is also an intermingling within the superficial fascia of the perforators emerging from the rectus sheath with the branches of the superficial epigastric vessels, a component of the vascular 'cartwheel' arising in the groin, just below the inguinal ligament in the femoral triangle (Fig. 4.8). The main 'spokes' of the cartwheel are the

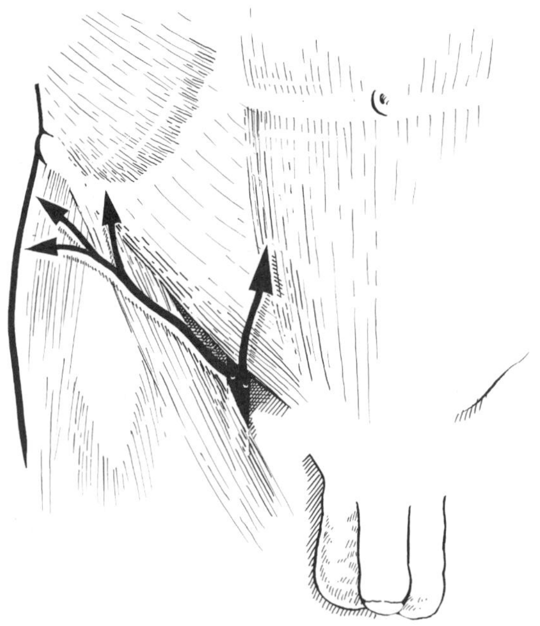

Fig. 4.8 The perfusion sources of the skin of the hypogastrium.
These are formed by elements of the vascular 'cartwheel' in the groin, the superficial epigastric and the superficial circumflex iliac vessels which combine with the perforating system shown in Figure 4.7.

superficial circumflex iliac and the superficial epigastric vessels. The superficial circumflex iliac vessels run laterally parallel to the inguinal ligament and provide the vascular basis of the *groin flap* (p. 92). The superficial epigastric vessels pass upwards and medially superficial to the rectus sheath. In addition to anastomosing with the perforators emerging from the rectus sheath in the hypogastrium they provide the vascular basis of the *hypogastric flap* (p. 94). Both sets of vessels run in the superficial fascia, becoming more superficial as they course towards their peripheral extent.

In the **limbs**, the deep fascia is a clearly defined structure and provides the 'skeletal' background on which the blood supply to the skin relies and through which it is distributed. It encircles the limb as an investing layer, fusing with the periosteum where bony surfaces lie directly under the skin, and continuous with the intermuscular septa.

In relation to flap design, it is the fascia of the forearm and the lower half of the upper arm, and of the leg below the knee, which are of greatest importance. Despite certain differences, particularly their comparative strength and relative flexibility, and the directional layout of their fibres, they have the same structural basis and vascular relationships.

A plexus of small vessels covers the fascial layer on both its superficial and deep surfaces, communicating between its fibres. It is fed from

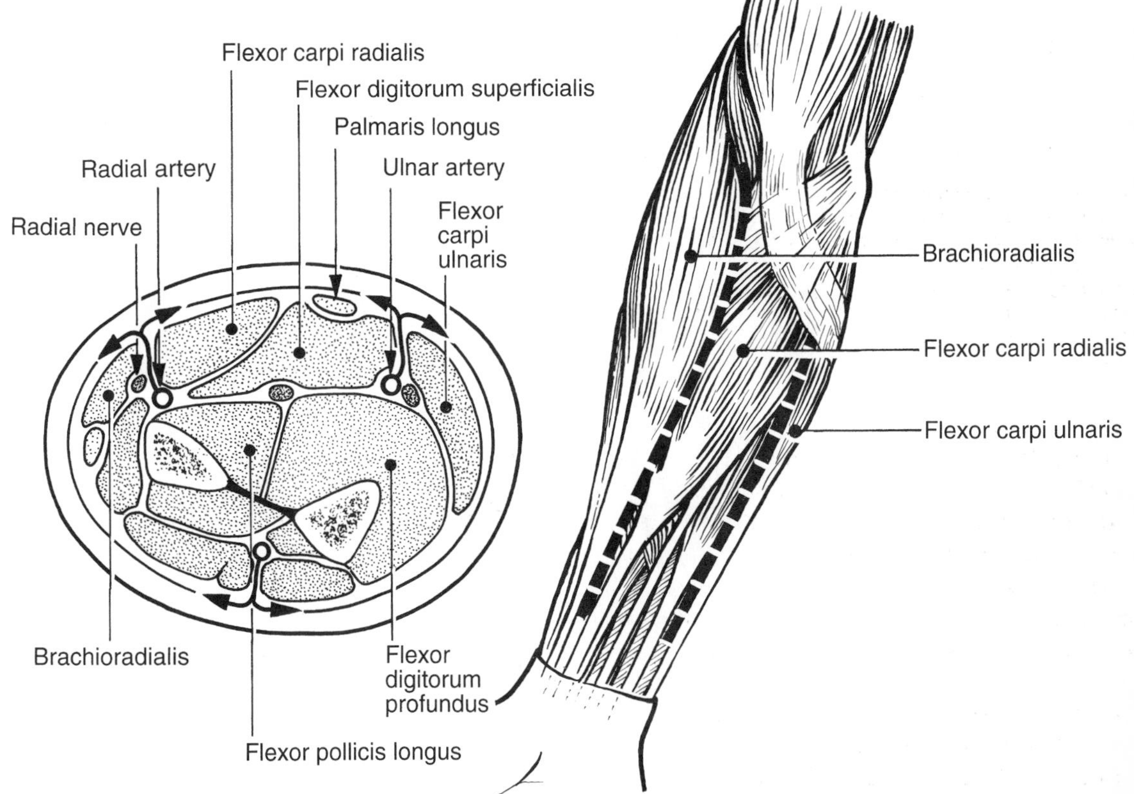

Fig. 4.9 The perfusion sources of the forearm skin.
These are derived from the radial and ulnar vessels on the flexor aspect, and the posterior interosseous vessels on the extensor aspect. Along the course of these vessels, perforating branches pass superficially in the intermuscular septa and form a plexus in the investing layer of the deep fascia from which the skin is perfused. The perforating vessels derived from the radial artery pass superficially in the septum between brachioradialis and flexor carpi radialis, the ulnar derived perforating vessels emerge lateral to flexor carpi ulnaris, and those from the posterior interosseous vessels emerge between extensor carpi ulnaris and extensor minimi digiti.

branches of the major vessels of the limb which pass towards the surface largely in the intermuscular septa. These branches, like those in the trunk, are referred to as perforators and the sites on the limb where they emerge are relatively constant. Occasional contributing vessels emerge from the muscles, but, like their counterparts in the trunk, these are primarily concerned in the perfusion of the muscles through which they have passed, though they contribute also to skin perfusion.

In the **forearm** (Fig. 4.9) the investing fascia is a fine, flexible structure. In the sites where fasciocutaneous flaps are raised the muscles are freely mobile within the sheath created by the fascia and intermuscular septa, and the fascia can be elevated easily because there are no perforating vessels crossing the plane. The closeness of the radial and ulnar vessels to the surface means also that the perforators have a short course within the intermuscular septa.

The perforators arising from the radial artery lie along the line of the intermuscular septum which separates brachioradialis from pronator teres proximally and from flexor carpi radialis longus distally, and they provide the vascular basis of the *radial forearm flap* (p. 111). The perforators arising from the ulnar artery lie along the line of the intermuscular septum lateral to flexor carpi ulnaris, between it and flexor digitorum superficialis, and they provide the vascular basis of the *ulnar forearm flap* (p. 114).

In the **upper arm** (Fig. 4.10), the lateral intermuscular septum is attached to the humeral

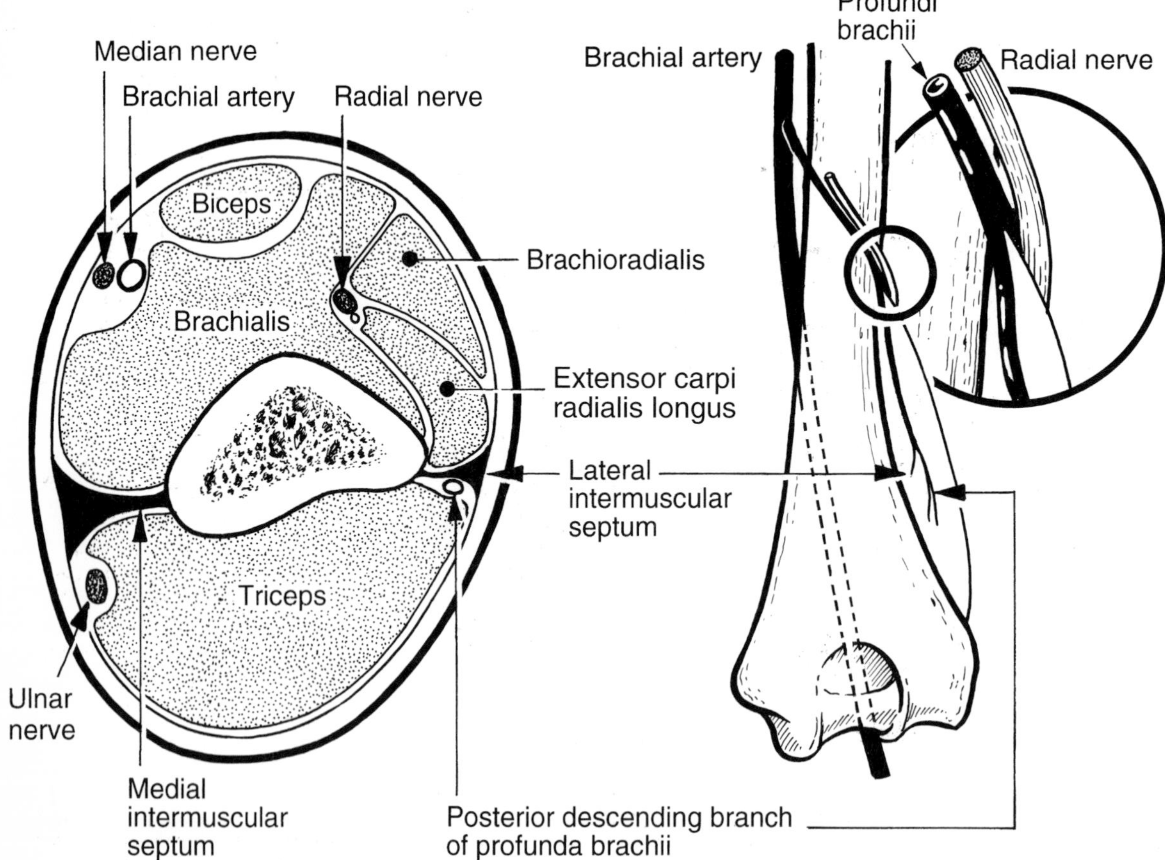

Fig. 4.10 The perfusion source of the skin of the lateral aspect of the upper arm below the insertion of deltoid.
The posterior descending branch of the profundi brachii, also referred to as the middle collateral artery, one of its terminal branches, passes distally between the lateral intermuscular septum and triceps, giving perforating branches which pass superficially to reach the investing layer of deep fascia and perfuse the overlying skin.

shaft, and between the elbow joint and the lower border of deltoid it separates brachioradialis and, more proximally, brachialis from triceps. This septum carries the posterior descending branch of the profunda brachii artery, and its branches perfuse the investing fascial layer and through it the overlying skin. It provides the vascular basis of the *lateral upper arm flap* (p. 114).

In the **leg between the knee and the foot** (Fig. 4.11), the investing layer of deep fascia is a strong, inextensile structure with a strictly limited degree of flexibility. In addition to the contribution it makes to the skin circulation, both it and the intermuscular septa also provide areas of origin to the muscles. This is seen most strikingly proximally, the fascia fusing with the aponeurotic covering of the muscle, a mixture of features which has resulted in its being referred to as an exoskeleton.

The anterior and posterior tibial, and the peroneal vessels, which provide the main perforating systems, lie deep in the substance of the limb, each within its own muscle compartment, and the perforators have a relatively long course in the intermuscular septa before they reach the overlying fascia. The muscle bulk of gastrocnemius and soleus creates a considerable volume imbalance in that part of the limb, with an absence of intermuscular septa, and there the system of perforators using intermuscular septa is replaced by a series of branches of the posterior tibial vessels passing directly through soleus and gastrocnemius to emerge and join the fascial plexus in the calf.

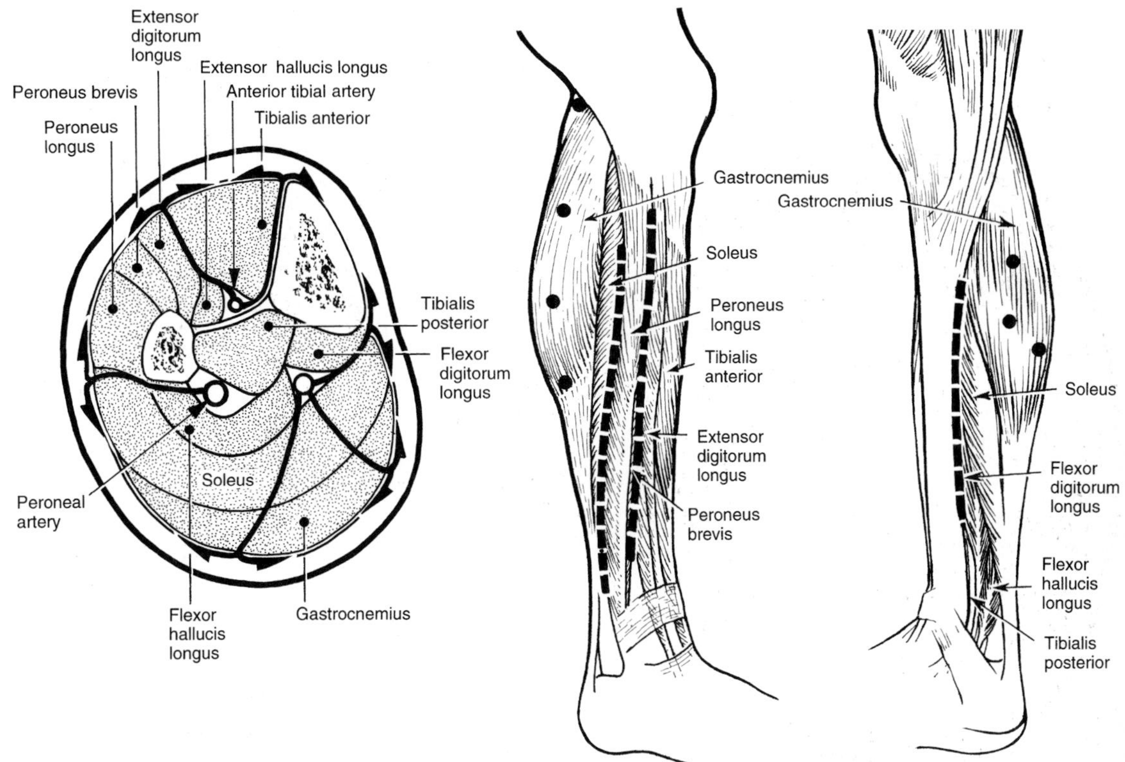

Fig. 4.11 The perfusion sources of the skin of the leg between the knee and the ankle.
Perforating vessels from the three main arteriovenous systems pass towards the surface in the intermuscular septa to reach the investing layer of deep fascia forming a plexus from which branches pass superficially to perfuse the skin. This results in linear patterns of perforators emerging at intervals along the septa which separate the major muscle groups, extensor, flexor and peroneal, and where the flexors abut on the subcutaneous border of the tibia. Where intermuscular septa are absent over a large area, as in the calf, vessels, predominantly from the posterior tibial vessels, pass directly through soleus and gastrocnemius, to reach the deep fascia.

The perforating branches of the anterior tibial vessels emerge in a linear fashion along the anterior border of the subcutaneous surface of the tibia, and also along the line which separates the anterior tibial and peroneal muscle compartments. The branches of the peroneal vessels emerge along the line separating the peroneal and posterior muscle compartments. From the vessels in the posterior compartment, branches pass medially in the intermuscular septum between flexor digitorum longus and soleus, emerging in the line just behind the posterior border of the subcutaneous surface of the tibia. Branches of the posterior tibial vessels also pass backwards through the substance of soleus and gastrocnemius to emerge in the midline between the two bellies of gastrocnemius, and also midway between the midline and the lateral and medial margins of gastrocnemius.

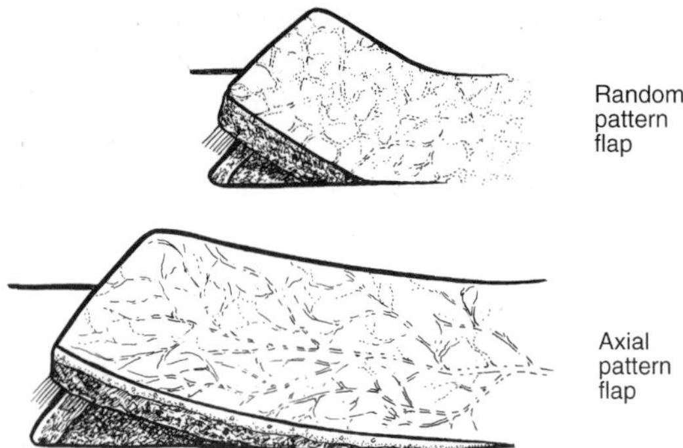

Fig. 4.12 Random and axial pattern flaps.
The presence of the axial arteriovenous system in the axial pattern flap determines the length : breadth ratio which is safe, compared with the random pattern flap where the absence of an axial vascular system generally limits it to a safe length : breadth ratio of 1 : 1.

FLAP TYPES

On the basis of their anatomical content and the nature of their vascular patterns flaps can be categorised into **skin** and **fasciocutaneous**, **muscle** and **myocutaneous**, and **free flaps**.

Skin and fasciocutaneous flaps

These flaps rely virtually entirely on the pattern of blood vessels running horizontally in the superficial fascia, reinforced in many body sites by the rich plexus of small vessels in relation to the general investing layer of deep fascia.

With this as their vascular background, three categories of flaps — **axial pattern flaps**, **random pattern flaps**, and **fasciocutaneous flaps** — are recognised, each with a distinctive geometry imposed by its vascular anatomy and each with its individual characteristics and behaviour patterns.

Axial pattern flaps (Fig. 4.12) are designed along pre-existing anatomically recognised arteriovenous systems. Such a system running along the length of the flap allows it to be constructed as long as the territory of its axial artery with minimal regard to considerations of breadth.

Random pattern flaps (Fig. 4.12) have insufficient pre-existing bias in the pattern of their arteries and veins to be of any value in design of the flap. *The term random pattern flap was originally introduced in order to distinguish it from axial pattern flaps, but the extent to which current knowledge of the patterns of blood supply to the skin is harnessed in the design of flaps has greatly reduced the number of flaps which can confidently be considered to have a truly random pattern. It is increasingly difficult to define such a flap other than in negative terms. Local and direct flaps which do not include the fascial layer, and the tubed flap where thinning has removed the fascial layer, may well be the only ones to which the term can properly be applied. Because of the random nature of the vascular pattern of such a flap, it is subject to limitations in dimensions, particularly in its permissible length:breadth ratio.*

The difference in the circulatory dynamics of the two flap types is strikingly shown in the skin colour of each. The healthy axial pattern flap shows extreme pallor with virtually no circulation apparent in the skin. The healthy random pattern flap is pink, blanching on pressure with return of skin colour as quickly as in the surrounding skin.

Fasciocutaneous flaps have had their maximum relevance in the limbs, where the role of the investing layer of deep fascia in improving flap perfusion has been most striking. Length : breadth ratio limitations were always recognised to be particularly stringent in skin flaps raised on the limbs. It has been in this respect that the situation has been markedly altered by the inclusion of the underlying investing layer of deep fascia, making the flap fasciocutaneous, and in the process significantly improving its vascularity and safety. The effect has been to free limb flaps to a considerable extent from the length:breadth ratio limitations to which they were previously subject.

It has also been found in practice that axial pattern flaps are regularly raised which extend beyond the demonstrated territory of their axial arteriovenous system. The area outwith the axial territory found safe approximates to a square, and it can be viewed as being in the nature of a 'random pattern flap' on the end of the true axial pattern flap.

Muscle and myocutaneous flaps

The principle of moving a muscle as a flap to manage the problem of a surface which is unsuitable for skin grafting by covering it with the highly vascular muscle belly, on top of which a skin graft can be applied, has proved extremely effective, but in carrying out such a transfer certain points of technique have to be observed scrupulously if consistently satisfactory results are to be achieved.

The transfer must be made without tension or compression of the muscle belly if its blood supply is not to be compromised. Embarrassment of the circulation shows in the appearance of the muscle fibres, with slight darkening in colour where the blood supply is inadequate. The need to avoid tension and compression means that tunnelling of the muscle through deep fascia or under skin to reach its destination has to be used with extreme discretion. In the lower limb, the deep fascia is strong and unyielding, and is more likely to be the source of tension or compression than the skin. There should be no hesitation in dividing the fascia widely, and even excising areas if necessary, in order to provide the muscle belly with a free passage to its destination. Allowance also needs to be made in planning for a degree of swelling of the muscle belly in the early phase after transfer. Muscle does not tolerate sutures which exert significant tension or crush the fibres, and any sutures should only be of a tacking nature, used to hold the muscle over the defect without exerting traction. Associated aponeurosis or tendon should be used wherever possible for holding sutures, and it is for this reason that wherever possible a fringe of tendon is taken with the muscle when it is detached in preparation for transfer.

When the transferred muscle is being covered with a split skin graft, exposed grafting is desirable to avoid applying pressure to the muscle bed. Delayed exposed grafting (p. 54) may be used, the area of exposed muscle in the interval being dressed. Alternatively, the graft may be meshed (p. 57) and applied primarily. Meshing allows any exudate from the muscle belly to escape without dislodging the graft, and the gaps between the strips of meshed skin heal quickly.

The clinical usefulness of the muscle flap has been increased greatly by including the overlying skin in the transfer, the skin element being perfused from the underlying muscle through the vascular connections between the two. In such a transfer the skin generally becomes the *raison d'être* of the procedure, the muscle reduced to the status of carrier.

When they were first introduced, myocutaneous flaps were raised with the skin extending over the entire length of the associated muscle so that the skin element had the benefit of its own intrinsic blood supply as well as that reaching it from the muscle. It is now recognised that the skin element can safely rely entirely on the underlying muscle for its blood supply, and it is now generally transferred with the muscle as an island. The attachment between the skin and the muscle is not always a strong one, and care has to be taken during transfer of the composite flap to avoid shearing strains and tension generally on the blood vessels passing between the two.

The combination of skin and muscle is the one most frequently used but the attachment between muscle and bone has also been successfully exploited to allow transfer of vascularised bone.

Free flaps

The free flap technique involves the transfer of a flap whose perfusion source is concentrated into a single arteriovenous system. With the flap raised and isolated on its vascular pedicle, the pedicle is divided and the flap is transferred to the recipient site. There the divided vessels are joined to suitable vessels, re-establishing effective perfusion. When the method was used initially the flaps were the axial pattern flaps recognised at the time. It soon became apparent that they were not suited for the purpose because of the unpredictability of the presence, length and calibre of their vascular pedicles. The free flaps in general use today have a larger calibre of vessel and a longer vascular pedicle, both factors which make for greater technical ease and more consistent success.

The principle of free tissue transfer has also been extended to certain of the myocutaneous and fasciocutaneous flaps where the perfusion source is particularly well concentrated, with a calibre and length which makes anastomosis relatively easy. The principle has also been extended to include bone in certain circumstances. Where suitable, nerves present in the flap have also been sutured to a suitable recipient nerve, motor as well as sensory, depending on the local circumstances.

In free flap transfers vascular input and outflow are confined to the vessels which are anastomosed, and in this respect they contrast with their skin flap counterparts, where the pedicle attachment provides an additional perfusion source. The flap must therefore stay very strictly within the territory of the artery. The safe extent of the various flaps which are used in clinical practice is now well established, and will be described in discussing individual flaps.

FLAP GEOMETRY

Tension at any stage in the transfer of a flap has an adverse effect on tissue perfusion, and steps to avoid it begin at the planning stage. When the flap has an anatomically recognisable arteriovenous system, it is on that element that attention is particularly focused, regardless of whether the transfer is as a pedicled or as a free flap. In flaps without a recognisable arteriovenous system, tension must be avoided throughout the flap as a whole.

Planning the flap with a margin of reserve is an additional way in which tension can be avoided. Skimping, making the flap just neat, is unwise, and it must not be sutured under greater than normal tension. If anything, tension should be a little less than normal. It is easy to trim an excessively large flap, but difficult to add to one, once begun.

Wherever possible, the position of the **pivot point** of the flap should be established at the outset. This point is the centre of the arc around which the flap is moving in its transfer. The general principle that the distance between the pivot point and each point of the flap *prior to transfer* must not be less than the distance between the pivot point and the position which the point will take up *after transfer* holds good for flaps of all types.

In the case of a muscle or myocutaneous flap the pivot point is the site of the neurovascular hilum. In the case of a skin flap its position is less predictable, and this issue is discussed in relation to the individual flaps.

In the case of distant flaps and in certain instances where a local flap is jumping over intact skin, pivot point planning is inappropriate and **planning in reverse** is used instead. With a piece of fabric to represent the flap, a mock transfer is carried out in reverse through the various stages of the transfer from completion with the flap in the recipient site to the beginning on the skin area from which it is to be transferred. In this way the patient is not given an impossible position to maintain at a critical stage of the transfer and the surgeon avoids a flap which is too small, too short, or liable to kink during transfer. The flap types which require planning in reverse are decreasing in popularity and the method is not often required.

The exigencies of the blood supply of the flap may dictate dimensions, shape and thickness which would not be necessary otherwise, and subsequent trimming, thinning and Z-plasties may have to be carried out after completion of the transfer in order to achieve the best result.

VASCULAR INSUFFICIENCY

In the case of skin and fasciocutaneous flaps, **mechanical tension** and **kinking** are two of the more frequent causes of vascular insufficiency. The avoidance of tension has already been discussed. The effect of kinking is to create a partial or complete bar to the passage of blood across the line of the kink, and where the site involved is the base of the flap the entire flap is put at risk. It tends to be most serious when the flap lacks flexibility.

In the case of a muscle or myocutaneous flap, **compression** of the muscle is the most frequent cause of insufficiency, with kinking of the pedicle as an alternative possibility. Compression is generally the result of passing the muscle through a tunnel which is too tight. Deep fascia and skin can each be responsible for the tightness, the former the more likely offender where the investing layer of deep fascia is strong and unyielding.

The skin island of myocutaneous flaps is particularly vulnerable to relatively minor degrees of compression of its muscle pedicle, sloughing on occasion, even although the muscle may survive.

In free flaps, vascular insufficiency is virtually invariably due to problems at the site of the anastomosis in the immediate postoperative period. Its occurrence, recognition and management are an essential element in the postoperative care of free flaps and are discussed in that context.

FLAP NECROSIS

In a *random pattern skin flap*, developing necrosis presents clinically with the skin acutely congested and cyanosed, blanching momentarily on pressure, but with vessels rapidly filling again. As the condition progresses, blanching on pressure becomes less and less definite until there is clearly no active circulation. At this point the margin of the affected area is seldom well demarcated and the process tends to extend until a skin area is reached whose vascular capacity is able to cope not merely with ordinary metabolic needs, but also with the added vascular burden arising from the inflammatory reaction resulting from the adjacent necrosis. The whole process is acute, settled one way or the other in 1–2 days.

In an *axial pattern flap*, the sequence is different, and the vascular pathophysiology underlying the sequence of clinical events is not fully understood. Necrosis takes several days to develop and during this period it is difficult to be sure whether the flap is going to recover or not. Instead of the pallor indicating a healthy flap, the area of concern is slightly cyanosed with what appears to be a sluggish circulation. The signs are not gross and can easily be missed in the early stages. For several days the appearance remains virtually unchanged, transient improvement often occurring temporarily, until finally necrosis becomes definite. The slow way in which the whole sequence evolves often gives time for the margin of the flap to become revascularised from the surrounding tissues, and the area of final necrosis, instead of being the entire distal flap, is an island in its centre. Once seen, the premonitory slight cyanotic colouration is easily recognised and its appearance usually means inevitable necrosis, although several days may elapse before it is acknowledged as such.

In a *myocutaneous flap*, the sequence of events is more complex because two tissues are involved. Not infrequently the skin island alone necroses leaving the muscle bare but viable. When this happens the surface presented may be suitable for the application of a split skin graft. This is most likely to be the case when the flap has been used to provide skin cover. When the flap has been used to reconstruct an intraoral defect, it is rarely possible to graft the muscle surface, and spontaneous healing from the surrounding mucosa has to be allowed. In the intraoral environment this occurs surprisingly quickly and the result when healing is complete can be unexpectedly good.

The sequence of events which ends up in necrosis of a *free flap* is closely bound up with postoperative management and is discussed on p. 110.

PREVENTION OF NECROSIS

The most important steps to prevent necrosis are taken at the stage of designing the flap. In the case of a random pattern flap, it concerns such factors as its length:breadth ratio and making allowance for the normal increase in tension with the temporary phase of oedema generally seen in such a flap. In the axial pattern flap, design is particularly concerned with ensuring that the flap includes its axial arteriovenous system and does not extend beyond its recognised safe length. These factors all vary in the different flaps and will be discussed in relation to each.

When random flaps were in universal use the **delay principle** was regularly used to improve the vascular efficiency of the flap when it was considered to be inadequate. With the reduction in the use of random pattern flaps it is required much less frequently, though even with axial pattern flaps it is occasionally required. The techniques involved are discussed in greater detail on p. 77.

Postoperatively the development of a haematoma is prone to initiate the cycle of events which leads to necrosis. This complication occurs less frequently if planes of surgical cleavage have been used when the flap is being raised, the vessels traversing these planes being large, relatively few in number, and more readily controlled. The use of exposure of the flap coupled with suction drainage has also contributed to the reduction in the incidence and severity of the problem, exposure by allowing continuous monitoring of flap perfusion, suction drainage by closing the flap/bed interface. Closed suction can certainly cope with a minor ooze, but the flap must still be watched carefully for the local bulge indicative of significant haematoma due to bleeding beyond the capacity of the suction drain. If this occurs, the flap must be elevated, the clot evacuated, and haemostasis achieved.

In the past, many of the flaps in routine use

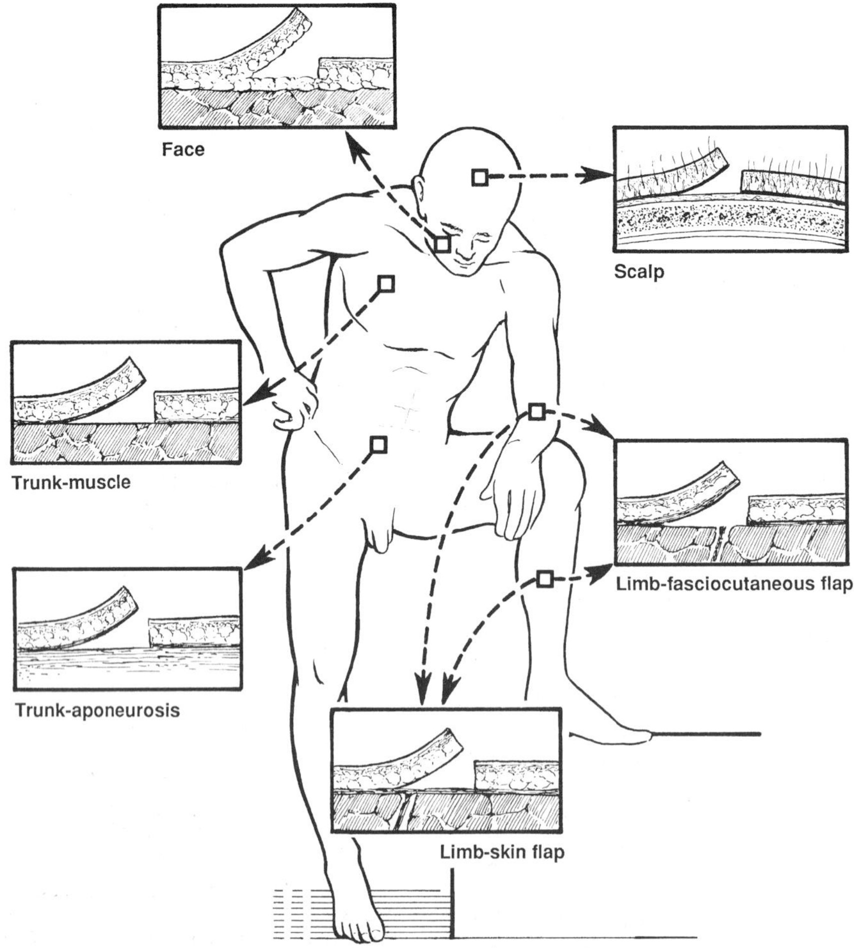

Fig. 4.13 The levels at which skin and fasciocutaneous flaps are normally raised in the scalp, face, limbs and trunk. The difference in level on the limbs depends on whether the flap is being raised as a skin or as a fasciocutaneous flap.

had a small margin of safety and necrosis was an everpresent hazard. It is not surprising therefore that methods were described for managing the flap showing signs of circulatory embarrassment, such as cooling 'in order to reduce the metabolic rate', infusion of low molecular weight dextran, hyperbaric oxygen, and others. In practice none were effective.

The increase in the use of axial pattern and myocutaneous flaps has reduced the frequency of the problem. There is also a wider acceptance of the fact that once any obvious cause of the necrotic cycle has been treated the surgeon is largely powerless to influence the course of events.

In managing free flaps, willingness to intervene at the earliest stage of concern over the state of the flap has been a major factor in the improvement in their salvage rate. This topic is discussed as part of the postoperative management of free flaps (p. 110).

SKIN AND FASCIOCUTANEOUS FLAP PRACTICE

Raising a flap (Fig. 4.13)

In the **trunk**, the plane in which a flap is raised lies between the deep fascia and the underlying muscle or aponeurosis. In the **limbs**, it is possible to raise flaps immediately superficial or deep to the investing layer of fascia, but the added safety which the fascial layer provides has resulted in its almost invariable inclusion. The **face** has no comparable natural plane and one has to be artificially created when raising the flap. The level chosen is the fat just deep to the dermis. This leaves the flap with the rich subdermal circulation present in facial skin, while not disturbing the facial nerve or muscles. In the **scalp**, the plane lies between the galea aponeurotica and the pericranium, virtually no vessels crossing the interface. In the **forehead**, the standard plane is superficial to the pericranium, but smaller flaps are often raised in the plane between the skin and the frontalis muscle.

All the surfaces exposed when flaps are raised in these planes will accept a graft if this is required to manage the secondary defect.

Thinning a flap

When a flap is thinned, it is usually in order to match the thickness of the defect, or to allow it to be tubed without tension. With the decrease in the usage of random pattern flaps, formal thinning of the flap (Fig. 4.14) is less often required, though it is still often desirable to trim the fat along its margin. Lobules of fat tend to bulge over the skin edge and their presence there makes a neat suture line, marginal or along a tubing seam, difficult to achieve. The amount of thinning which flaps tolerate safely varies greatly in different sites and with different flap types.

In the **face** the well-developed subdermal plexus allows the smaller flaps to be thinned considerably, removing the greater part of the fat. With the larger flaps thinning is rarely required,

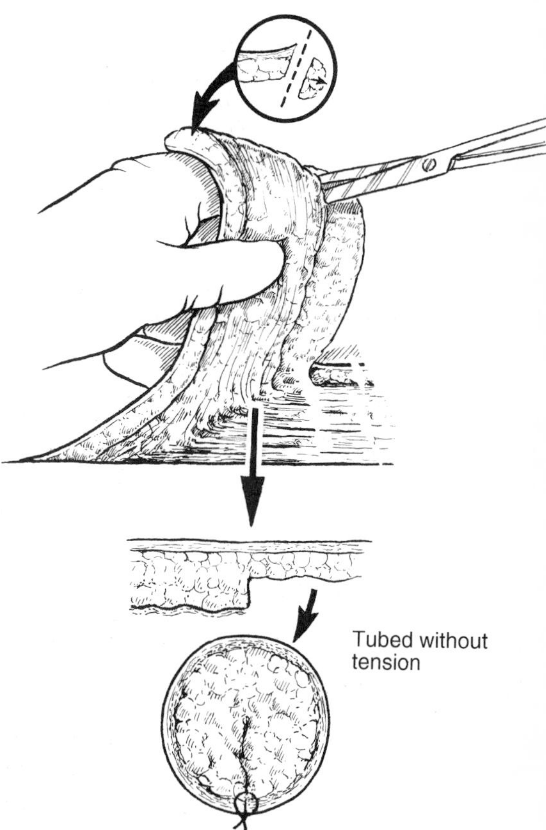

Fig. 4.14 Thinning a skin flap, including trimming of the margins, to allow it to be tubed without tension.

In the case of an axial pattern flap, such thinning may require to be carried out with considerable care to avoid incidentally dividing the axial artery in the process.

their initial thickness approximating usually to the final thickness. **Scalp** flaps are raised at the subgaleal level and the physical character of scalp is such that thinning is not practicable. In the **limbs**, flaps are seldom if ever thinned — fasciocutaneous flaps because the investing layer of fascia which is forming their deep surface carries the blood vessels crucial to their survival, skin flaps because the layer of subcutaneous fat is not thick enough to warrant it.

In the case of an axial pattern flap in the **trunk**, the problem varies with the site of the flap and the sex of the patient. In most males the chest and upper abdomen are not adipose and thinning is not often needed. Trimming of the fat along the margin of the flap may suffice. The presence of the breast in the female complicates matters when the flap encroaches on it, particularly where the breast is large and pendulous. There should be no hesitation about thinning the flap to make its overall thickness correspond to that of the part of the flap outwith the margin of the breast. The problem of thinning is less easily solved when the flap is being raised from the lower abdomen or groin. This is a notoriously fat site in many adults, and indeed the presence of fat in excess may be a valid reason for selecting an alternative site when a flap is being planned. This topic is discussed in relation to the groin and hypogastric flaps on p. 93.

When a flap is being thinned, the hand holding the flap for thinning should be used to judge the amount required. Touch gives a much more accurate measure of the uniformity of the thinning than vision alone.

Avoidance of infection

Many flaps have a less than entirely satisfactory vascular reserve, and unnecessary demands on the circulation are to be avoided. A particularly undesirable addition to the normal circulatory load is an inflammatory reaction, and two steps are taken to avoid it — **prevention of haematoma** and **avoidance of raw areas**.

Prevention of haematoma

Assuming careful haemostasis at operation the most effective measure which can be taken postoperatively to prevent haematoma is the use of suction. The larger the area of the surfaces apposed by the transfer of flap the greater the need for suction drainage to ensure that the surfaces are not separated by haematoma, but adhere quickly.

Where wall suction is available a wide-bore catheter with additional openings works well; alternatively, commercially produced suction drains can be used. The drain (Fig. 4.15) may be placed under the flap, either through the marginal suture line or via an independent stab incision. If the bridge segment of the flap has been tubed the drain can be inserted along its length to lie under the distal end of the flap.

In addition to the potential it creates for infection, haematoma has the further adverse effect of preventing rapid and effective adhesion of a flap to its bed, adding to the time required for the flap to settle in and soften.

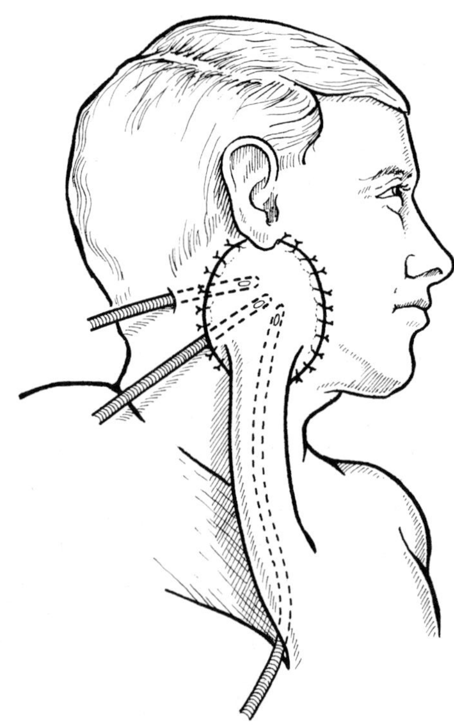

Fig. 4.15 The ways of inserting a suction catheter deep to the distal end of a flap to ensure that the flap adheres deeply – by the use of a separate incision, through the marginal suture line of the flap, by passing the catheter along the length of the tubed bridge segment.

Elimination of raw surfaces (Fig. 4.16)

The raw surfaces involved are the defect left by the raising of the flap and the deep surface of the flap itself. In each instance the raw surface of the secondary defect is eliminated by direct closure or, when this is not possible, by split skin grafting.

Secondary defects on the face can generally be closed directly because of the laxity of the skin locally. Elsewhere on the body, the size of the flaps usually raised and the relative absence of skin laxity frequently preclude the use of direct closure, many defects having to be split skin grafted.

The raw surface of the flap which is involved is usually its bridge segment, and it is closed whenever feasible by converting it into a tube. With flaps raised on the trunk tubing is usually possible, but virtually never with flaps in the face and scalp. Fortunately the vascular reserve of most flaps raised on the face and scalp enables them to cope with the added load of a raw surface, and infection from this source is seldom a problem. In the case of a flap raised on a limb, the raw surface involved is its bridge segment, and it is unsuitable for tubing because it is short and wide. Instead, the skin graft used to close the secondary defect is extended to cover the bridge segment also.

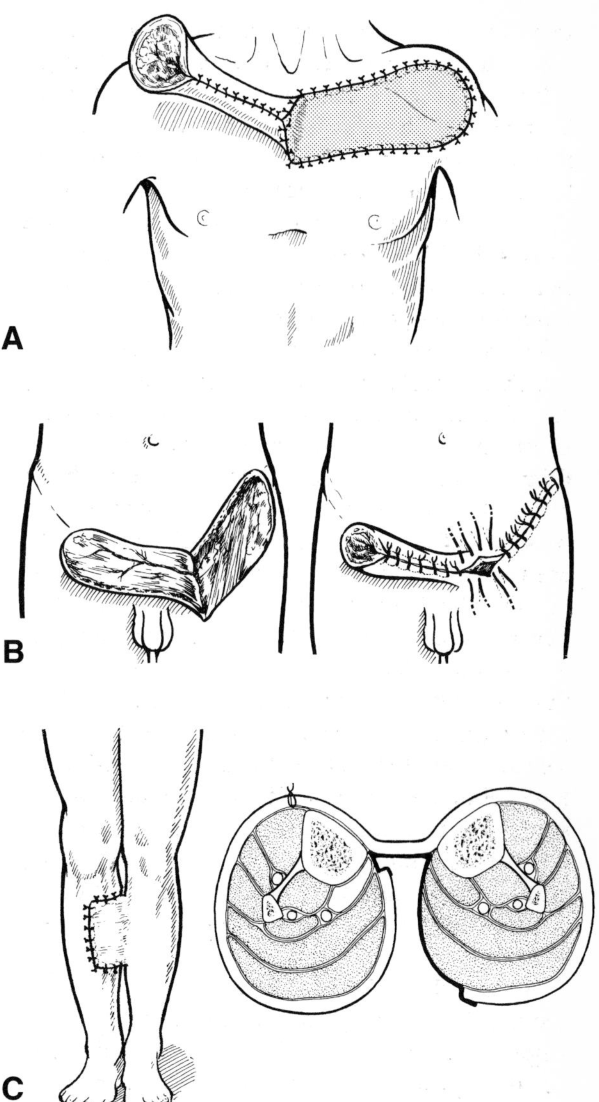

Fig. 4.16 The methods used to avoid the presence of raw surfaces during the transfer of the various types of skin and fasciocutaneous flaps.

A Transfer of a deltopectoral flap. The bridge segment has been tubed, and the secondary defect on the chest has been split skin grafted, with extension of the graft to meet the tubed segment of the flap.

B Transfer of a groin flap. The bridge segment of the flap has been tubed, and the secondary defect has been closed directly.

C Transfer of a cross-leg fasciocutaneous flap. The secondary defect has been split skin grafted, and the graft has been extended to line the bridge segment of the flap.

The technique of lining the bridge segment of a flap with a split skin graft, as in ***C****, is used when the shortness of the flap in relation to its breadth makes tubing technically impossible.*

Use of delay

The original use of a delay (Fig. 4.17A) was to allow a random pattern flap to have a more advantageous length:breadth ratio. With the advent of the axial pattern flap, the technique has also been used to extend the basic flap beyond its recognised safe length. The purpose of a delay is to restrict the flap to the blood vessels on which it will have to rely at the time of the transfer, without adding the strain of the actual transfer itself, in this way 'training' it to rely on these vessels, presumably by inducing in them a degree of axial reorientation, though this is unproven.

As originally used, an incision was made along the line across which the surgeon wished to cut off the blood supply. The blood vessels crossing the line were divided, the wound was resutured

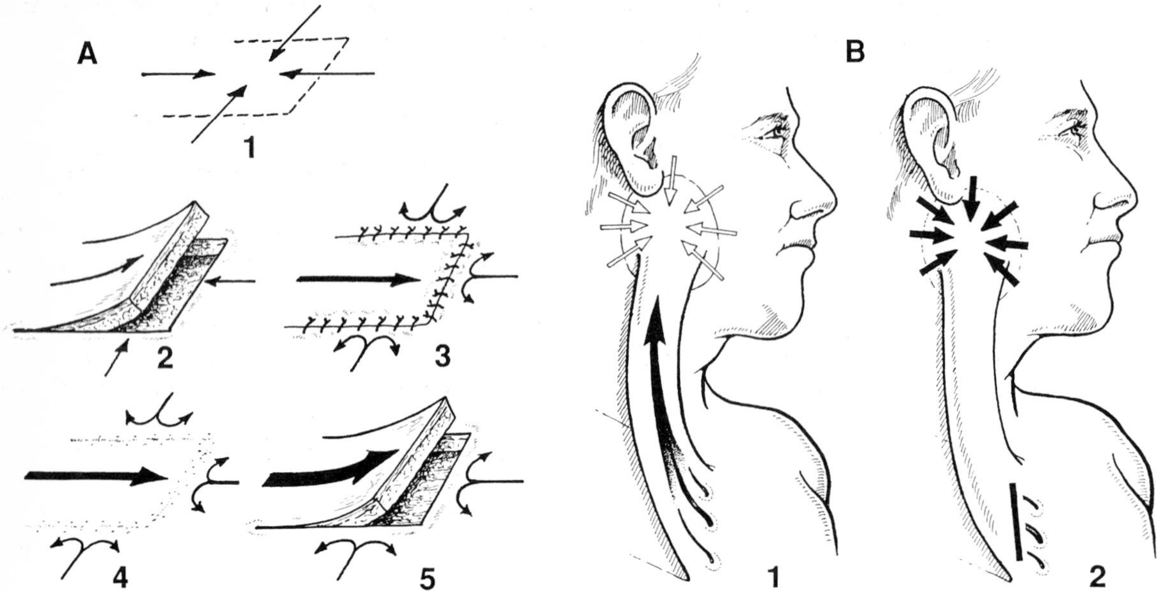

Fig. 4.17 The usage of the delay procedure.

A The delay is being used to allow the safe transfer of a random pattern flap with a greater length:breadth ratio than 1 : 1. The flap, outlined (**1**), with its blood supply coming from all directions, is raised (**2**), dividing the marginal blood vessels other than those entering and leaving its base. The flap is sutured back in position, and 10–14 days later is raised for transfer. During the interval (**3,4**), its blood supply remains restricted to that reaching it through the base and this supply increases in efficiency so that it is capable of perfusing the flap effectively during the actual transfer (**5**). *For clarity the blood supply entering the deep surface of the flap has been omitted.*

B The delay is being used to enhance the flow of blood across the distal attachment of an axial pattern flap, in this case a deltopectoral flap. (**1**) shows the vigorous axial vascular flow and the poor blood flow across the distal attachment prior to delay, in contrast with the situation (**2**) following the delay in which the axial vasculature has been divided, the effect being to enhance the blood flow across the distal attachment.

and allowed to heal. This divided only the marginal vessels, and if the blood supply entering the deep surface was also being cut off the flap was elevated in addition. In a difficult situation, the flap might be delayed in stages at intervals of 7–10 days.

When the delay is used to extend an axial pattern flap beyond its accepted safe length a similar technique is employed, elevating the extension to leave its sole attachment to the distal end of the basic flap. The axial pattern flap, together with its extension, is then transferred in the usual way. In such circumstances the added segment is described as having been **delayed** on to the end of the parent flap.

A delay may also be needed at other stages of flap transfer (Fig. 4.17B), particularly in the case of axial pattern flaps. When such a flap has been attached to a wrist carrier, or has been inset as part of a waltzing transfer, the next stage involves division of the base of the flap, i.e. its pedicle. Division of the pedicle has the effect of cutting off its axial vascular flow, and the flap is immediately downgraded to the status of a random pattern flap. Division also means that the flap is immediately dependent on the vascular through-flow which has been established through its carrier or waltzing inset, and this may not be adequate to ensure its survival. The efficiency of its pre-existing axial arteriovenous system is such that there has been little encouragement for the flap to develop an effective new vascular attachment at the inset, and its efficiency must be enhanced before it can be judged capable of sustaining the entire flap. This is achieved by carrying out a delay of the pedicle with the aim of reducing the axial blood flow passing through it, rather than cutting it off completely.

The delay is carried out by *partially* dividing the pedicle but, more importantly, by making sure that the axial vessels, particularly the axial artery, are divided in the process. The effect is to alter the vascular dynamics of the flap by reducing the perfusion pressure through its base, and encouraging flow through the wrist or waltzing inset. Such a delay is usually carried out 3 weeks after the initial transfer to the wrist or the waltzing inset. Full division of the pedicle is carried out a week later.

Failure to stage division in this way is likely to result in substantial flap necrosis. Staging of the division even of a random pattern flap may also be advisable if the adequacy of blood flow across an attachment is regarded as doubtful.

TUBED FLAP AND DIRECT FLAP PRACTICE

Tubed flaps and direct flaps are both pedicled, but they differ in their geometry and their vascular patterns. The typical tubed flap has an axial vascular pattern, and this allows it to be long in relation to its breadth, making it possible to tube its bridge segment. The typical direct flap has a random vascular pattern, and so has to be short in relation to its breadth. As a result it cannot be tubed. With both flap types the transfer from the donor site to the recipient area generally involves more than one stage.

Mechanisms of tubed flap transfers

When a tubed flap is raised and its bridge segment is tubed in preparation for transfer, tubing is stopped towards its distal end, leaving an area of raw surface which is used to re-attach the flap in its new site. A raw surface similar in shape and size is created in the new site, and the two raw surfaces are apposed to one another. Closure of the skin edges eliminates both raw surfaces and creates the new attachment.

The tubed flaps which are used with any frequency are the deltopectoral and groin flaps. The deltopectoral flap is virtually always 'waltzed' to its destination, a method of transfer which involves pivoting of the flap on its pedicle to reconstruct a defect within its reach, usually in the lower face or neck. With the groin flap, waltzing is also used when the defect is in its vicinity, for example the hypogastrium or opposite groin. Defects of the hand and lower forearm can also be brought within the range of the groin flap, and transfer to reconstruct defects further afield is possible by making use of a wrist carrier.

In a **waltzing transfer** (Fig. 4.18) an estimate

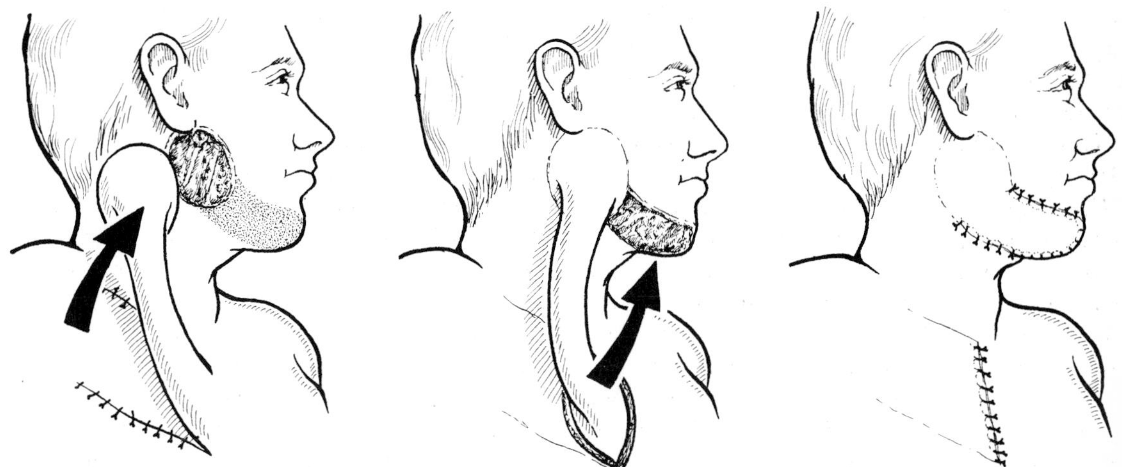

Fig. 4.18 Transfer of a tubed skin flap by waltzing.
This form of transfer is used when, for technical reasons, the entire defect cannot be covered by the flap in a single procedure. At a first stage, part of the primary defect is covered by the flap, the remainder being covered at a second stage.
If such a transfer is to be completed without necrosis, it is essential that the second stage is preceded by a formal delay stage, as shown in Figure 4.17B.

is made of the proportion of the recipient site which it will be possible to cover at the first stage of the transfer, and the raw surface left on the distal end of the flap is designed to match it. The pedicle is usually divided 3 weeks later, and the unused segment of the flap is untubed and returned to its original site. This aspect of the transfer, the need to use a delay, and possibly also stage division of the pedicle before insetting, are discussed below.

When the flap is transferred using a **wrist carrier** (Fig. 4.19), its distal margin is designed as a semicircle so that when tubing is stopped the raw surface is circular. A similarly circular raw surface equal in size is created on the wrist by elevating a semicircular trap-door of skin and superficial fascia, the effect being to maximise the area of raw surface contact between the flap and its attachment to the wrist, and hence the speed and effectiveness of the vascular link-up.

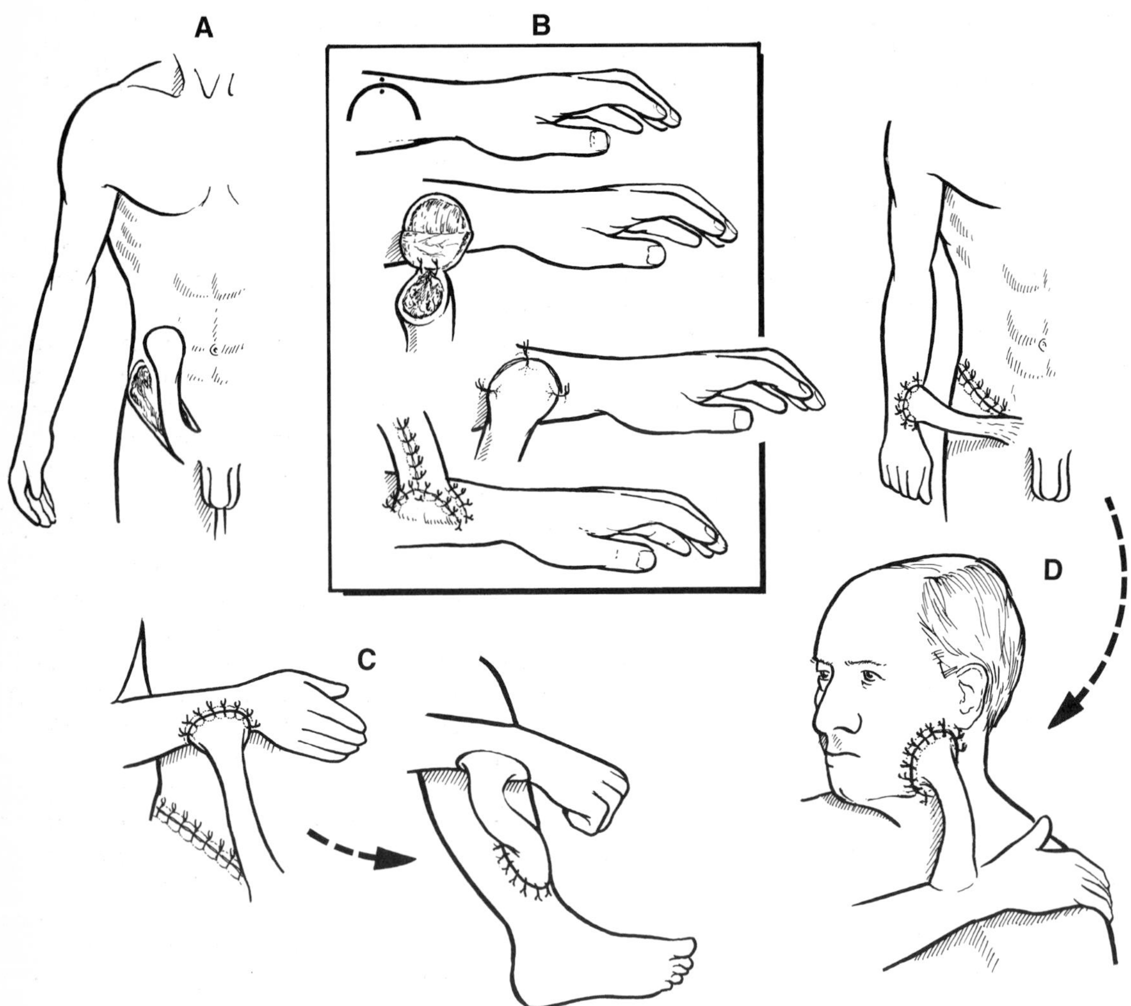

Fig. 4.19 Transfer of a tubed skin flap using a wrist carrier.
When the single pedicled flap (**A**) is tubed, a circular raw surface is left when tubing is completed. A semicircular trap-door (**B**) is outlined and raised on the side of the wrist. The effect is to create a circular raw surface corresponding in shape and dimensions to the raw surface left on the flap, as seen in **A**. The circular raw surface at the distal end of the flap is then sutured to the corresponding raw surface on the wrist. Depending on the destination of the flap, whether in a downward or upward direction, the attachment is made to the ulnar or the radial side of the wrist. The tubed flap is then detached at its base after a delay, as shown in Figure 4.17B, and carried on the wrist to the site of the planned reconstruction, where it is sutured to the defect, of the leg in **C**, of the masseteric area in **D**.

The size appropriate for the trap-door can be ascertained easily by making a blood-stained imprint of the raw surface of the flap at the site of the planned attachment, and its site is the ulnar or radial margin of the wrist, depending on the plan of the transfer. It should be positioned on the wrist margin so that the turning back of the trap-door leaves the raw surface in one plane. In this way the trap-door lies smoothly back when suturing is complete, and the attachment as a whole runs cleanly off the limb. The other variable is the angle of attachment of the flap to the forearm. Consideration of how arm and wrist are going to lie at the next stage of the transfer will decide this. The 'hinge' along which the trap door is raised will be perpendicular to the desired direction of the flap.

The next stage of transfer on a carrier involves division of the flap at its base. If the flap has an axial vascular pattern, division must be preceded by a delay at the base for the reasons discussed on p. 78, usually 3 weeks after transfer to the wrist carrier. The base is formally divided 1 week later, leaving the tubed flap hanging free from the wrist.

With the flap moved to the recipient site a length of the tubing is undone sufficient to provide the necessary raw surface for the inset into the recipient site, where a similar amount of skin is removed, the two raw surfaces then being sutured together. Three weeks later the transfer is completed by detaching the flap from the wrist and closing the defect there, and completing its insetting at the recipient site.

Mechanisms of direct flap transfer

The shortness of the standard direct flap makes it necessary to bring the defect into close proximity with the donor site of the flap in order to allow the transfer to take place. When the defect is of the arm or the hand, it is brought to the donor area, to the upper abdomen for example (Fig. 4.21A); when the transfer is to the leg or foot from the other leg, as in a cross-leg flap (Fig. 4.20), the limbs are approximated to one another, and a comparable sequence is involved in the transfer of a cross-finger (Fig. 11.19) or cross-arm flap (Fig. 11.15). It is with the two sites, donor and recipient, brought into close proximity that the detailed planning of the transfer is carried out.

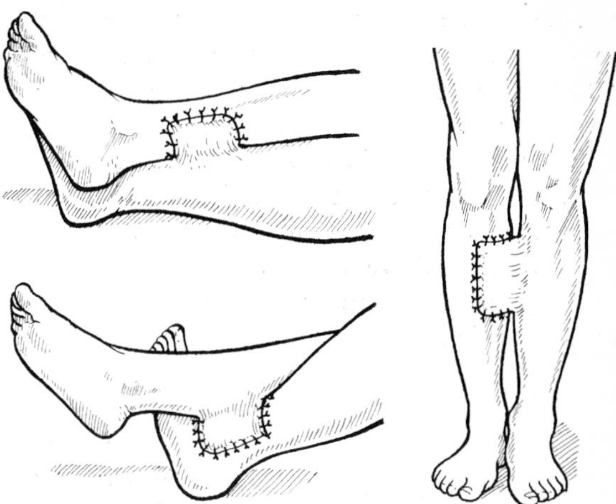

Fig. 4.20 Examples of cross-leg flap positions used in clinical practice.

The 1 : 1 length:breadth ratio of the standard direct flap imposed by its random vascular pattern, although mitigated a little by its conversion to a fasciocutaneous flap, still has the effect of making the planning of the transfer a critical phase of the technique if flap necrosis is to be avoided. Planning in reverse, described on p. 72, is the method used, and extreme care is needed to avoid tension, shearing and kinking of the flap, and to ensure that the patient is given as comfortable a position as possible to maintain during the transfer, immobilisation in that position being crucial to the success of the transfer.

The donor site defect left when the flap is raised and sutured to the defect on the recipient area is split skin grafted, and the graft is extended to line the short bridge segment of the flap, so that unnecessary raw surface is avoided.

Immobilisation of the upper limb, to ensure that traction on the flap and shearing are prevented, makes use of Elastoplast (Fig. 4.21A) in conjunction with sand-bags and pillows, and the position which was set up on the operating table has generally to be adjusted when the patient is returned to bed.

When the transfer is to the lower limb, immobilisation by plaster of Paris is usual (Fig. 4.21B), though it imposes its own discipline on

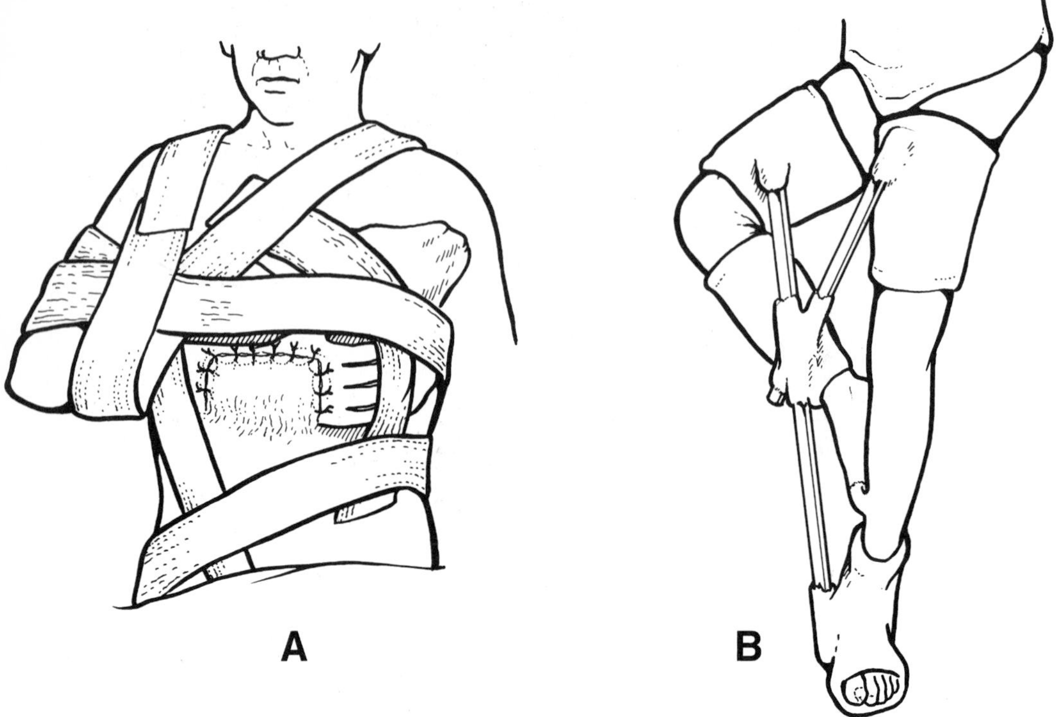

Fig. 4.21 Elastoplast immobilisation used during transfer of a direct flap to the hand (**A**), and prefabricated plaster fixation used during the transfer of a cross-leg flap (**B**).

the surgeon, and it must be used with care. It can be applied at the time of operation, but prefabrication has undoubted advantages. Preoperatively, with the limbs in the position to be maintained postoperatively to permit accurate moulding of the plaster to the muscular contours, lengths of encircling plaster can be applied at strategic points, and strutted together postoperatively, e.g. with lengths of broom-handle, to hold the system rigidly immobile in its correct position.

With the limbs involved immobilised for the necessary 3 weeks the flap is divided, an aspect discussed below.

A problem with direct flaps in general is the joint stiffness which results from the unavoidable immobilisation for 3 weeks. In the young patient this clears up quickly when the fixation is removed, but in the older age group the possibility of permanent limitation of movement has to be seriously taken into account in weighing up the pros and cons of the method.

Flap division and insetting

When a pedicled flap is transferred, at least 3 weeks have to elapse before its new vascular attachment is capable of perfusing the flap entirely on its own, and it is ready for the next stage of the transfer. Various tests have been introduced over the years, aiming to assess the efficiency of the vascular attachment in the hope of reducing this time. Each in turn has been discarded. The question more often should be whether the transfer is safe at 3 weeks. In such an assessment, the extent of the area of the attachment in relation to the length of the tubed segment to be left lying free after division of the pedicle, is the most important consideration, but the presence of surrounding scarring, the speed of healing, the relative absence of induration and vascular reaction locally, are also factors used in assessing the adequacy of the vascular throughput, and deciding whether or not it is safe to divide the flap.

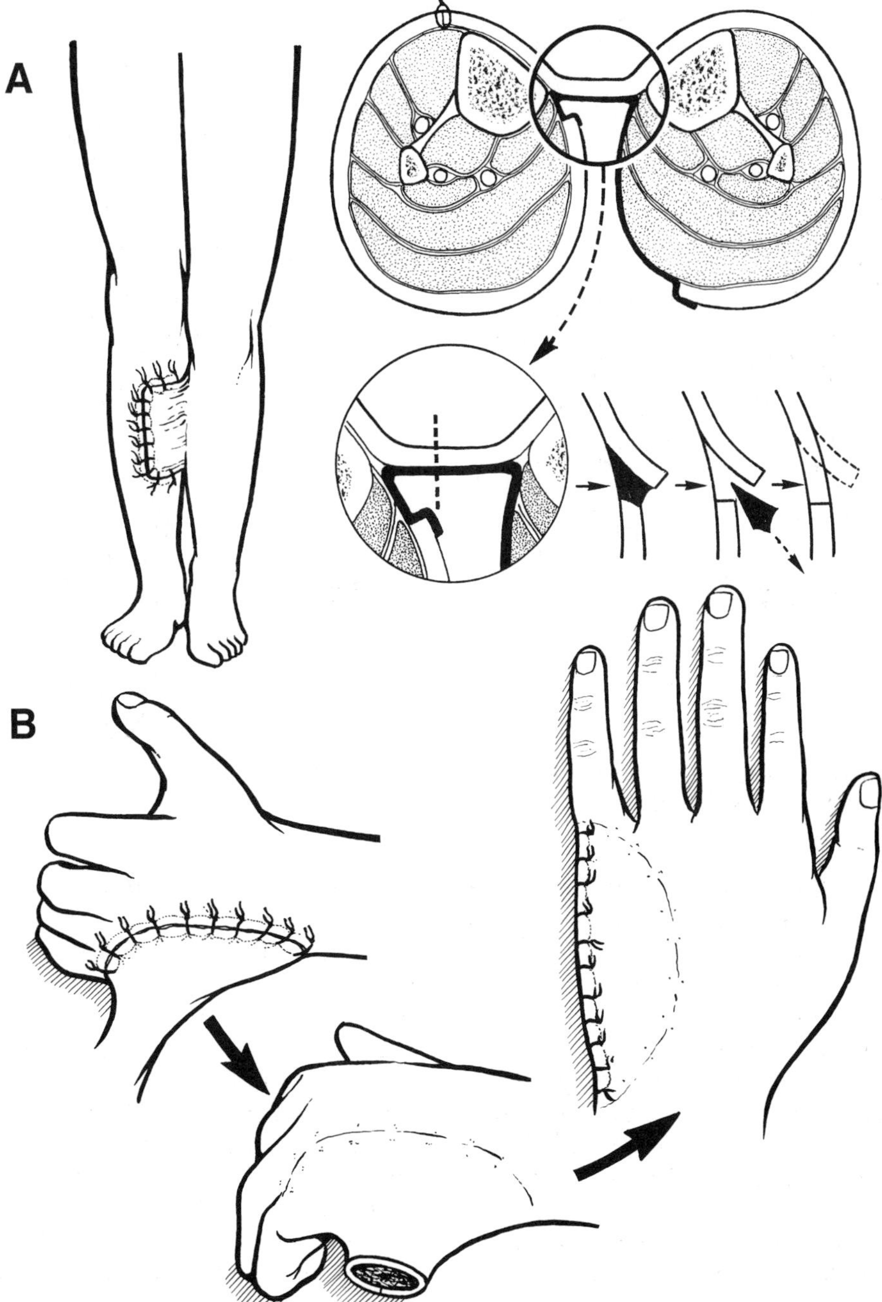

Fig. 4.22 Staging of division and insetting.

A Staging as used with a direct flap. An angle of fibrous tissue is built up at the junction of the flap and the recipient site, and this has to be excised to allow the flap to sit into the remainder of the defect. The flap is divided at the end of the third week, but excision of the wedge of fibrous tissue and insetting are postponed for a further week.

B Staging as used with a tubed flap. The pedicle of the flap is divided at the end of the third week, but insetting is postponed for a further week.

The dissection involved in division and insetting in both instances has an adverse effect on the blood supply of the flap margin and, unless the two procedures are staged, rim necrosis is liable to result. The excellent blood supply of the head and neck area makes staging of division and insetting in this way less often necessary.

When the pedicle is being divided prior to insetting it is frequently safer to separate division and insetting into two distinct stages, even when only a fringe of the flap remains to be inset. In the case of a direct flap (Fig. 4.22A), a wedge of fibrous tissue builds up at the junction of the recipient area and the flap, and it has to be dissected off the defect and excised to allow the flap margin to be inset neatly. With the tubed flap (Fig. 4.22B), even when the length of the flap lying free is short, untubing is similarly required. The dissection involved in each instance may appear to be minor, but it has an adverse effect on the blood supply of the segment of the flap which has been elevated, and the margin is liable to slough, creating 'rim necrosis'. Rim necrosis is less of a hazard in the head and neck, where the rich blood supply makes it safer to divide and inset immediately, but even there the least doubt should mean a staged division and inset.

When a greater length of the flap remains to be inset, it is essential to carry out a delay at the base of the flap (Fig. 4.17), as described on p. 78, a week before formally dividing the pedicle and completing insetting, making sure that the axial vessels are divided. In a particularly difficult situation an additional precaution can be to postpone for an additional week the final insetting of the flap after division of its pedicle.

Clinical usage

The 'waltzing' method of transfer is regularly used, as is the cross-finger flap reconstruction. Cross-arm flaps are occasionally used. The other forms of transfer have only a tiny role. Faster and safer alternatives which make fewer demands on the patient's tolerance are available today, and they are used only when these alternatives have failed. With the number of alternatives available today this is a rare occurrence.

TRANSPOSITION AND ROTATION FLAP PRACTICE

In order to cover a defect which the surgeon considers unsuitable for grafting it may be possible to move the tissue adjoining it in the form of a local flap. Such a transfer usually leaves a secondary defect, and this is closed either by direct suture or a free skin graft.

When the flap moves laterally into the primary defect it is called a **transposition** or **transposed flap**, and when rotated into the defect it is called a **rotation flap** (Fig. 4.23). Many of the flaps used in practice combine both principles in varying degrees, and a particular flap tends to be called then by the principle which predominates.

At the outset it must be stressed that these flaps are not procedures to be embarked upon lightly. The surgeon using such a flap should remember always that a major vascular disaster is liable to leave a deformity far greater than the one the flap was designed to correct. They cannot adequately be described fully in print, for every flap is an individual problem. In the face particularly, judgment in selection and imagination in design come with the experience born of surgical apprenticeship. Present discussion is concerned primarily with explaining the principles which underlie their construction.

These flaps depend to a considerable extent on the elasticity of the tissues, but in planning this

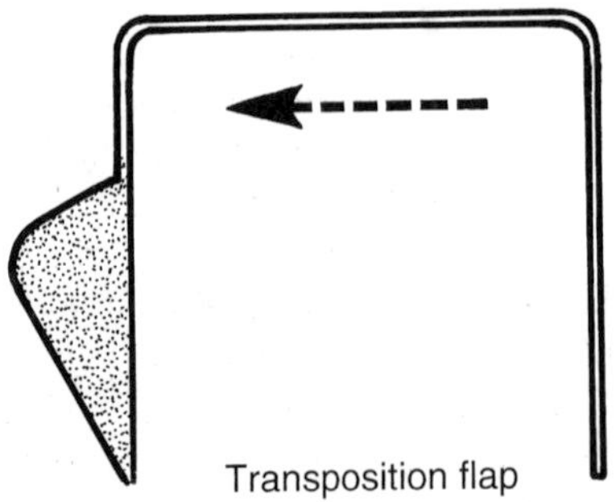
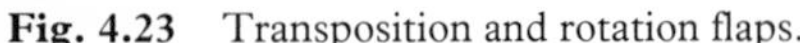

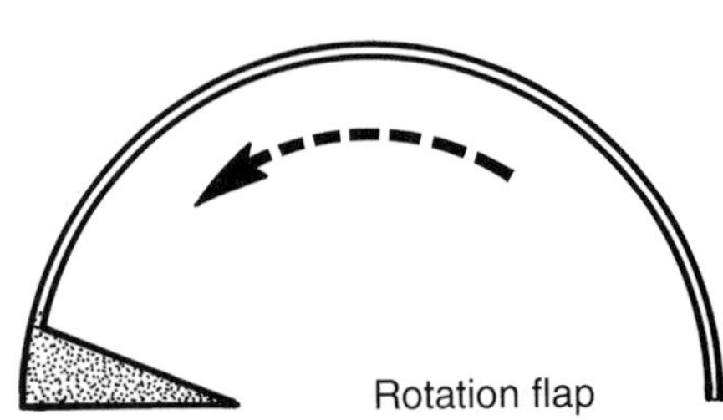

Fig. 4.23 Transposition and rotation flaps.

should not be relied upon. Rather it should be viewed as an added insurance. They are geometrical manoeuvres, and treated as such they are more likely to be trouble-free in practice.

Planning the flap

The guiding principles (Fig. 4.24) to be laid down apply to transposed and rotation flaps in their classical forms.

With either type of flap the first step is conversion of the defect into one with the shape of an isosceles triangle — **triangulation of the defect** — a step which generally involves the sacrifice of some normal tissue around the defect. In constructing the flap one of the equal sides of the triangle acts also as a side of the flap, and the effect of the transfer is to move that side across to the other side of the triangle, closing the defect.

The shape of the initial defect generally determines the shape of the triangle, its apex and its base, though with a long narrow defect it may be possible to plan the triangle placing its apex at either end. The base of the flap will be alongside the apex of the triangle, and therefore the end should be chosen as the apex which will provide the better flap base from the point of view of tissue availability and blood supply.

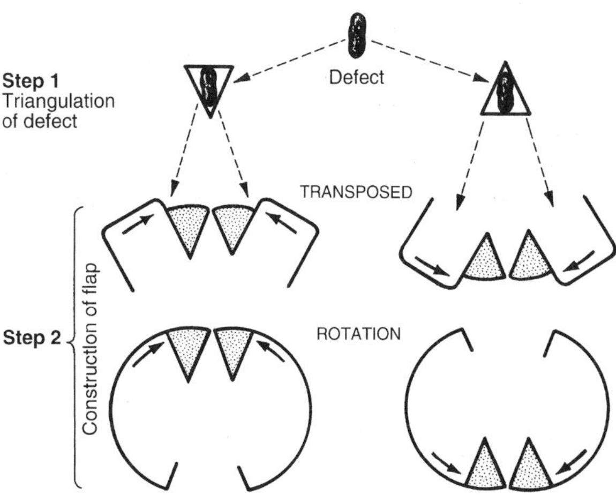

Fig. 4.24 The steps in planning a transposition and a rotation flap.
Step 1 selects the direction of the base of the flap, whether transposition or rotation.
Step 2 selects the side of the defect on which the flap is to be designed, and from which it is transferred.

With the triangle defined, the side with the greater area of available skin is likely to provide the best flap.

TRANSPOSITION FLAP

The transposition flap is classically designed as a square immediately adjoining the triangulated defect, and its movement laterally closes the defect. Transfer has the effect of opening up a secondary defect which is of greater size than the primary defect. It is generally closed with a split skin graft.

Although the classic outline of the flap is square, the ratio of its length to its breadth considered to be safe depends to a considerable extent on the vascularity of the site from which the flap is raised, whether the flap is truly random or has an axial element, and whether it is a skin or a fasciocutaneous flap.

In the *face and scalp*, the richness of the skin circulation, even in the absence of an anatomically recognised axial system, permits length: breadth restrictions to be somewhat relaxed, frequently allowing the flap to be planned as a rectangle (Fig. 4.25), rather than as a square.

In the *trunk*, the possibility also exists of harnessing knowledge of the exit points of perforators, and their inclusion will obviously enhance the safety of the flap, though in practice their usage has been restricted by the popularity of other reconstructive techniques.

In the *limbs*, the length: breadth ratio limitation of 1 : 1 applies with particular stringency when the flap does not include the investing layer of fascia, and even then such flaps have a bad reputation for necrosis. Raised as fasciocutaneous flaps, their safety is considerably enhanced, and it has been found possible to relax the length: breadth requirements somewhat. Although this may simplify the transfer technically, it does not alter the need to adhere to the geometrical aspects of planning the flap. An additional aspect of this added freedom is the surgeon's awareness of the lines along which the perforating vessels emerge, and the possibility of incorporating one in the flap, a possibility enhanced when the Doppler probe is available to help in the search. They are discussed further on p. 94.

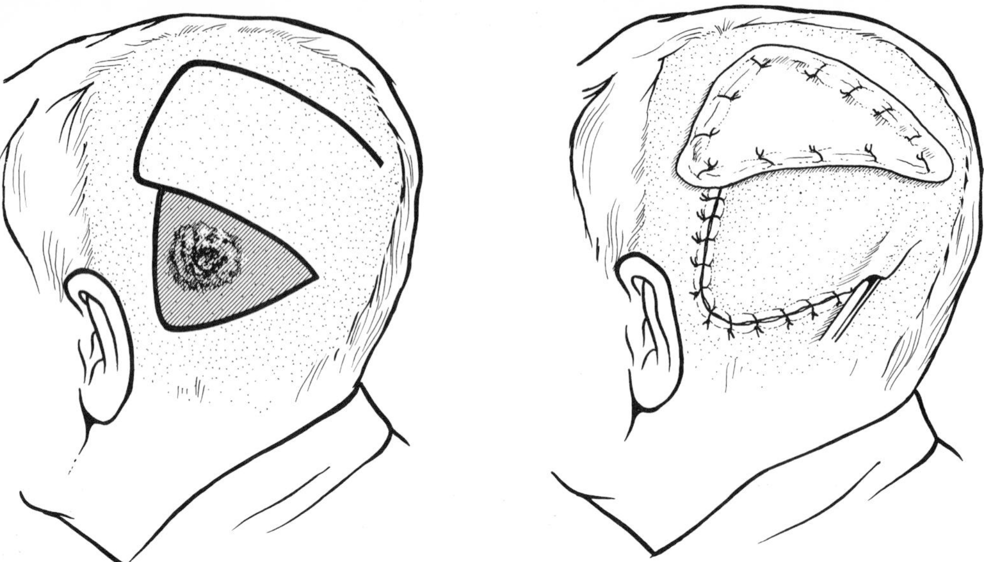

Fig. 4.25 The use of a transposition flap following excision of a tumour of the scalp where excision left the bony vault of the skull exposed.

The excellent vascularity of the scalp permitted the flap to be designed with a ratio of length : breadth significantly greater than 1 : 1, rather than the square design which is standard in other sites unless the flap is recognised to have an axial pattern.

The **geometrical aspects of safe planning** involve recognition of the fact that the point around which the transposed flap pivots in its transfer is not the apex of the triangle forming the defect, but is the other side of the base of the flap. In designing the flap, and before any incision is made, the pivot point must be clearly defined, and the distance from it to each point of the flap compared with its estimated distance to the same point when transposition is complete. The diagonal length of the flap from the pivot point is the one particularly liable to be short, and is the one on which attention should be concentrated (Fig. 4.26).

The effect of these planning requirements is that the flap is generally considerably larger than might otherwise be expected. In particular, the side which is also part of the defect has to be made longer than the side of the triangulated defect so that the diagonal length of the flap before and the estimated diagonal length after transfer are at least equal.

If the size of the flap is inadequate (Fig. 4.26), it will be found when transfer is attempted that a tension line develops along the diagonal of the flap. At best this makes the flap vulnerable to vascular insufficiency; at worst it may make the transfer impossible. The use of a back-cut across the base of the flap is likely then to be needed to allow the transfer to be completed, its effect being to alter the position of the pivot point to a more advantageous site from the viewpoint of reducing tension. Unfortunately its effect is also to reduce the breadth of the base of the flap and hence its vascular safety. When it is unavoidable, such a back-cut should at least be made as small as possible.

In making such a cut it may be possible to reduce the tension without significantly reducing the vascularity of the flap by cutting only the actual tissue responsible for the tension, at the same time leaving the blood vessels intact. In skin with a good thickness of superficial fascia, for example, section of the skin alone may give enough relaxation; in the scalp, cutting the galea aponeurotica may have the same result. In general, however, the need for a back-cut is the result of poor planning, and its use is distinctly hazardous as regards flap survival.

The clinical role of the transposition flap is confined to situations where a secondary graft is not contraindicated for cosmetic reasons and so

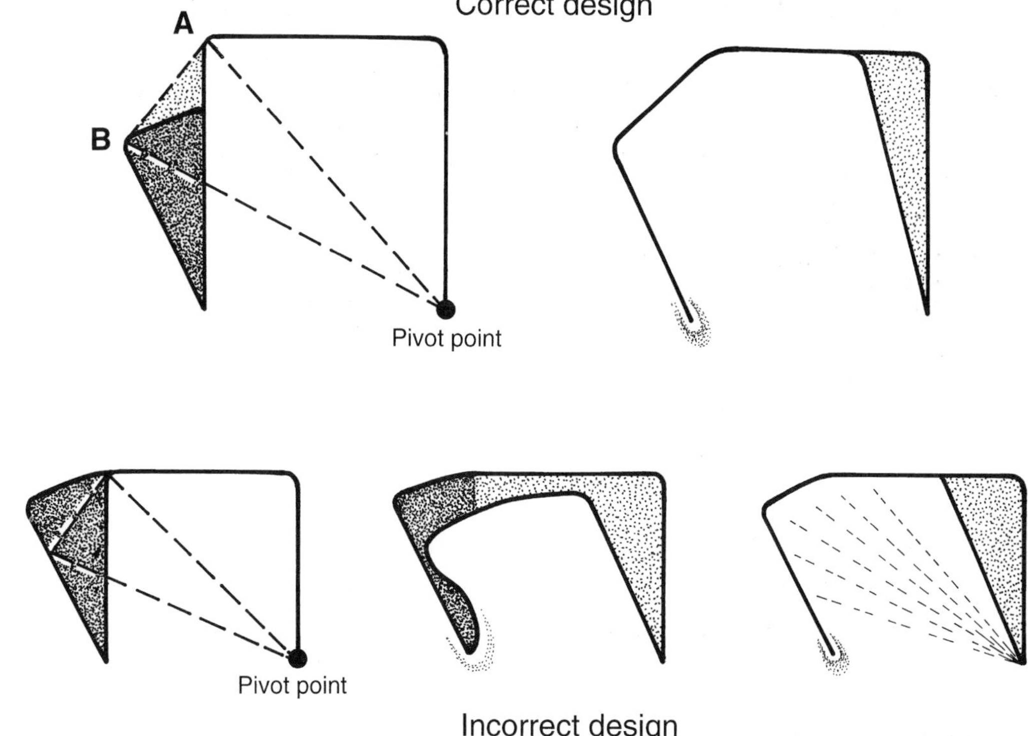

Fig. 4.26 The design of a transposition flap.
In the correctly designed flap, the distance from the pivot point to **A** equals the distance to **B** and the transfer is carried out without tension. In the incorrectly designed flap, the distances are unequal because the flap is too short, and the transfer can only be achieved with the flap under tension.

it is used mainly outside the face. The secondary defect is larger than the primary defect, but any attempt to close it, or even reduce it in size by suture, is undesirable. It should be covered with a split skin graft.

The graft can be applied either primarily, using pressure methods, or delayed, using exposed grafting. If it is decided to use primary grafting, it is essential to make sure that the tension on the tie-over dressing is not transmitted to the flap. This can be achieved by ensuring that the tie-over sutures which pass through the margin of the flap include the deep tissues in their bite, and so anchor both the flap margin and the graft to the deeper tissues (Fig. 4.27). This manoeuvre allows the flap to be managed independently of the graft from the point of view of suction, pressure dressings, etc. Delayed exposed grafting

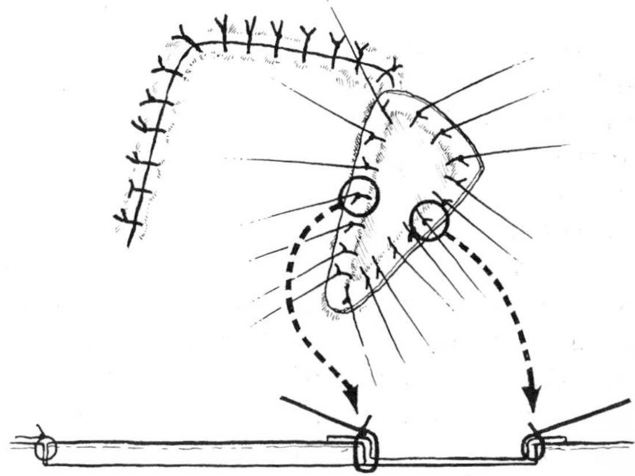

Fig. 4.27 Isolation of the transposition flap from the graft by the use of sutures which anchor both the graft and the flap to the deeper structures, preventing tension from being transmitted from the graft to the flap, and allowing them to be managed independently of one another.

has the virtue of ensuring that any haematoma collecting under the flap can freely drain into the secondary defect without creating tension in the flap itself.

ROTATION FLAP

The rotation flap is classically illustrated as a semicircle of which the defect is a segment. In reconstructing the defect the curve of the flap rotates along the corresponding curve of the other side of the incision outlining the flap.

With such a design, the pivot point lies at the extremity of the semicircle opposite the defect (Fig. 4.28A), and in the absence of local tissue laxity sufficient to absorb any tension difference, attempted rotation of the flap results in lines of tension spreading from the pivot point which may be sufficient to prevent the transfer from taking place. A partial solution to this impasse has proved to be the use of a back-cut made along the diameter line of the semicircle (Fig. 4.28B). Its effect is to move the site of the pivot point towards the centre of the semicircle outlined by the flap, and this reduces the tension lines built up when the flap is transferred.

In practice, the larger the flap in relation to the defect the more likely the flap is to be transferred successfully without a back-cut, even when tissue laxity is minimal. With a large flap the relative amount of rotation required to close the defect is reduced, and there is a corresponding reduction in the amount of tension generated (Fig. 4.29). Even so, successful transfer of a rotation flap without requiring a back-cut, shown in Figure 10.5, indicates the presence of local tissue laxity sufficient to absorb the tension which would otherwise build up. In such a situation the position of the pivot point is extremely vague since the tissues along the entire base of the flap are in some degree taking part in the rotation process (Fig. 4.30).

In assessing the suitability of a defect for reconstruction using a rotation flap the degree of local tissue availability and general laxity must be estimated, and the likelihood of the need for a back-cut considered, particularly in relation to the effect it may have on the vascular safety of the flap.

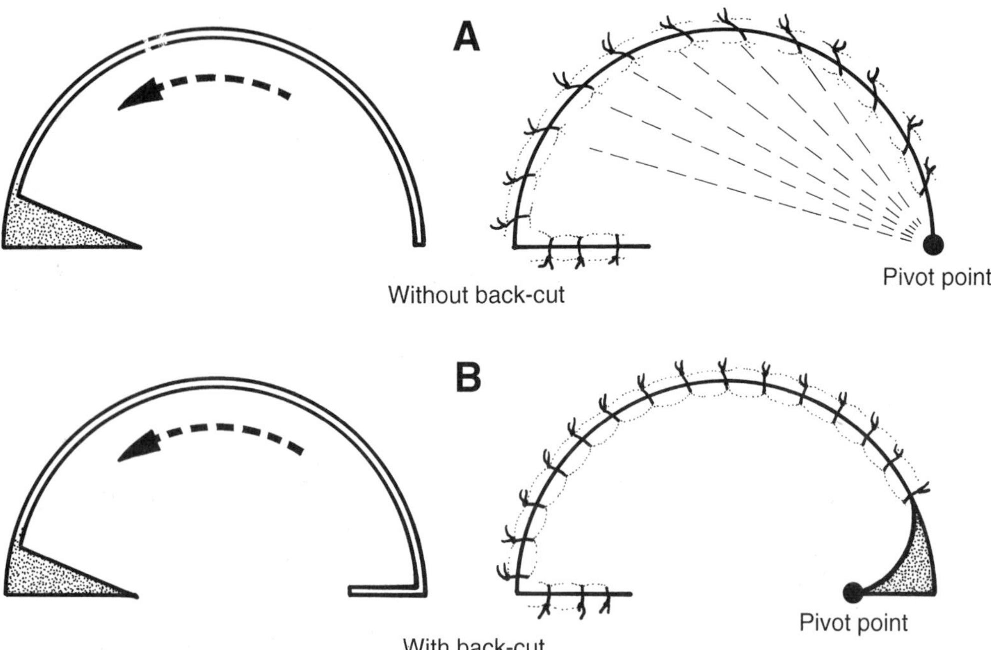

Fig. 4.28 Tension in a rotation flap.
The flap (**A**) without, and (**B**) with a back-cut, showing how the back-cut has altered the position of the pivot point and reduced the tension created by attempting to rotate the flap.

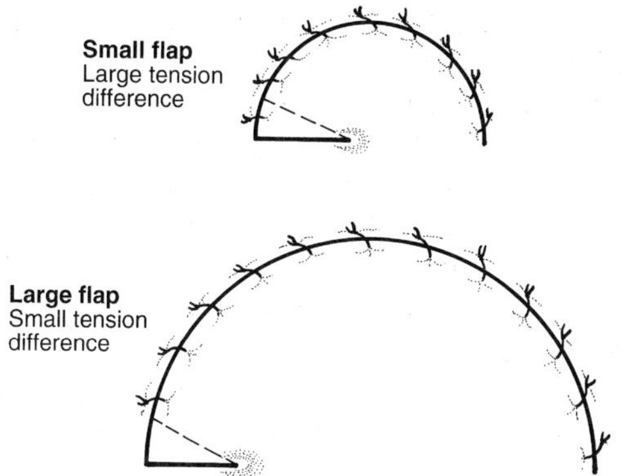

Fig. 4.29 Increasing the size of the flap in relation to the defect and its effect on reducing the tension of the transfer.

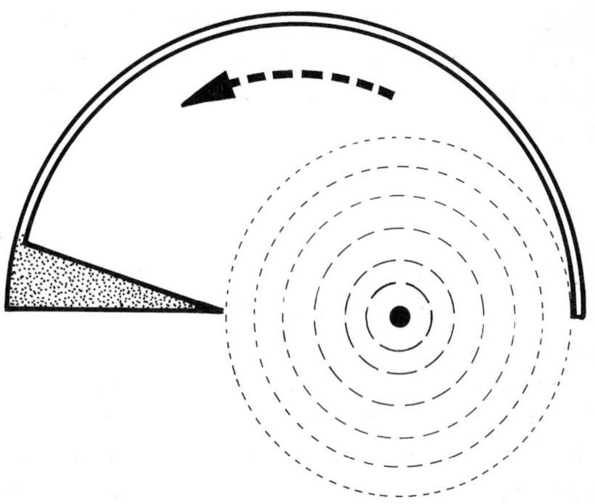

Fig. 4.30 The vagueness of the pivot point when the flap is raised in an area of skin laxity. An example of this situation in clinical practice is shown in Figure 10.5.

The relationship of the size of the defect to that of the flap required to reconstruct it is also a critical factor in planning. Most of the errors made in practice are in the direction of making the flap too small. Such an error is less likely to be made if the outlines of the triangulated defect and the flap are formally drawn out on the skin before any incision is made, the laxity of the local tissues is dispassionately assessed, the position of the pivot point is sited as accurately as possible, and the relevant lengths from it are carefully measured.

The management of the defect created by the opening up of the back-cut depends on the degree of laxity of the local tissues (Fig. 4.31). If

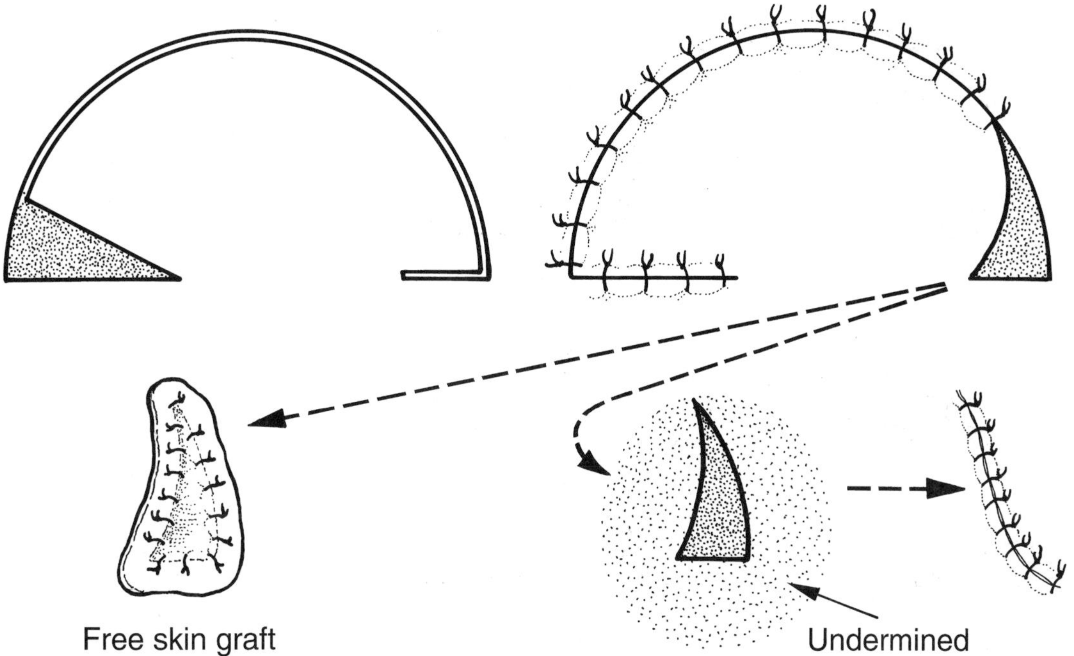

Fig. 4.31 Closure of the secondary defect created by the use of a back-cut following transfer of a rotation flap, by skin grafting, and by direct suture.

The form which direct suture takes must not have the effect of recreating the tension which the back-cut was used to relieve.

it proves possible to close the defect directly, care should be taken to see that closure does not create tension across the base of the flap sufficient to jeopardise its blood supply. The head and neck areas apart, tissue laxity is seldom adequate to allow complete closure and split skin grafting is necessary.

An alternative method of managing the problem of a back-cut is sometimes used when the flap is raised on the cheek. With the flap rotated into the defect, the margin of the flap is shorter than the margin to which it is being sutured, and the two lengths are equated by excising a triangle of tissue opposite where the back-cut would normally be (Fig. 4.32). In practice, as suturing of the flap in its rotated position proceeds, it becomes obvious that there is a redundancy on the outer side of the suture line and eventually a dog-ear develops. Excision of the dog-ear leaves the two sides equal in length. The use of this method in clinical practice is illustrated in Figure 10.4.

The dog-ear of the triangulated defect

If the pivoting took place round the apex of the triangulated primary defect the resulting suture line would be quite flat, but with the pivot point elsewhere both in the transposition and rotation flaps, a dog-ear tends to be present at the apex of the triangle when the transfer is complete. It usually settles with time, but in any case it is best left for subsequent revision if its removal at the time of the transfer would in any way jeopardise the blood supply of the flap.

CLINICAL USAGE

For their effective use both the transposition and rotation flaps require a reasonably extensive surface area unencumbered by any anatomical features which might interrupt the geometrical outline of the flap.

In the *side of the face and submandibular area*, the site where the rotation flap has been exploited most effectively, the mandibulomasseteric area of availability must be assessed carefully, since it is its presence which allows successful use of the flap. In the older age group tissue laxity of the face generally, and of the mandibulomasseteric area in particular, is generally sufficient to permit

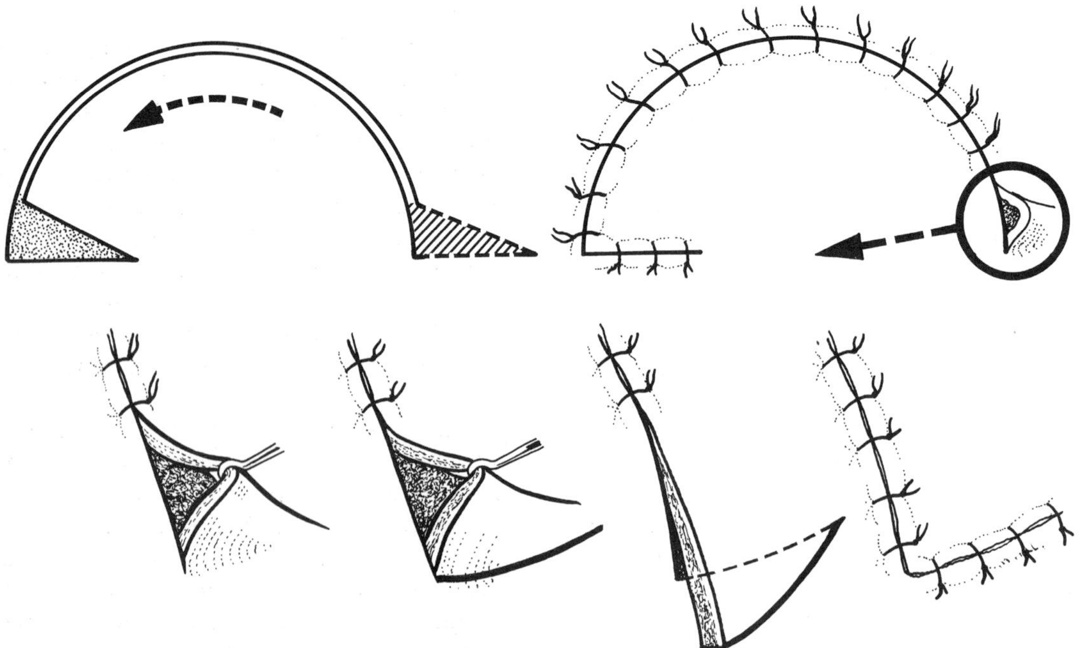

Fig. 4.32 A method of avoiding a secondary defect following the transfer of a rotation flap, which can sometimes be used when the skin is lax, and tissue is available locally. Figure 10.4 shows the method used in a clinical context.

use of the flap, but this does not absolve the surgeon of the need to make the assessment. Depending on the site and shape of the defect, the flap may be based inferiorly (Fig. 10.4) or superiorly (Fig. 10.5).

In the *scalp*, the extent of unimpeded surface available makes it an excellent site for using both transposition and rotation flaps, but its rigidity and inextensibility makes care in the geometrical planning of rotation flaps imperative, and a back-cut can rarely be avoided. The rich vascularity of the scalp permits transposition flaps which are considerably narrower than their length to be transferred successfully (Fig. 4.25), but their geometrical design limits still need to be observed scrupulously.

In the *trunk*, it is possible to add to the vascular safety, particularly of transposed flaps, by using the knowledge of the sites and the subsequent course of the perforating vessels in their design. The potential inclusion of perforators, however, should be regarded as a means of enhancing the safety of the flap rather than a method of circumventing the geometrical aspects of flap planning.

In the *limbs*, the inclusion of the investing layer of the deep fascia has added greatly to the safety of the local flaps designed in the leg, particularly between the knee and the ankle, the area where there is the greatest clinical demand. Their design and usage are discussed on p. 94.

AXIAL PATTERN FLAPS

The axial pattern flaps which have become established are the **deltopectoral** and **groin** flaps.

DELTOPECTORAL FLAP

The deltopectoral flap (Fig. 4.33) runs horizontally across the anterior chest wall towards the shoulder tip from its base along the border of the sternum. Its upper border is formed by the line of the clavicle, its lower border is at the level of the anterior axillary fold. The first three perforating branches of the internal mammary vessels provide its axial vascular basis.

Clinical experience has shown that, raised deep to the investing layer of fascia and stripping the underlying muscles bare, it can be extended

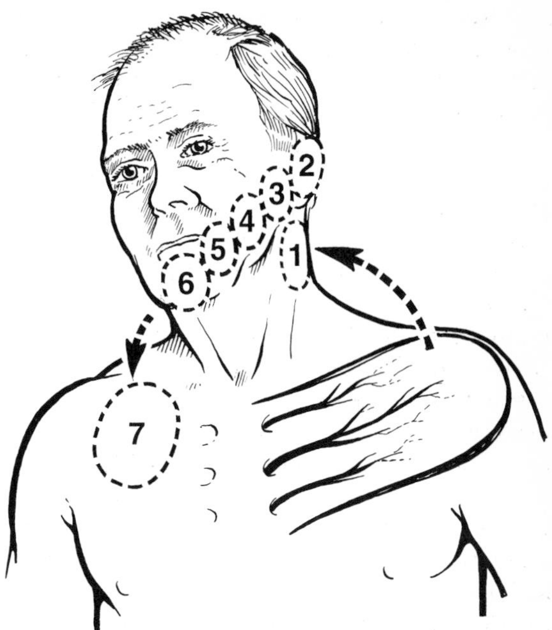

Fig. 4.33 The outline of the standard deltopectoral flap, and sites on the head, neck and chest where it can be used for reconstruction. The flap can also be used to reconstruct defects inside the arc formed by these sites.

laterally without preliminary delay almost as far as the midlateral line on the deltoid muscle, and can safely be raised almost to the sternal margin where the axial vessels emerge into it, one in each intercostal space. The only artery of size regularly met in raising the flap is the deltoid branch of the thoraco-acromial artery. On the basis of comparative size, the second perforating branch of the internal mammary artery is the most important of the arteries incorporated in the flap.

The flap is generally reliable, but any extension beyond the midlateral line is unsafe, unless preceded by a scrupulous delay, and even then problems of viability of the extension must be expected.

The secondary defect created by its transfer is split skin grafted, and the site is an ideal one for delayed exposed grafting. The defect is an extensive one and, grafted in its entirety, leaves a considerable area of grafted skin to be excised when the bridge segment is returned to its preoperative site following division of the pedicle 3 weeks after the initial transfer. There is a good deal to be said for grafting only the area which will finally be left on the deltoid area as the permanent secondary defect. The remainder can be treated as a temporary raw surface and merely dressed (Fig. 4.34).

Transfer to its destination is generally by waltzing, and the bridge segment is tubed. If suction drainage is being applied to its distal attached segment it is usually convenient to insert the catheter along the length of the tubed segment.

The deltopectoral flap is most often moved upwards in a quarter-circle, waltzed on its sternal attachment (Fig. 4.35) to resurface defects within its arc — mastoid region, ear, parotid, cheek, mouth and chin. It is capable of reaching about as high as the zygomatic arch. The zygomatic arch is actually higher than planning measurements would appear to permit, taking the pivot point to be the medial end of the lower border of the flap. This anomaly is explained by the fact that the lower border lies along the anterior axillary fold where there is a large amount of slack skin available, taken up when the arm is abducted. The inequality in length between the two borders of the flap which this slack creates means that any tension line developed during transfer tends to be along the shorter upper border and not the longer lower border. In planning, therefore, the effective length of the flap should be measured along the upper border with the pivot point at its medial end (Fig. 4.35).

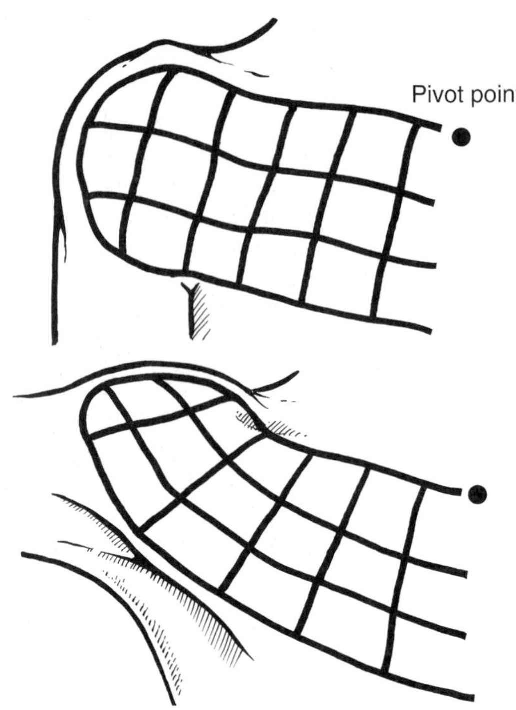

Fig. 4.35 The slack skin available along the anterior axillary fold, taken up when a deltopectoral flap is transferred upwards, explains its anomalous pivot point. It also explains the unexpectedly long reach of the flap when it is transferred in an upward direction.

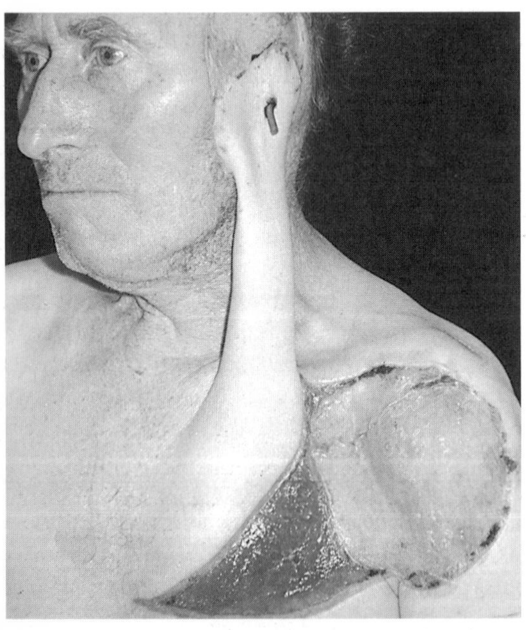

Fig. 4.34 A deltopectoral flap used to resurface the defect left following the amputation of the ear for squamous carcinoma, showing the extent of the upward reach of the flap, and restriction of the graft to the area which will form the final secondary defect.

Although the most common transfer of the deltopectoral flap is upwards it can also be transposed to any area on the chest and upper abdomen within its reach.

The planning of the various stages of its transfer and their management are discussed on pp. 79–81.

GROIN FLAP

The groin flap (Fig. 4.36) is based medially and lies along the line of the groin, using as its arteriovenous axial system the superficial circumflex iliac vessels. The artery arises 2–3 cm below the inguinal ligament, usually from the femoral

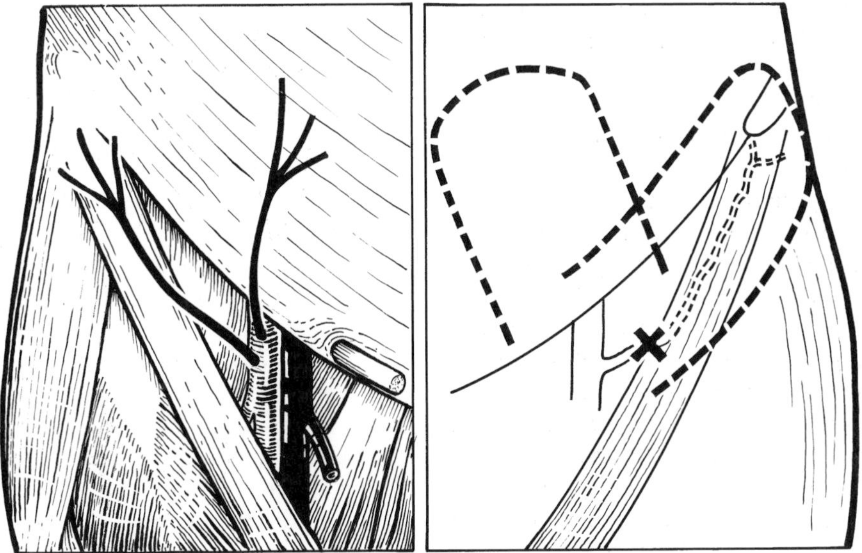

Fig. 4.36 The vascular anatomy of the inguinal region, showing the vessels which provide the axial basis of the groin and hypogastric flaps, and the skin markings which are used when either of these flaps is raised in clinical practice.

artery, occasionally from the superficial epigastric artery at its origin. It runs laterally, parallel to the inguinal ligament, and at the medial border of sartorius gives a deep branch. From that point onward it gradually becomes more superficial, passing into the tissue which would be raised as a groin flap. Lateral to the anterior superior iliac spine it divides and is no longer regularly identifiable. The corresponding vein has a general pattern parallel to the artery ending at the saphenous opening which is very close to the origin of the artery.

In planning the flap, the anterior superior iliac spine, the pubic tubercle, and the intervening inguinal ligament are marked on the skin. The line of the femoral artery can be palpated, and on it 2.5 cm below the inguinal ligament, the origin of the superficial circumflex iliac artery is marked. The line of the vessel is then drawn parallel to the inguinal ligament, and its point of entry into the flap can be marked where the vessel crosses the medial border of sartorius. With these skin markings, the flap can be planned to include the artery, although it is not essential that it should lie along the central axis of the flap. The usual width is 10 cm but extremes of 6 cm and 19 cm in an adult, and 14 cm in a child, have been used successfully. The safe maximum length is difficult to define since the lateral extent of the vascular territory is not known with certainty, but experience would suggest that if the flap is raised beyond the anterior superior iliac spine, the part of the flap beyond this should be square, i.e. with a 1 : 1 length : breadth ratio.

The flap should be raised to include the deep fascia. In making the upper marginal incision the superficial epigastric vessels are usually divided, and they provide an excellent guide to the plane in which the flap is raised. If the flap is raised through a plane deep to these vessels, it is certain to include its own axial vessels since the two sets of vessels, superficial epigastric and superficial circumference iliac, lie in the same plane. In raising the flap, a key point is the virtually constant branching of the artery at the medial border of sartorius. When the sartorius muscle is reached, it should be exposed and stripped bare to just short of its medial border. Dissection can usually stop there in the knowledge that the artery is safely out of the way.

Unless the flap is broader than average the secondary defect can usually be closed directly, though it may be necessary to flex the hip to reduce tension during the actual closure. If grafting is unavoidable, the method to be used depends on whether or not the secondary defect is overlaid by the flap. When the flap overlies the defect, primary grafting with a tie-over dressing is unavoidable; if the defect is not overlaid by the flap, delayed exposed grafting can be used.

The clinical usage of the groin flap is as a tubed flap to resurface the hand, as a local flap waltzed to a destination within its reach, and, as an extreme rarity, transferred further afield on a wrist carrier or as a free flap.

The **hypogastric flap** (Fig. 4.36) is raised on the lower abdomen with its axis passing upwards from the inguinal ligament along the line of the superficial epigastric arteriovenous system which it uses as its axial vessels. It has been used as an alternative to the groin flap, mainly for resurfacing the hand.

Subsequent stages of transfer

The modes of transfer of these flaps, their planning and management, have been described on pp. 79–81.

FASCIOCUTANEOUS FLAPS

The vascular basis of fasciocutaneous flaps consists of a plexus of small vessels ramifying on the superficial surface of the general investing layer of deep fascia, fed by perforating vessels which reach it from larger deeper arteries. The system is best developed in the limbs, where the fascia is a well-defined structure, and it has been most fully investigated in the lower leg and the forearm.

In the *trunk*, an investing fascial layer is less obviously present, but when flaps are raised in the plane which exposes bare muscle or aponeurosis a layer is exposed with a clearly visible plexus of small vessels. This corresponds in general terms to the system in the limbs, although it has not been investigated with the same thoroughness, probably because the other vascular systems which form the basis of axial, myocutaneous and free flaps have greater relevance in design of flaps generally in the trunk. Nonetheless, in raising axial flaps, the fascial layer is generally included, taking advantage of the additional vascular efficiency which it provides.

In both the *lower leg* and *forearm*, the vascular pattern is basically similar, with individual perforating vessels passing outwards from the main vascular trunks in the septa between the muscle groups to supply the plexus of the investing fascial layer. This results in lines of perforators along the axis of the limb (Figs 4.9 and 4.11).

Transposed fasciocutaneous flaps, proximally based, have been the ones used most frequently in the lower limb, but it has also been shown that the safety of cross-leg flaps is increased if they are raised to include the fascial layer, and fasciocutaneous flaps have been raised and transferred with a distant pedicle. Their major use has been to cover defects at various levels in the lower leg, most often its lower half, a site incidence probably related to the fact that defects there, particularly those exposing the tibia, are not readily managed in any other way.

The vascular basis of these flaps is medial perforators from the posterior tibial vessels, or lateral perforators from the peroneal vessels. The site of emergence of the perforators can be identified in the line of the intermuscular septum, by the use of a Doppler, but it should be appreciated that identification gives no quantitative information about the size of the vessel or its flow rate. Flaps transferring skin and deep fascia from the calf areas medial and lateral to the defect on a long, relatively narrow, pedicle have been successful, transposed through up to 180°, and constructed as large as 18 cm × 8 cm, although the average size is nearer 15 cm × 6 cm.

Rigidity of the fascia tends to hinder transfer of the flap and, since the presence of the perforating vessels feeding the flap and the fascia with its vascular network are providing the basis of success in its transfer, the use of a fascial back-cut to allow easier transposition must be carefully judged if it is to be used at all. As a result careful geometrical planning is essential. The limb also tapers towards the ankle, and in its distal third the subcutaneous border of the tibia takes on an increasing proportion of the limb circumference. This has the effect of reducing the size of the defect which can be covered from either side, and it becomes increasingly difficult to design a flap of suitable size which can be transposed into the defect.

The secondary defect in all fasciocutaneous transfers in the lower limb is split skin grafted. The result is a rather unsightly lower limb, in which skin integrity has been achieved at the expense of considerable contour abnormality. This limits the usage of the technique, particularly in women.

Flaps of the transposed type can be raised on the flexor aspect of the forearm and their transfer is accomplished much more easily than in the leg because the fascial layer does not hinder movement of the flap. This, however, is not the commonly used form of transfer. The presence of two arteriovenous systems, one of which, judging from the experience of dialysis, can be sacrificed with impunity, and the shortness of the perforator vessels, have made it feasible to raise skin and fascia together with the radial vessels and the intervening system of perforators as a single package, perfused effectively from the radial artery. Such a flap can be transferred as an island on a pedicle confined to either the distal or proximal radial vessels depending on the geometry of the transfer. Elevation of the flap is similar in essence to that used in raising it as a free flap, and is described on p. 111 *et seq.* A comparable flap based on the ulnar vessels is also possible but it would appear to offer no special advantages.

MUSCLE AND MYOCUTANEOUS FLAPS

The muscles which are used as flaps, either muscle or myocutaneous, have a localised neurovascular hilum, as opposed to a segmental supply, which acts as the pivot point around which they move in transfer. When they are used as free flaps, it is their hilar vessels which are anastomosed in the recipient site. In addition to these anatomical features the characteristics common to those flaps in routine use are that they fill a regularly recurring need, are simple to use, have been found reliable and safe, and leave a minimum of disability from loss of function of the muscle component. They fall into two categories — those which have established themselves for regular use, and those which are recognised to have a valuable clinical role, but one which is strictly limited and largely occasional. The first group alone will be considered in the present discussion. The second group will be discussed as part of the management of the clinical situations in which they are liable to be used.

Latissimus dorsi and gastrocnemius are the most frequently used muscle flaps; pectoralis major, latissimus dorsi, and rectus abdominis are transferred more commonly as myocutaneous flaps. Latissimus dorsi and rectus abdominis are also used as free flaps, both as muscle and myocutaneous flaps.

GASTROCNEMIUS

Flaps using gastrocnemius (Fig. 4.37) have proved of particular value in covering defects in the region of the knee and the upper third of the tibia. Each head of the muscle has its own neurovascular hilum close to its origin and the two bellies remain separate until they insert into an aponeurosis, common to both, on their deep surface. This aponeurosis, although in contact with the aponeurosis covering soleus, is quite separate from it until the two fuse below to form the tendo Achillis.

These anatomical features make it possible to dissect either muscle belly free of the other, divide its distal attachment, mobilise it towards its origin, and swing it around to its destination, using the neurovascular pedicle as its pivot point. The medial head is capable of reaching the upper third of the medial aspect of the tibia and the corresponding portion of the knee joint. The lateral head, less often required, can cover the upper fibula and lateral aspect of the knee joint.

In the case of an acute injury, the skin incisions required for exposure, mobilisation and transfer of the muscle are usually dictated by the site and size of the exposed bone and/or open joint and any associated skin loss. In the absence of clear-cut indications, the muscle can be exposed by an incision in the lower popliteal fossa curving downwards and medially or laterally according to the muscle belly to be used.

Gastrocnemius is easily separated from soleus using finger dissection and the line between its two muscle belles is easily felt through the

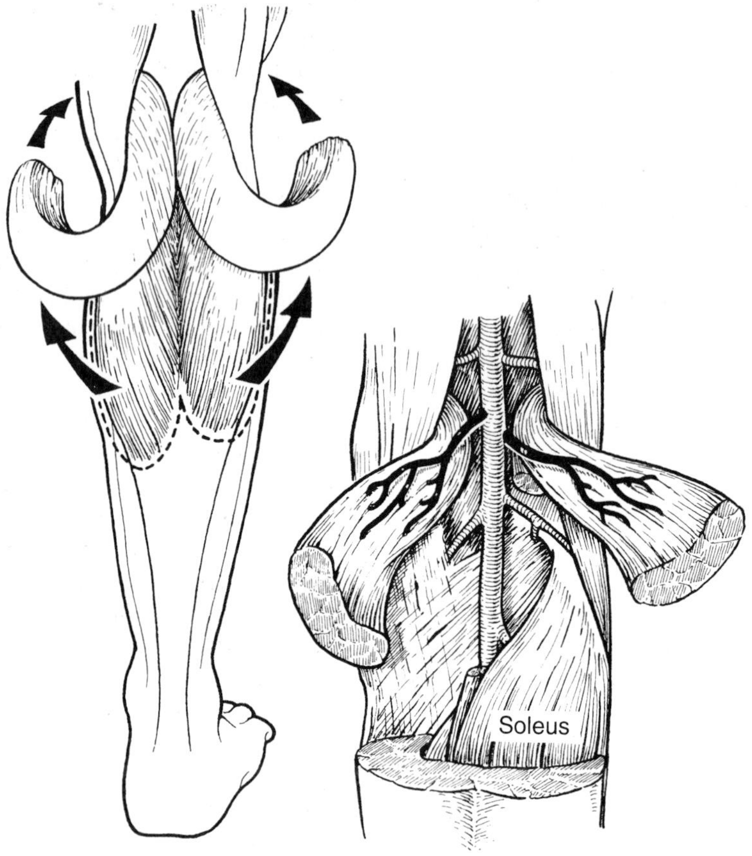

Fig. 4.37 The gastrocnemius muscle flap.
Gastrocnemius has two well-defined dominant perfusion sources, both derived from the popliteal vessels, and one of which enters each head of the muscle close to its origin from the femur. Their sites of entry are used as the pivot points of the respective bellies when they are transferred as muscle or myocutaneous flaps.

aponeurosis which covers its deep surface and holds the bellies together. Mobilised deeply as far as the tendo Achillis, the insertion of the particular muscle belly can be divided keeping a fringe of tendon on the muscle. Splitting of the aponeurosis on the deep surface in a proximal direction allows the muscle belly to be mobilised towards the popliteal fossa as far as required.

Gastrocnemius can also be used as a myocutaneous flap, either medial or lateral, like the muscle flap from which it is derived, but it is not often used in this form.

The functional deficit which results from its use is made up quite quickly by the other muscles of the flexor compartment.

LATISSIMUS DORSI

From its tendinous insertion into the upper humeral shaft the fibres of latissimus dorsi (Fig. 4.38) fan out to form a flat muscle with an origin which extends from the posterior part of the iliac crest upwards to the midthoracic spine. The arteriovenous system which perfuses it during transfer in its various forms is the subscapular, and it derives from the axillary vessels as they cross in front of the tendon. The vessels pass downwards on the posterior wall of the axilla towards the muscle belly, giving off the circumflex scapular vessels about 4 cm below their origin, and continuing downwards for a further

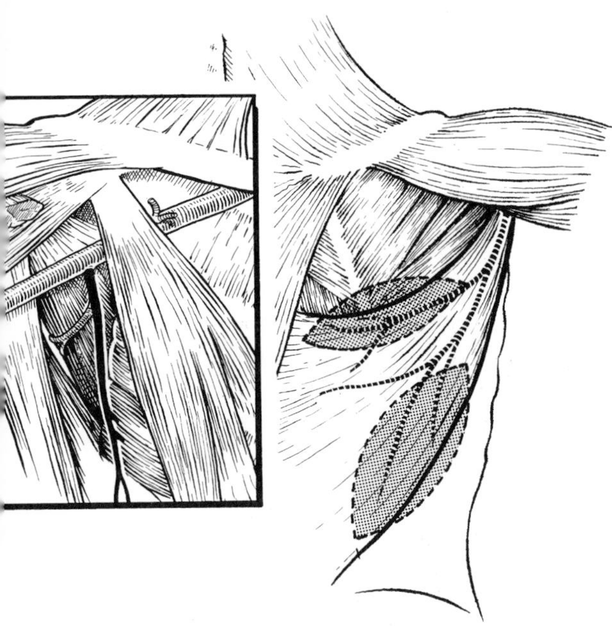

Fig. 4.38 The latissimus dorsi flap.
The vascular basis of this flap is the thoracodorsal branch of the subscapular artery with its associated veins and it is on the point of origin of these vessels that calculations of its pivot point are made. Used as a myocutaneous flap, the skin island is most frequently placed near one of its borders, upper or anterior.

6 cm as the thoracodorsal vessels before entering the substance of the muscle. Within the muscle the branching vessels have a course which is generally parallel to the muscle fibres.

In raising it as a myocutaneous flap, an appropriately sized skin ellipse overlying the muscle is chosen, its long axis directed along the line of the fibres as they fan out from the tendon. Depending on the circumstances of the transfer the ellipse is sited over the upper part of the muscle, lying almost horizontally, or more vertically along the anterior border of the muscle. The skin island taken from the anterior border can be extended anteriorly beyond the muscle, the safe extent depending on the size of the island.

The pivot point of the transfer is close to the point of origin of the subscapular artery. Over its initial 10 cm both the artery and its accompanying vein are lying free of the muscle, and the length of the vascular pedicle which this allows makes it possible for a skin island placed at the far end of the muscle to be transferred safely over a much greater distance than is usual with such flaps.

In dissecting the pedicle proximally the vessels on its deep surface can be visualised by retracting the muscle and this makes it possible to tailor the pedicle safely, dividing the various arterial and venous branches of the parent vessels as the flap is mobilised towards the axilla. Dissection is continued proximally only as far as the geometry of the transfer dictates, but if need be the entire muscle component of the pedicle can be divided. With a pedicle reduced to the vessels alone it becomes essential to avoid all traction during and after transfer of the flap.

When the flap is designed as an almost vertical ellipse over the anterior border of the muscle it can be raised and transferred with the patient supine. Flaps taken from other areas of the muscle generally require turning of the patient to a suitable position. Depending on its size and site the secondary defect is closed directly or split skin grafted.

The steps involved in raising of the flap for transfer as a free flap are basically similar to those for myocutaneous transfer, apart from the dissection of the proximal vessels where they are completely free of the muscle. The subscapular vessels at their origin have a substantial calibre and the length of the free vascular pedicle is considerable, both factors which make for a technically easier transfer.

In its various clinical roles the most important virtues of the latissimus dorsi flap lie in the large area of skin which is available for transfer, and the distance over which it can be transferred with its vascular pedicle intact. The functional deficit which follows its use is also remarkably small. The initial bulk of the flap is liable to be considerably greater than is ideal, but the denervated muscle element diminishes in volume relatively quickly, and the final result may be much more acceptable than the early appearance would have suggested.

PECTORALIS MAJOR

The vessels which provide the vascular basis of the pectoralis major myocutaneous flap (Fig. 4.39) are the pectoral branch of the thoracoacromial

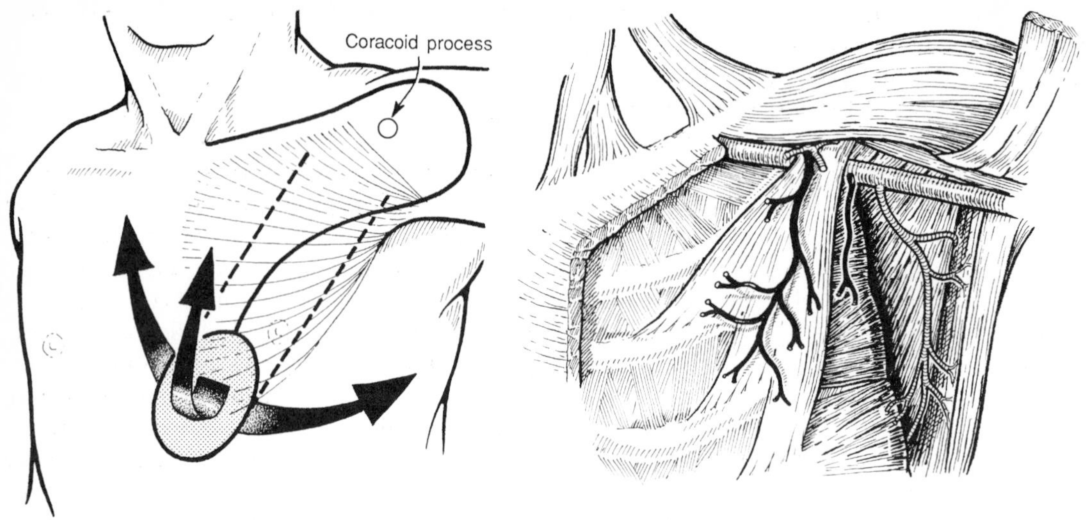

Fig. 4.39 The pectoralis major flap.
The perfusion sources of this flap are the pectoral branch of the thoraco-acromial artery and the lateral thoracic artery, although the latter source is not essential for its survival. The 'defensive' approach to the flap, making use of the skin incision used in raising a deltopectoral flap, leaves the latter flap available as a back-up technique should the myocutaneous flap run into problems. The placing of the island which is shown is probably used most frequently, but variations in the site have been described. The muscle pedicle is generally made as broad as the skin island.

artery and its associated veins. These, together with the lateral pectoral nerve, emerge from the clavipectoral fascia 2–3 cm medial to the attachment of pectoralis minor to the coracoid process. The lateral thoracic vessels also contribute to the blood supply of the muscle, reaching it lateral to pectoralis minor. The vessels do not enter the muscle immediately but run in a generally downward and medial direction over its deep surface, branching as they go, entering the muscle and continuing in its substance. The pivot point of the flap based on pectoralis major is the neurovascular hilum of the muscle but, depending on the geometry of the transfer, it is sometimes possible to avoid dividing the lateral thoracic vessels.

The skin island which is usually transferred is placed below and medial to the nipple, about the level of the 6th rib. In this area the amount of skin which precisely overlies pectoralis major is quite small, and the island is usually extended beyond the strict confines of the muscle. How far beyond it is safe to carry the extension is not precisely known, but 3–4 cm is generally regarded as the extreme, and the aponeurosis overlying rectus abdominis is raised as part of the extension. In the female the breast is a significant factor in siting the island below the inframammary fold, and in determining the direction of any extension, which may have to be medial.

As part of the preliminary skin markings it is useful to mark out the pivot point in relation to the coracoid process. Its surface marking of the hilum is 2–3 cm medial to the coracoid process, the bony prominence readily felt below the clavicle near the junction between its middle and outer third. The skin island to be transferred is then incised down to muscle or aponeurosis. The most direct approach to the muscle pedicle would use a skin incision passing directly from the pivot point to the skin island, but such an incision precludes simultaneous or subsequent use of a deltopectoral flap, a point which may or may not be regarded as important depending on the circumstances of the transfer. The alternative incision, following the outline of a deltopectoral flap, and turning down to meet the skin island, leaves it still available in reserve if needed. With the muscle exposed over the length and breadth of the pedicle, its fibres are incised and the composite of skin and muscle is elevated from the chest wall, exposing the ribs, intercostal muscles and pectoralis minor. The muscle pedicle is usually made as wide as the skin island, although as the flap is raised and its arteriovenous network becomes visible the pedicle can sometimes be narrowed. It becomes apparent in raising the muscle off the deeper structures that many vessels enter it from other sources, but the arteriovenous system to which it is restricted during transfer appears to be adequate. Elevation is continued as far up as the coracoid process, disturbing the hilar vessels as little as possible in the process. With the lateral pectoral vessels intact, a trial of the transfer can be carried out and, depending on the tension produced, the vessels are left intact or divided.

It is often possible to close the secondary defect in the female by moving the breast without giving rise to unacceptable asymmetry. In the male split skin grafting is generally required.

The major uses of the flap have been in intraoral and pharyngeal reconstruction, and in resurfacing defects of the lower face and neck. It has the incidental but not inconsiderable virtue that its muscle pedicle is able to cover and protect the major vessels in the neck, and this may be of particular value when these vessels are at risk as a result of previous irradiation.

RECTUS ABDOMINIS (Fig. 4.40)

The rectus abdominis muscles run vertically on each side of the midline from the xiphisternum and adjoining costal cartilages to the pubic crest, enclosed within the anterior and posterior layers of the rectus sheath, formed by the aponeuroses of the other abdominal muscles, external and internal oblique and transversus abdominis. Along its medial border the two layers of the sheath fuse with one another and with their fellows on the opposite side in the linea alba, a largely avascular structure. The formation of the sheath differs in the upper and lower abdomen. In the upper two-thirds, the aponeurosis of internal oblique splits to form its anterior and posterior layers, the anterior layer being reinforced by the aponeurosis of the external oblique, the posterior layer by the aponeurosis of transversus abdominis. In the lower third the aponeuroses of all three muscles pass superficial to the rectus muscle, forming the anterior sheath. The posterior sheath is replaced

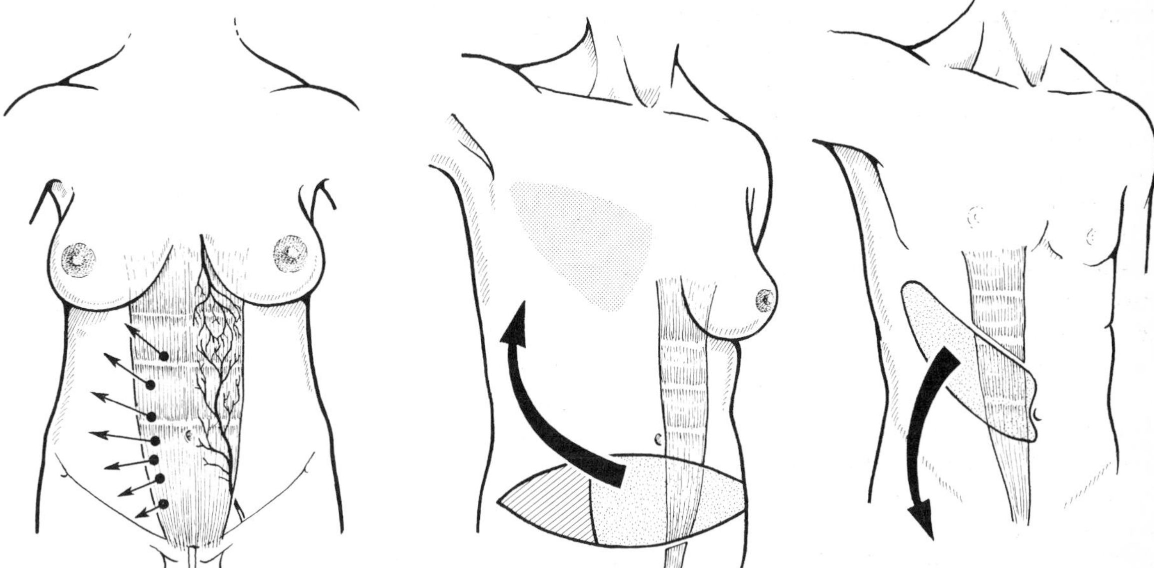

Fig. 4.40 The rectus abdominis flaps.
These flaps are based on the vertical vascular pattern running on its deep surface and within its substance, together with the system of perforating branches which pass laterally in the directions shown. The superiorly based flap is used most frequently in postmastectomy reconstruction of the breast. The inferiorly based flap, with its long axis reflecting the predominantly upward and lateral direction of the vascular pattern in the upper abdomen, can be used as a free flap, or transferred as pedicled flap to the upper thigh and groin areas.

by a layer of fascia, the transversalis fascia, and the junction line of the lower border of the posterior sheath and the fascia is referred to as the arcuate line. The rectus muscle has three tendinous intersections which are adherent to the anterior sheath; posteriorly it lies free within the sheath.

Accompanying the segmental nerves which supply the rectus muscle, a pattern of arteries and veins, running in the plane between internal oblique and tranversus abdominis, reaches the muscle by piercing the posterior sheath. The communication between the subclavian and the external iliac vessels through the superior and inferior epigastric vessels provides an additional vascular pattern, the inferior usually the larger of the two. In approaching one another from above and below, each set of vessels runs vertically on the deep surface of rectus abdominis inside the rectus sheath for several centimetres before entering the substance of the muscle, anastomosing with its fellow at about the level of the umbilicus, and with the segmental vessels.

Branches are given off from the combined system which supply the muscle and the overlying skin, the latter by a series of segmental perforators (p. 66) which reach the superficial fascia by piercing the anterior layer of the rectus sheath, and on which is superimposed a pattern of perforators, distributed around the umbilicus in the form of a cartwheel. The background plexus of small vessels in the superficial fascia (Fig. 4.1) receives a further contribution to the perfusion of the skin below the umbilicus by the superficial inguinal vessels, superficial epigastric and superficial circumflex iliac.

The directions in which the perforators run in the superficial fascia following their emergence from the anterior sheath determine to a considerable extent the shape of the skin islands which are designed to exploit them. Around the umbilicus the axis is oblique, extending upwards and laterally in the general direction of the axilla; below the umbilicus the direction is horizontal. The pattern of perforators does not extend medially, but it has been found safe in practice to prolong skin islands for some 4 cm across the midline.

The presence of a vascular input from both ends of the muscle allows rectus abdominis to be used as a **muscle flap**, based either above or below. The concept underlying its use as a **myocutaneous flap** is that if the muscle belly with its associated vessels is transected and elevated along with an island of overlying skin with the perforating vessels joining the two, both the muscle and the skin will continue to be effectively perfused via either the superior or the inferior epigastric vessels, depending on the level of the transection.

When the flap is destined for transfer to the chest, the level of transection and the site of the skin island would be the lower abdomen, with the superior epigastric the perfusing system. When the flap is intended for the groin, perineum and upper thigh, the corresponding transection level would be in the upper abdomen, perfused by the inferior epigastric vessels.

Transfer as a **pedicled myocutaneous flap** with a superior muscle pedicle is used in chest wall reconstruction, most frequently to reconstruct the breast, postmastectomy. Transferred with an inferior muscle pedicle, it is used most frequently to reconstruct defects of the groin or perineum. With each transfer the flap can be turned through an arc of up to 180°. Transfer as a **free flap** uses the inferior vascular pedicle.

Difficulties are encountered in the raising and transfer of the flap, arising from the fact that the muscle is enclosed within an aponeurotic sheath. The flap in its myocutaneous form consists of skin, anterior rectus sheath and rectus muscle with the perforating vessels which connect them. To ensure the presence of as many perforators as possible, the maximum breadth of the skin paddle should directly overlie the rectus muscle, though it may extend beyond the sheath medially and/or laterally. The long axis of the skin paddle should also follow the direction taken by the perforators after they emerge from the sheath, towards the axilla at the level of the umbilicus and above, horizontal below the umbilicus.

Above the arcuate line, this design leaves the posterior rectus sheath intact and strong enough, even in the absence of the anterior sheath, to require no reinforcement. Split skin grafting is capable of providing adequate cover of the secondary skin defect if it cannot be closed directly.

Below the arcuate line, the rectus sheath is lacking posteriorly, and a different approach is required, designed to conserve as much of the anterior sheath as possible, and allow the defect in it to be closed directly if at all possible, reducing the likelihood of subsequent hernia. To achieve this, the sheath is incised vertically medial and lateral to the line of emergence of the perforating vessels, leaving the strip of sheath between, containing the perforators, to be raised with the muscle and the skin island. The perforators are identified as they emerge from the anterior sheath, and approached carefully both from the medial and lateral aspect, allowing the width of the segment of the sheath which is transferred with the muscle and skin to be reduced to a minimum.

When a superior pedicle is used the skin is raised as a horizontal island, its level on the abdomen determined by the geometry of the transfer, its pivot point being a little below the costal margin in the line of the rectus muscle. Designing the flap in this way allows the skin island to coincide with the skin normally discarded in the standard abdominoplasty, and it is outlined and initially raised on the lower abdomen to leave a symmetrical defect, suitable for direct closure, even although a considerable part of the contralateral element may be discarded in the event because effective perfusion across the midline is limited in its extent. The part of the flap which extends across the midline is elevated as far as the linea alba and the ipsilateral segment is elevated as far as the lateral margin of the rectus muscle. The effect is to leave the skin island attached to the anterior rectus sheath.

The anterior sheath from the level of the island upwards to the xiphisternum is divided in the paramedian line and dissected off the muscle, freeing it from each of the tendinous intersections. The segmental blood vessels approach the muscle from its lateral aspect, and this anatomical fact can be exploited to achieve a more avascular dissection by mobilising the muscle, together with the vessels on its deep surface, along its medial margin and working laterally, dividing and ligating each neurovascular bundle as it is met. Below the arcuate line which marks the lower free border of the posterior sheath the inferior epigastric vessels and the muscle diverge making it possible to divide the muscle at the level of the lower border of the skin island in preparation for the transfer without dividing the vessels at the same time. The effect is to leave the rectus and the skin island perfused from below as well as above until everything is ready for the transfer.

At the level of the xiphisternum it is generally necessary to excise a segment of the anterior sheath so that the muscle pedicle will not be restricted when the transfer has been completed. When the flap is being used to reconstruct a breast defect it may in fact be preferable to design the flap on the contralateral rectus in order to reduce the arc through which the flap has to rotate in the transfer upwards to its destination.

When an inferior pedicle is used, the steps taken to raise the flap are similar in principle although there are some differences in detail. The site of the upper division of the rectus muscle is determined very much by the geometry of the transfer and the size of the skin island required. A long pedicle or a large island requires an oblique construction of the island in order to make use of the periumbilical perforators. A shorter pedicle permits the use of a lower abdominal island. The fact that the inferior epigastric vessels diverge from the rectus abdominis below the arcuate line makes it possible to retain part of the lower rectus intact, using as part of the flap only the segment of the muscle where the vessels are in contact with the muscle and providing perforators. Within the sheath, medial retraction of the muscle exposes the inferior epigastric vessels, passing upwards and medially over the fascia transversalis to enter the sheath at the arcuate line. Their mobilisation is technically straightforward, though branches pass directly to the peritoneum, and care is required to avoid accidentally avulsing one.

The inferiorly based myocutaneous flap can be converted to a free tissue transfer with a pedicle length of 10 cm and a vessel diameter of 3 mm.

Both the superiorly based and the inferiorly based transfers involve a significant amount of skin mobilisation, the superiorly based flap considerably more than the inferiorly based, and drainage following closure of the secondary defect is essential.

The problems created by the need to restore the integrity of the anterior abdominal wall depend on the width of the defect of the sheath, and whether it is above or below the arcuate line. Above the arcuate line, the continuing integrity of the posterior sheath ensures that direct closure of the anterior defect, though desirable, is not essential to avoid weakness of the wall. Below the arcuate line whether direct closure will be possible depends on the width of the strip of sheath resected as part of the flap. This depends on a favourable pattern of perforators, and it cannot be reliably predicted preoperatively. Failing this, a sheet of a synthetic mesh, such as Marlex, is used to reinforce the wall. The use of the contralateral anterior rectus sheath as a 'turn over' flap has also been used, but experience is that they result in a weak anterior abdominal wall in a proportion of patients.

The standard design of the pedicled myocutaneous flap based on the superior epigastric vessels, or the free flap based on the inferior epigastric vessels, uses the pattern of skin island usually used in an abdominoplasty, and this allows the secondary skin defect to be closed directly, mobilising the abdominal skin and advancing it downward, as in abdominoplasty.

The effectiveness of the perfusion of the skin island using the superior pedicle, and based on a single rectus abdominis muscle has been found to be unpredictable. The skin of the island which directly overlies the muscle is the best perfused, while the skin most distant from the muscle has the poorest safety record. This skin area is often surplus to requirements and can be discarded, but if its survival is essential, its perfusion can be improved in one of two ways. In both, the lower half of the other rectus muscle is raised, including the perforators to the skin, and with it the inferior epigastric vessels. These can be anastomosed to an artery and vein at the receptor site, the technique referred to as **supercharging**. Alternatively, the inferior epigastric artery on the pedicled side can be anastomosed to the inferior epigastric artery on the non-pedicled side, referred to as **recharging**. The latter technique relies on the fact that a considerable proportion of blood flow through the rectus muscle is shunted past the skin island and reaches the inferior epigastric artery. Venous drainage is via the cutaneous circulation, and this as a rule appears adequate but, if doubt exists, the inferior epigastric vein can be anastomosed to a vein at the flap receptor site.

The main factors which mitigate against the use of the flap in any of its forms are obesity, because of problems resulting from fat necrosis, and pre-existing midline and paramedian scars, because these interfere with the skin circulation derived from the vessels which reach it from the muscle.

FREE FLAPS

As part of the planning of a free flap transfer a knowledge of the local vascular anatomy is essential, with a clear idea of which vessels are likely to be used in the receiving site as well as their probable normality. If the flap is required as a result of trauma, the effect of the injury on the vascular anatomy, and the degree of damage which the vessels have sustained, also need to be assessed, since local scarring makes dissection more difficult, reduces the mobility of the vessels, and makes their inadvertent injury more likely. In making such an assessment, arteriography is only of limited value. It provides no information on flow volume, on the state of the vessel wall, and the severity of the scarring. A healthy vessel wall and an adequate pulse volume must be demonstrably present. Similar considerations apply if the area has been previously irradiated. In both situations it may be necessary to move beyond the field of damage to find a vessel with a healthy wall which is suitable for anastomosis, and make use of a vein graft to bridge the gap. The presence of infection in the vicinity of the planned site of the anastomosis is an absolute contraindication to the use of a free flap. Thrombosis is inevitable.

The vascular anatomy of the free flaps in current use is well established, and in raising the flap it is safe to postpone exposure of the vascular pedicle until it is convenient. The calibre of their arterial component is also such that the adequacy of input of blood to the flap does not pose a problem. The corresponding factors regarding venous outflow are less well established, but a reasonable rule of thumb is that the vein which is used should be at least as large as the artery, and a second vein is often anastomosed in addition if it is available. The vessels selected for anastomosis in the recipient site should also be no smaller in calibre than the flap vessels to ensure adequate circulation through the flap.

During the transfer, the total operating time can be reduced by preparing the recipient site and raising the donor flap simultaneously. The time which elapses between division of the axial vessels of the flap and restoration of perfusion is referred to as the **ischaemia time**. To minimise its adverse effects, the operative sequence should be organised to reduce it to an absolute minimum by maintaining flow through the vascular pedicle of the flap until the last minute before transfer.

Vessels may be anastomosed by attaching the flap vessel to an opening made in the wall of the donor vessel in the recipient site — **end-to-side** anastomosis. Alternatively the donor vessel in the recipient site may be divided and anastomosis carried out **end-to-end**. The presence of collateral circulation in most body sites allows diversion of an artery to act as the donor vessel for a free flap without compromising tissue viability in its vicinity, and end-to-end anastomosis is quite safe. Following trauma, however, vessels can become virtual end-arteries, and division is then liable to result in ischaemia of the region they normally supply. End-to-side anastomosis, which preserves the pre-existing flow pattern of the artery, then becomes essential.

When the surgeon is in a position to choose the form of the anastomosis, the relative diameters of the vessels being joined together usually determines the method chosen. When vessel diameters are similar it is usual, although not obligatory, to use end-to-end anastomosis. If the diameters are nearly equal, gentle dilatation of the narrower lumen will still allow end-to-end anastomosis to be carried out. When inequality is greater, end-to-end anastomosis may be technically possible, but turbulent blood flow with thrombosis is then likely, and end-to-side anastomosis should be used.

Much less is known about the venous side of the circulation, but the criteria used for arteries in deciding whether to use end-to-end or end-to-side anastomosis have been found to be effective also for the veins.

Instrumentation

The instruments used to dissect the vessels free, prepare them for anastomosis, and carry out the anastomosis, are modified versions of instruments designed for other purposes, such as jeweller's forceps, or for other surgical disciplines, such as ophthalmology. They are relatively few in number — a spring-handled needle holder; spring-handled scissors, straight to cut vessels, curved to dissect, trim periadventitia from the vessels, and cut sutures; forceps, generally straight but with a curved version, useful when access to a vessel is awkward, and also modified with blunt tips, used as a vessel dilator to overcome vessel spasm. The instruments are held and manipulated using the 'pencil holding grip' (Fig. 4.41), and in the case of the needle holder making sure that the needle is held at its mid-point.

Microclamps of various designs are used to occlude the vessels during anastomosis. They share the characteristic of exerting just enough closing pressure to maintain vessel occlusion without damaging its intima. Double clamps are available which also hold the vessels in position

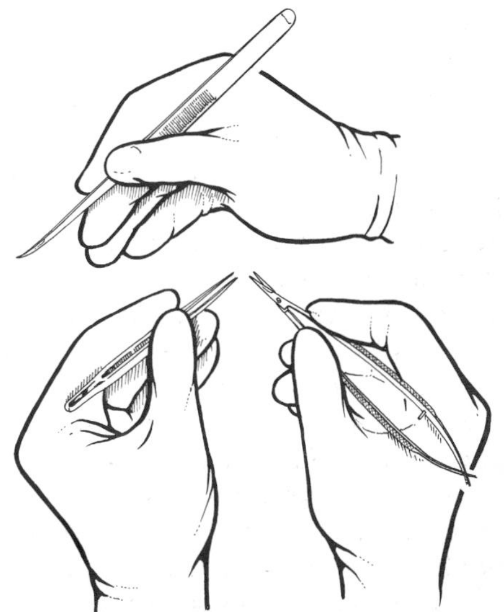

Fig. 4.41 The 'pencil holding grip', used in manipulating microvascular instruments.

for anastomosis, but individual clamps allow greater flexibility in use, making it easier for the surgeon to control the degree of tension of the suture line, and ensure that there is an absence of torsion of either vessel.

VESSEL SELECTION AND PREPARATION

The vascular pedicle of the flap, both arterial and venous, must be long enough to reach the donor vessels in the recipient site with a comfortable margin and correctly orientated, to ensure that there is a positive absence of tension, kinking, and torsion, each of which is a cause of turbulent flow and increases the likelihood of thrombosis. A healthy vessel wall and atheroma-free intimal lining, with no branches, and in the case of veins no valves, in the vicinity of the anastomosis are also essential. Each of these is likely to create turbulence.

Vessel handling

When handling the vessels, both of the flap and in the recipient site, before, during and after anastomosis, an atraumatic technique is essential. Stripping of the periadventitia is a powerful inducer of vessel spasm, and for this reason it is undesirable to dissect out the vessels cleanly at the outset. A cuff of periadventitia should be left around each vessel until it is being prepared for anastomosis under the microscope, and manipulation should be confined to pushing the vessels with closed forceps, or grasping periadventitial tissue. Any form of injury, whether crush due to application of forceps, heat due to careless use of bipolar coagulation, or stretch due to excessive traction, injures the vessel wall and may damage the intima, making the vessel liable to thrombosis. Side branches can be carefully coagulated using bipolar diathermy, but care must be taken to avoid the wall of the main vessel. Alternatively, ligation and division can be used, but the ligature should not interfere with the wall of the main vessel. It makes little difference whether dissection is by scissors or scalpel, provided the main vessels themselves are not handled directly.

During mobilisation of the vessels, even the most careful of handling may induce a degree of spasm, and it is common practice to irrigate the vessels with topical antispasmodic agents such as local anaesthetics, e.g. lignocaine or procaine, or alternatively, papaverine. There is no objective evidence that such irrigation is of real benefit, but clinical experience has been that no harm results.

Vessels in the recipient site should be dissected free over a length sufficient to allow easy delivery into the wound, and when anastomosis is to be end-to-side, delivery can often be facilitated by packing gauze swabs deep to the vessels in question. Prior to division of the vessels of the flap, as the final step in preparation for the transfer, it is customary to apply a microclamp to each, and careful note should be taken of its orientation so that the vessels are not twisted about their long axis. Twisting of a vessel leads to turbulent flow and is liable to result in thrombosis.

Flap transfer

When both the flap and the recipient site are ready, the flap vessels are divided at the preselected point, and the flap is transferred. Depending on the local circumstances, the flap may be sutured to the defect around its entire circumference or merely held in position with tacking sutures. The purpose is to secure the flap sufficiently firmly that the anastomotic site will not be disturbed during any subsequent suturing.

Only when the macroscopic preparations are complete, with the vessels orientated correctly, and approximated to each other in a tension-free position for easy anastomosis, is the microscope brought in. *In adjusting the microscope the comfort and ease of the surgeon has absolute priority, with the table at the correct height and the seat stable, and the surgeon's wrists and elbows supported. Positioned awkwardly, the surgeon quickly tires, and is more likely to make errors. Competent assistance is also highly desirable.*

Preparation for anastomosis

Formal preparation of the vessels should be thorough, and demonstrably complete, before any suturing is begun, so that there is no subsequent unnecessary delay in the re-establishment of the circulation. Under the microscope, as in manipulation with the naked eye, vessels may be pushed to and fro with closed forceps, but must not be handled or grasped other than by the periadventitia.

The presence of periadventitial tissue in the lumen of the vessel, either loose or attached to the wall, will induce thrombosis, and as part of the final preparation of the vessel for end-to-end anastomosis the periadventitial tissue is removed for 2–3 mm back from its cut end (Fig. 4.42). In preparing the vessel for end-to-side anastomosis, periadvential tissue should be removed over a 1 cm length of the receiving vessel (Fig. 4.43).

As a final step, it is customary to trim the cut end of the vessel to ensure that all traumatised tissue has been removed, leaving the margin smooth and healthy. Vessels may be cut obliquely or transversely according to personal preference, but crushing of the cut end of the vessel and contact with the intima should be avoided.

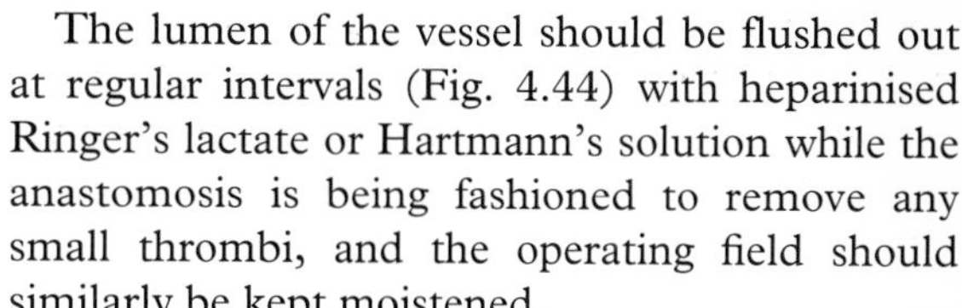

The lumen of the vessel should be flushed out at regular intervals (Fig. 4.44) with heparinised Ringer's lactate or Hartmann's solution while the anastomosis is being fashioned to remove any small thrombi, and the operating field should similarly be kept moistened.

Immediately before the anastomosis is begun, the vessel ends are dilated with forceps or the specifically designed vessel dilators. The instrument is introduced into the lumen with the jaws closed, and gently allowed to open, stretching the vessel slightly, opening its lumen and counteracting any spasm (Fig. 4.45).

Preparation for end-to-side anastomosis

If an end-to-side anastomosis is to be performed, microclamps are first applied to the receptor vessel on each side of the site chosen, and the opening is made on the same side as the flap,

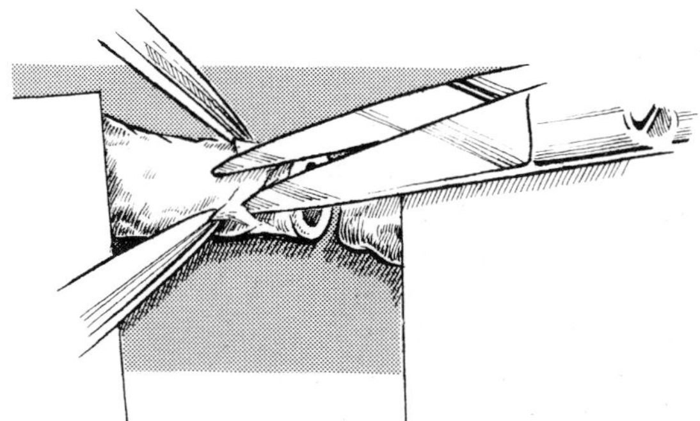

Fig. 4.42 Removal of the periadventitia in preparation for end-to-end anastomosis.
A background for the various microsurgical manipulations, provided by a strip of coloured plastic tape placed behind the vessels, is felt by some surgeons to improve visualisation of the anastomosis.

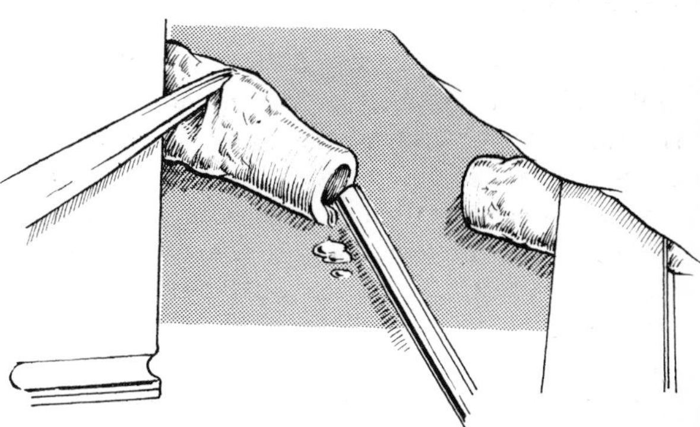

Fig. 4.44 Flushing out the lumen of the vessel.

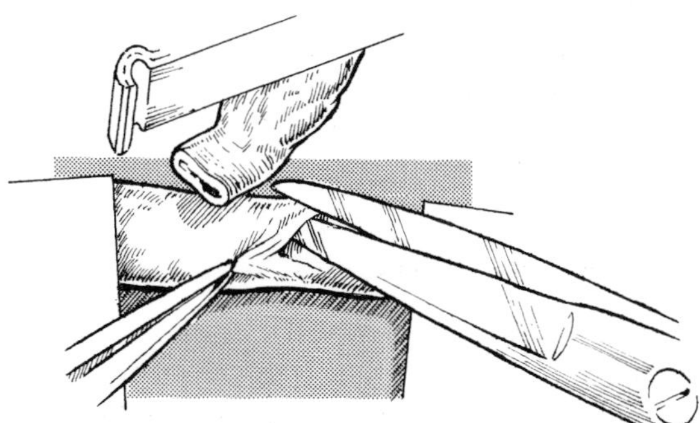

Fig. 4.43 Removal of periadventitia in preparation for end-to-side anastomosis.

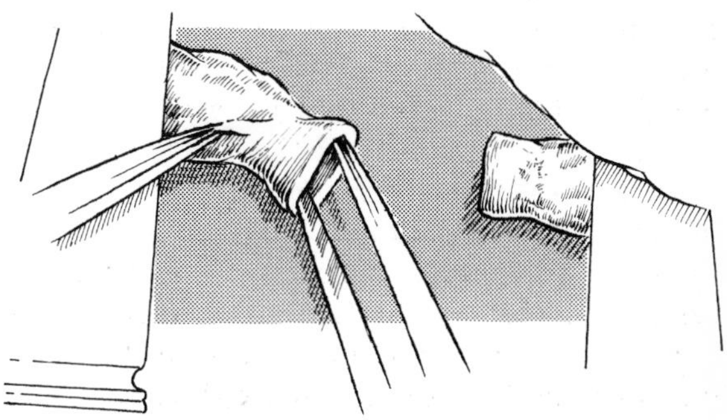

Fig. 4.45 The use of the vessel dilator to counteract spasm of the vessel.

either by incising the wall longitudinally with a scalpel, in which case the elastic fibres in the wall retract and form a round or oval opening or, more commonly, by excising a circular portion of the wall (Fig. 4.46). The making of such an opening, with its necessary smooth margin, can be technically quite difficult.

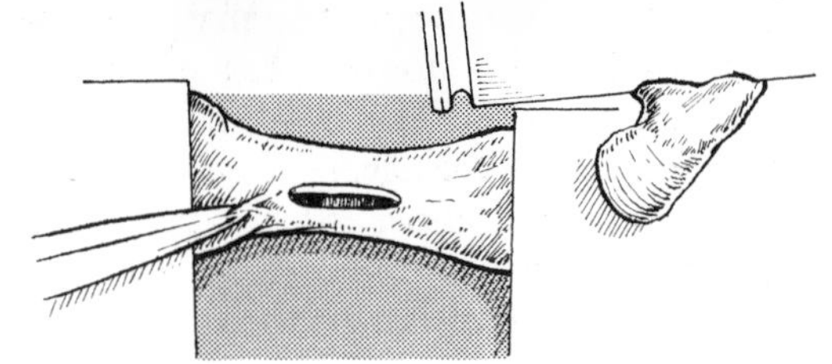

Fig. 4.46 Making an opening in the side of the receptor vessel in preparation for end-to-side anastomosis.

ANASTOMOTIC TECHNIQUE

Anastomosis is carried out using a fine monofilament suture, usually nylon, which can vary in thickness from 8/0 to 11/0 depending on the size of the vessels and the individual preference of the operator. Interrupted sutures are always used (Fig. 4.47), placed at regular intervals around the circumference with the needle inserted at a distance from the cut end of the vessel roughly equal to twice the thickness of its wall. The needle should be inserted vertically through the vessel wall, from the adventitia into the lumen in

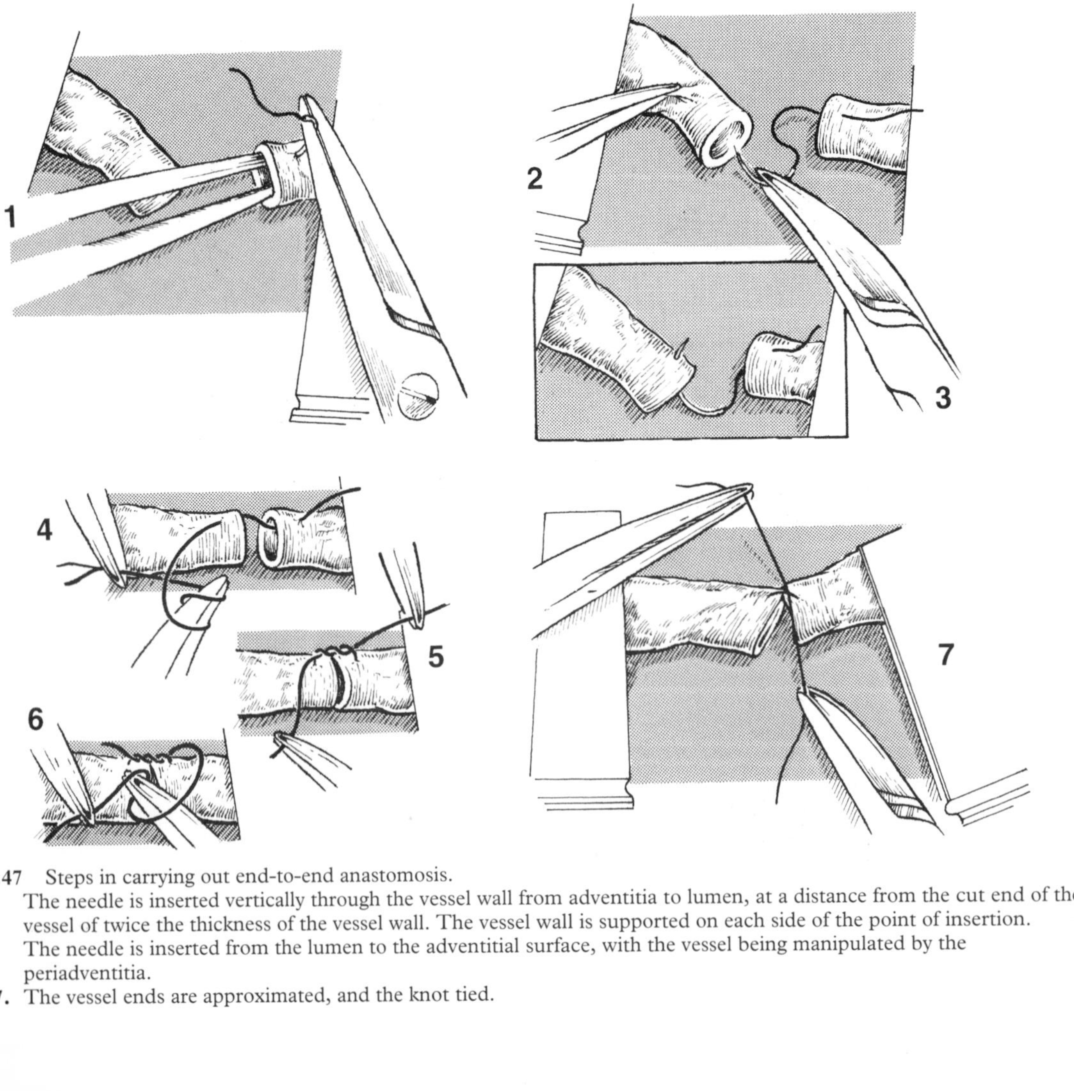

Fig. 4.47 Steps in carrying out end-to-end anastomosis.

1. The needle is inserted vertically through the vessel wall from adventitia to lumen, at a distance from the cut end of the vessel of twice the thickness of the vessel wall. The vessel wall is supported on each side of the point of insertion.

2,3. The needle is inserted from the lumen to the adventitial surface, with the vessel being manipulated by the periadventitia.

4,5,6,7. The vessel ends are approximated, and the knot tied.

a single smooth movement, stabilising the vessel wall with closed forceps inserted into the lumen and opened slightly. Pressed lightly against the intima on each side of where the needle will penetrate they exert gentle counter pressure. The needle is drawn through, and then inserted through the wall of the other vessel from intima outwards. The vessel ends are drawn together and the suture is tied with the knot on the outside of the vessel. The precise placement of the knot is not of great importance in end-to-end suturing, but in end-to-side anastomosis the knot should be placed on the flap vessel side as this helps it to 'snug down' in position.

Suturing sequence

The sequence in which the sutures are placed may vary, but the same technique is used foı each individual suture.

For *end-to-side anastomosis*, a suture is inserted at each end of the opening. The back wall is then sutured, followed by the front wall (Fig. 4.48).

For *end-to-end anastomosis*, the triangulation technique classically described by Carrel is standard. The technique involves the insertion of three key sutures at equal distances around the circumference of the line of the anastomosis, the

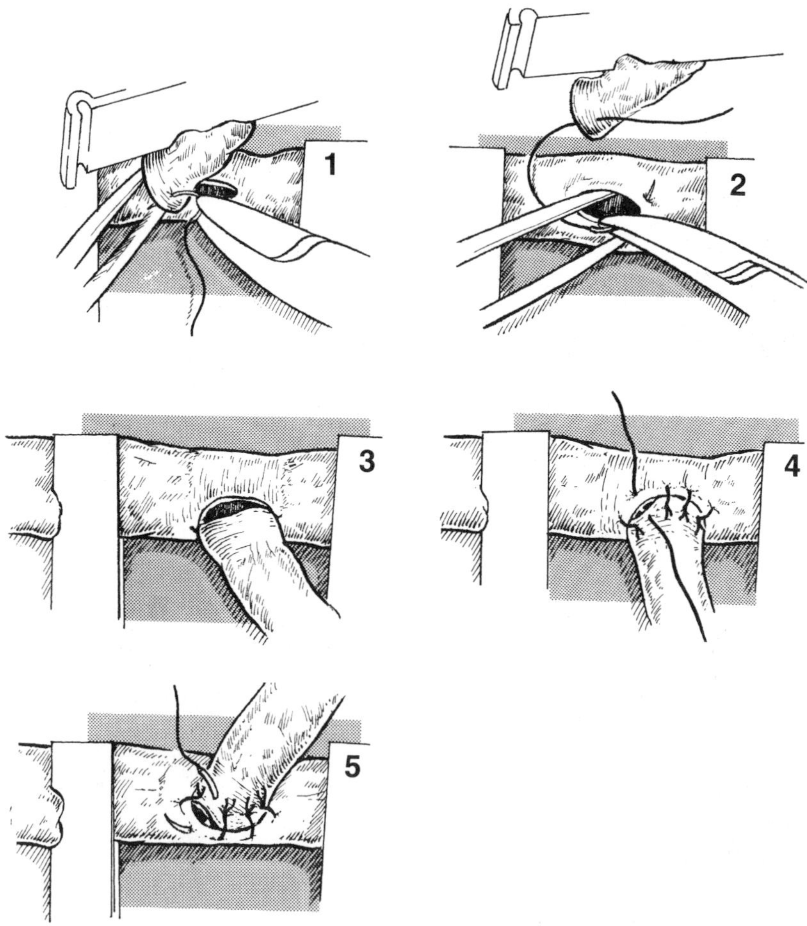

Fig. 4.48 The steps in end-to-side anastomosis, showing completion of the suturing of the back wall, followed by suturing of the front wall.

intervening gaps being filled in with additional sutures (Fig. 4.49).

The first two of the key sutures are inserted 120° apart, and the additional sutures inserted between. The vessels are turned over, and the third key suture is placed in the middle of the back wall equidistant from the first two. The intervening gaps are then closed. The distance between individual sutures should be such that the vessel ends are completely apposed leaving no holes between, through which blood can escape.

The sequence in which the vessels are anastomosed is to some extent a matter of personal preference, and is often dictated by the circumstances in the individual case. If one vessel lies deep to the other, the deeper anastomosis should be completed first.

In carrying out vessel anastomoses, a problem which the surgeon faces is what to do with the needle while the instrumental tying of each suture is being carried out. It is essential that it should be kept visible in the field, ready to be

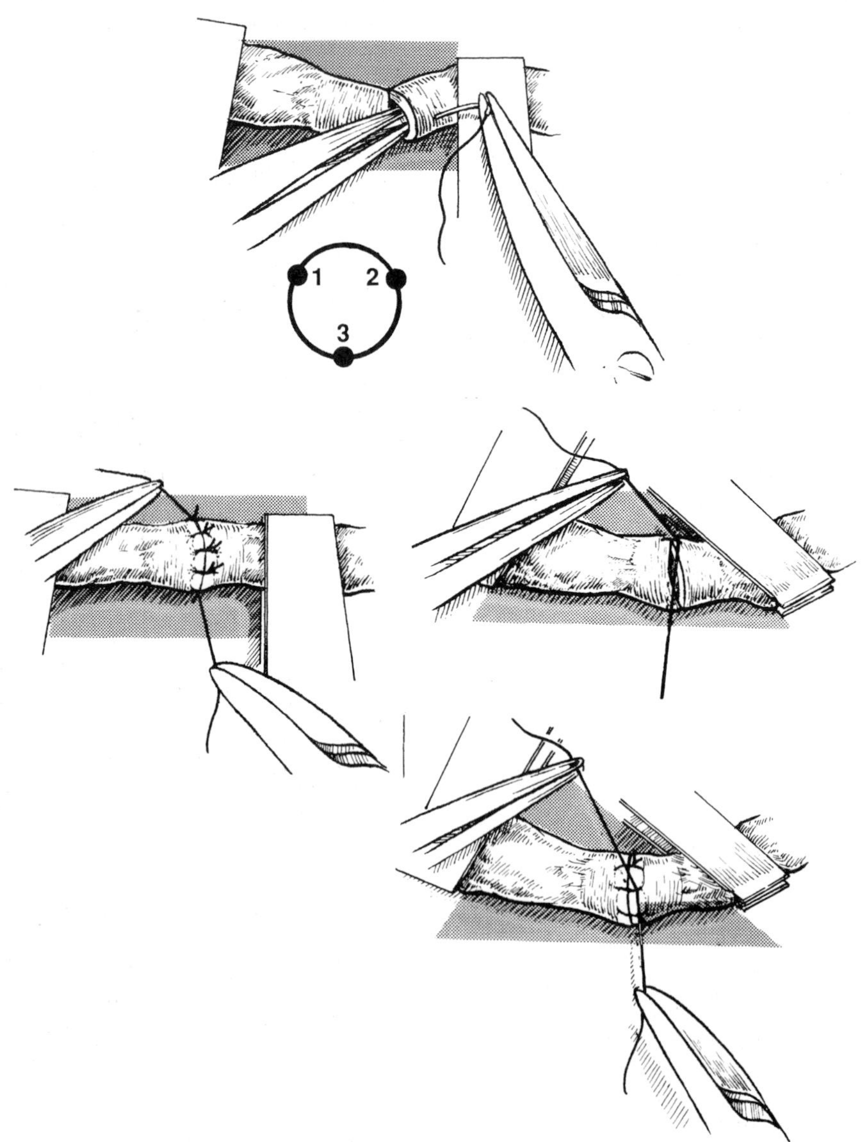

Fig. 4.49 The sequence which is used in end-to-end anastomosis, showing the insertion of three key sutures at equal distances around the circumference of the line of the anastomosis, and completion with sutures to close the intervening gaps.

picked up when the ends of the completed knot are cut. A solution is to insert its tip into the gauze swab usually in the field (Fig. 4.50), present to soak up excess irrigation fluid.

When both anastomoses, arterial and venous, are completed the circulation is restored by removing the microclamps, starting with the clamp distal to the venous anastomosis, working back against the direction of flow, and finishing with the clamp proximal to the arterial anastomosis. *The clamp distal to any anastomosis in the direction of flow should always be removed first, otherwise the build-up of pressure is liable to result in leakage of blood from the anastomosis, and thrombosis may result.*

When the clamps are opened, and blood passes across the anastomosis there may be a little bleeding from between sutures, but this subsides quickly. An obvious source of leakage calls for additional sutures. It may take a few moments for the flap to become pink, and the first sign of circulation is often filling of the vein. At first flow may be sluggish, but it usually picks up quickly. A bounding, pulsatile artery, a pink flap, and a full vein are signs of a healthy, satisfactory circulation. If this is not rapidly forthcoming, the cause must be sought. Arterial spasm can be corrected by topical application of a dilating agent such as local anaesthetic or papaverine, but if this fails it is better to take down or resect the anastomosis and refashion it. Expectant management merely postpones the inevitable. The same applies to venous problems.

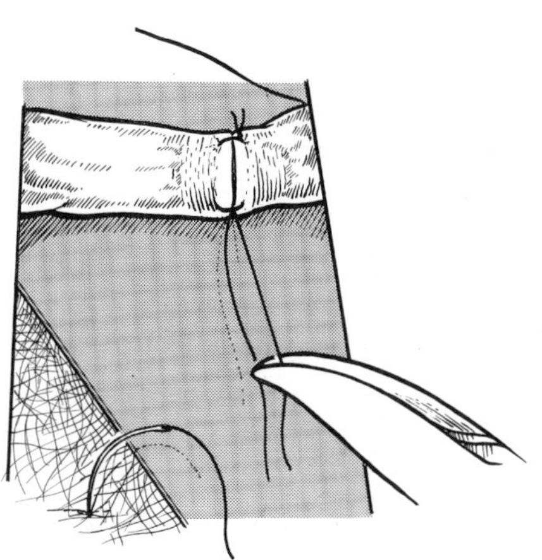

Fig. 4.50 The use of a gauze swab into which the needle can be inserted in order to keep it within the visual field while it is not being used.

Test for patency (Fig. 4.51)

If doubt exists, patency can be tested by occluding the vessel distal to the anastomosis with two microforceps placed side by side. Blood is milked distally by the distal forceps leaving an empty portion of vessel. The proximal forceps are opened and, if the empty portion fills, it means that the anastomosis is patent.

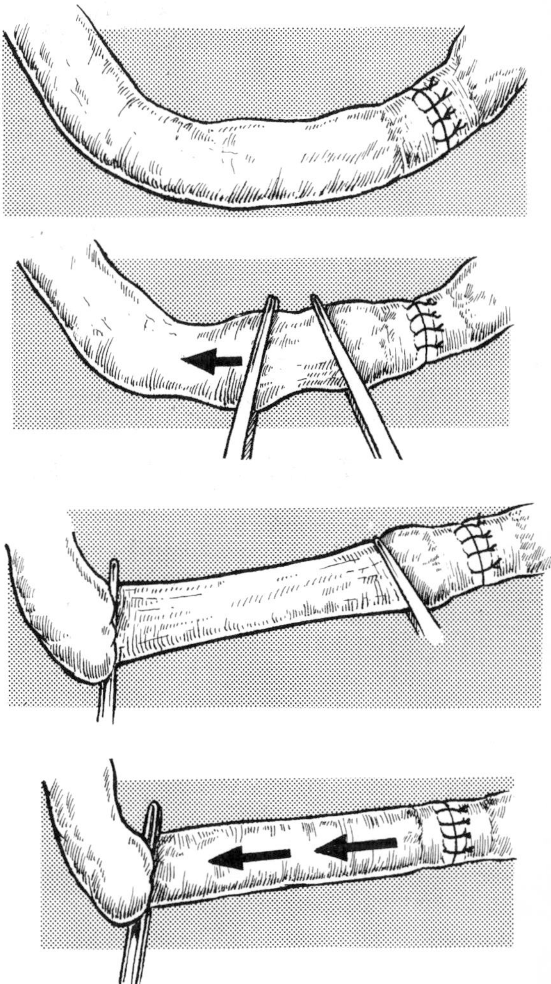

Fig. 4.51 The method of testing for patency of the vessel anastomosis.

With the anastomoses complete and functioning, the vessels usually take up a 'natural position' in which they curve or loop gently, but the surgeon must also see that there is no kinking or compression. The final step in the procedure is the insertion of a drain under the flap. If suction drainage is being used it should be applied at a distance from the site of the anastomosis, preferably fixed in position by using a transfixing suture through drain and skin.

POSTOPERATIVE MANAGEMENT

Free flaps are at their most vulnerable during the first 72 hours after operation, and most complications arise during this period. Things can go wrong later, but they do so sufficiently rarely that the first 3 days can be regarded as the danger period when observation should be most acute. Complications arising more than 3 days postoperatively tend to carry a bad prognosis, and appear to be little affected by surgical intervention.

The postoperative course of a successful free flap is not unlike that of a successful pedicled flap. Oedema is usual after 24–48 hours and it begins to settle after 72 hours. Transitory oedema is normal in pedicled random pattern flaps, but it is less marked than in the average free flap. Satisfactory progress is indicated by a flap with a definite pink colour, blanching on pressure, not unlike a healthy random pattern flap. Deviation from this pattern should give rise to suspicion that an anastomosis is not functioning properly.

A flap which looks 'collapsed and empty', fails to blanche on pressure and feels cold, is almost certainly suffering from arterial insufficiency, due either to spasm or thrombosis. These are distinguished clinically by stabbing the flap with a wide-bore hypodermic needle — if spasm is present, some bleeding will be seen, although reduced in quantity, but no bleeding occurs if the vessel is thrombosed. The distinction is essentially academic, arterial spasm almost invariably progressing to thrombosis at the anastomosis.

Excessive swelling of the flap, cyanosis, coolness, and venous stasis on pressure are indicative of venous thrombosis or insufficiency. Venous problems are much commoner than arterial problems.

Various attempts have been made to provide an objective continuous assessment of the circulatory state of free flaps, using plethysmography in its various forms, Doppler apparatus, temperature, and percutaneous oxygen tension measurements. None of these are entirely satisfactory, and they can, in fact, be misleading. The decision as to whether the anastomosis needs to be revised is essentially a clinical one, and the rule is simple. **When in doubt, re-explore.** Flaps do not suffer as a result of re-exploration. It is postponement of exploration and revision in the forlorn hope of spontaneous improvement which prejudices the survival of the flap, and may convert probable into inevitable flap loss.

The use of pharmaceutical agents to help maintain patency of the anastomoses and good perfusion of the flap has been described. Despite their theoretical virtues, little convincing evidence has been produced that they reduce the incidence of thrombosis. In the heyday of the tube pedicle a comparable pharmaceutical approach was recommended in the generally vain efforts to rescue the failing flap. With pedicled flaps the solution lay in designing safer flaps; with free flaps the solution lies in good anastomotic technique.

OMENTAL FLAP

The surgeon is occasionally confronted with a large defect which requires reconstruction without delay, which will not accept a free skin graft, and for which, for technical reasons, no flap is suitable, whether skin, fasciocutaneous, muscle or myocutaneous, pedicled or free. The sites most likely to give rise to such a problem are the scalp and the anterior chest wall. In the scalp area, the form the problem takes is how to provide cover as rapidly as possible for the defect with an extensive area of bare bone on the vault of the skull, and prevent it from progressing to sequestration of the outer table. In the chest wall, the problem concerns the extensive defect, usually from a combination of breast surgery and radiation, which is clearly incapable of granulating.

A possible solution in both situations may be to cover the defect with a tissue which will produce granulations rapidly and effectively, and provide a surface which will then accept a free skin

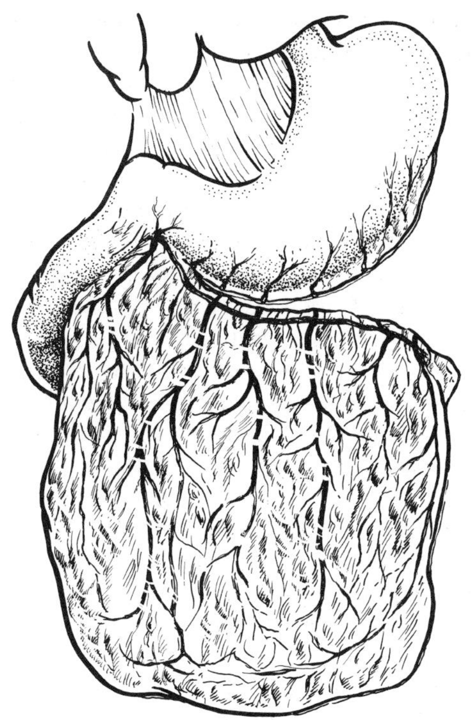

Fig. 4.52 The omental flap, pedicled on the right gastro-epiploic vessels.

graft. The omentum is such a tissue (Fig. 4.52), and it has the additional virtue of being able to fill a dead space with extremely vascular tissue, of particular value when the space is chronically infected, or the result of radiation injury.

In preparing the omentum for transfer, it is first freed from its avascular attachments to the transverse colon, leaving it attached along the greater curvature of the stomach. It is vascularised from branches of the epiploic vessels which form a series of loops in the direction of its free border. For transfer as a pedicled flap, it is usually pedicled on the right gastro-epiploic vessels, the larger of the two, though either can be used, the branches to the stomach being divided to allow it to be mobilised. Its looped vascular pattern allows it to be lengthened without losing its vascularity, and the calibre of its vessels makes its transfer as a free flap technically straightforward.

Used as a free flap, omentum can be transferred to the scalp area, using the superficial temporal vessels for anastomosis.

Used as a pedicled flap, it can be used to cover the anterior chest wall. It is harvested using a linea alba approach, leaving a gap in its upper end to allow its transfer.

Depending on the degree of adiposity of the patient the omentum can either be a substantial structure containing a proportion of fat, or apparently insubstantial. Regardless of which form it takes, when spread over the defect and tacked to its margins, it produces granulations with remarkable speed, and accepts a split skin graft readily.

The use of omentum has obvious disadvantages, with the need for a laparotomy, and the postoperative discomfort and degree of immobility of the patient which is inevitable. The amount of tissue the omentum can provide cannot be assessed preoperatively, nor can the effect on it of previous abdominal surgery. It is generally used only when every alternative has been considered and none has been found suitable. In such a situation its adverse factors have to be accepted.

RADIAL FOREARM FLAP

This flap, raised on the flexor aspect of the forearm, is perfused from the radial vessels. Their perforating branches supply the plexus of the investing layer of deep fascia, from which the blood is distributed to the overlying skin. The flap can be designed as a fasciocutaneous flap to transfer soft tissue alone, or in combination with a vascularised length of radial bone as an osteofasciocutaneous flap, and also transferring the fascia alone.

In the proximal part of the forearm, the radial vessels lie between the muscle bellies of brachioradialis and flexor carpi radialis, and their perforating branches reach the investing layer of fascia by passing along the intermuscular septum between the two muscles (Fig. 4.9). The tendons of the two muscles separate distally, and the vessels become more superficial, lying on flexor pollicis longus and pronator quadratus. The effect is to make the septum a less well defined structure, but the concept of perforating branches from the vessels reaching the fascial layer remains valid.

In the part of the forearm between the sites of insertion of pronator teres and brachioradialis the intermuscular septum, with its content of branches of the radial vessels, continues laterally over flexor pollicis longus towards the lateral surface of the radius. There the bone, over a length of approximately 10 cm, has a 'bare' area covered only by periosteum, with which the septum merges, its content of branches of the radial vessels forming a plexus on its surface, and supplying the underlying bone. Branches of the radial vessels also supply both the flexor pollicis longus and pronator quadratus muscles in addition to the flexor aspect of the radius from which they take origin, adjoining the 'bare' area.

The vessels passing superficially from the radial artery to reach the investing layer of fascia provide the perfusion source for the fasciocutaneous element of the flap; the vessels which continue laterally and deeply provide the vascular basis for the transfer of the segment of radius.

The fasciocutaneous element is generally constructed as an island and experience has shown that, *provided there is an adequate breadth of the investing layer of the deep fascia connecting the island to the intermuscular septum with its content of perforators and hence to the radial vessels*, it need not directly overlie the line of the vessels. The geometry of the transfer largely governs its site. A distal site allows a long proximal vascular pedicle, useful when the transfer is as a free flap; a proximal site allows a long distal pedicle, valuable when a pedicled transfer to the hand is planned. When the transfer is pedicled, the radial vessels provide the sole perfusion source; when a free flap is used, an additional superficial vein is generally retained, available for anastomosis should the need arise.

The flap is raised under tourniquet, and its outline, and the line of the radial vessels and a suitably sized superficial vein, generally the cephalic, are drawn out on the skin prior to its inflation.

Fasciocutaneous flap (Fig. 4.53)

The plane of elevation lies between the investing layer of fascia and the muscles, and the key to the dissection lies in identifying the intermuscular septum between brachioradialis and flexor carpi radialis. With these muscles and their tendons identified the septum is approached first from one side and then from the other, retracting the related structures to expose the radial vessels. The vessels are mobilised along with the flap and the intermuscular septum, dividing the multiple small branches to the surrounding muscles. Care should be taken to avoid damage to the terminal branch of the radial nerve which is a close lateral relation of the radial artery in the middle third of the forearm.

Additional skin incisions are made, proximally or distally as required, to allow further mobilisation of the vessels in creating the pedicle, and dissection free of the superficial vein. On the arterial side, the proximal limit is the origin of the anterior interosseous artery, which should be retained as a perfusion source for the distal forearm and hand; on the venous side, the proximal limit is the antecubital venous plexus.

Osteofasciocutaneous flap (Fig. 4.53)

The skin island is raised as already described as far as the mobilisation of flexor carpi radialis and brachioradialis from the intermuscular septum. Retraction of the flap medially, and brachioradialis laterally, exposes flexor pollicis longus and pronator quadratus, and the vessels entering them. An arbitrary line is drawn over the two muscles in the long axis of the radius between the insertions of pronator teres and brachioradialis, a length of approximately 10 cm, the line along which the muscles and the underlying bone will be sectioned. Medial to this line the vessels entering the muscles are divided as the flap is mobilised, but the vessels entering the muscles lateral to the line and reaching the 'bare' area are carefully preserved.

The line is selected so that the radial shaft is divided in a ratio of one-third lateral and two-thirds medial, the lateral element providing the bony component of the composite transfer. Along the line, the muscles are incised down to the underlying bone and the bone is sectioned using a power saw with a fine blade.

The segment of bone has also taken the form of a wedge, cut from the flexor surface of the bone or its lateral surface. All three forms of resection

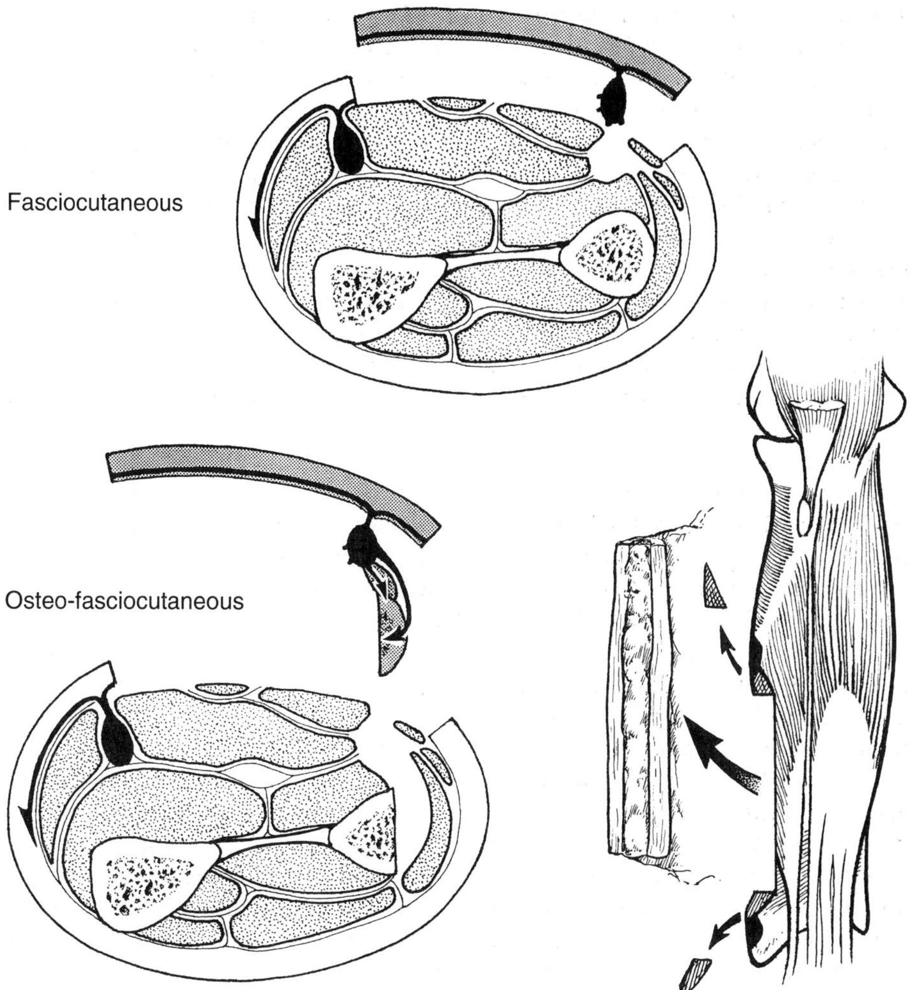

Fig. 4.53 The vascular basis of the radial forearm flap raised as a fasciocutaneous flap, free or pedicled, and as an osteofasciocutaneous flap, incorporating part of the thickness of the radius.

appear to result in a vascularised segment, as long as the muscles, and the periosteum covering the bare area, are maintained.

Removal of a rectangle of bone leaves a point of weakness at each end of the site of the resection, and this can be reduced if an additional triangle of bone is removed so that the sharp edge at each extremity of the defect is rounded off. Even so, a protective plaster of Paris is advisable for 4–6 weeks post-operatively.

Fascial flap

Vascularised transfer of the investing layer of deep fascia on its own has also been carried out in the form of a segment separated from the overlying superficial fascia and skin. It provides a vascularised sheet to reconstruct defects of the hand which has the virtues of thinness, and an ability to drape over an irregular surface, able to convert the defect into one capable of accepting a free skin graft.

Management of the secondary defect

The skin defect is split skin grafted, using a tie-over dressing. The defect almost invariably includes a considerable area of the visceral paratenon covering the tendon of flexor carpi radialis, and concentration on the raising of the flap is liable to divert the attention of the surgeon from the defect, allowing the paratenon to dry out. It must be kept constantly moist. Immobilisation, with the wrist held in extension in plaster of Paris to ensure good subsequent function of the hand, for 12-14 days is necessary to ensure that the graft is firmly attached before movements are allowed.

Fortunately, even if the graft fails, and an area of bare tendon is exposed, a final deficit in hand function is not inevitable. With a conservative regime of patience and bland dressings, making sure that a full range of finger and wrist movements is maintained throughout, the exposed tendon will be found to granulate slowly and heal spontaneously.

Clinical usage

Among free flaps, the radial forearm has an excellent safety record. It is technically easy to raise, and its popularity has added to this the virtue of familiarity. The skin which it provides is thin and pliable, capable of moulding to an irregular surface. Used as a fasciocutaneous flap, its only adverse factor of significance concerns the secondary defect, its appearance, and the potential for graft failure. Now that the reason for graft failure is understood and can be countered by maintaining an immobilised wrist until the graft is firmly attached, this is no longer an adverse factor. Used as a composite with bone, the perfusion sources spread along its length allow it to be osteotomised if necessary and, used to reconstruct mandible, this is an advantage. The cross-sectional area available, however, is not great. It cannot withstand major stress, and subsequent insertion of osseo-integrated implants is not possible.

ULNAR FOREARM FLAP

The perforating system of the ulnar forearm flap passes from the ulnar vessels to the investing layer of fascia in the septum between flexor carpi ulnaris and flexor digitorum superficialis (Fig. 4.9). The flap is generally sited towards the ulnar side of the forearm, but in other respects the techniques involved in its transfer are similar to those of the radial forearm flap in its fasciocutaneous form. The two flaps have a largely similar range of potential usage, but the radial form is more often used in clinical practice.

LATERAL UPPER ARM FLAP

This fasciocutaneous flap (Fig. 4.54) is raised on the lateral aspect of the upper arm, just above the lateral epicondyle of the humerus, using as its vascular basis the posterior branch of the radial collateral artery and its venae comitantes. It can also be transferred as an osteofasciocutaneous flap by including a segment of the underlying humeral shaft.

The parent vessel of the perfusion system is the profunda brachii artery. This vessel runs alongside the radial nerve, deep to triceps, in the spiral groove, and reaches the lateral intermuscular septum between triceps and the insertion of deltoid. There it divides into two branches, anterior and posterior. The anterior branch, small and not always present, accompanies the radial nerve as it passes distally in the groove between brachialis and brachioradialis. The posterior branch, with an external diameter of 1.5–2 mm, is consistently present, with associated venae comitantes, running distally in the intermuscular septum between triceps and the brachialis–brachioradialis muscle group. In the intermuscular septum it gives off branches which reach the investing layer of deep fascia and the overlying skin. Additional multiple small vessels pass from it into the surrounding muscles, and also reach the humeral periosteum to which the intermuscular septum is attached.

The lower lateral cutaneous nerve of the arm supplies sensation to the skin area and is available for suture in the recipient area if a sensate flap is desired. Division of the nerve, and of the posterior cutaneous nerve of the forearm which arises in common with it, leaves an anaesthetic area distal to the flap site.

Raising the flap

The flap, designed astride the intermuscular sep-

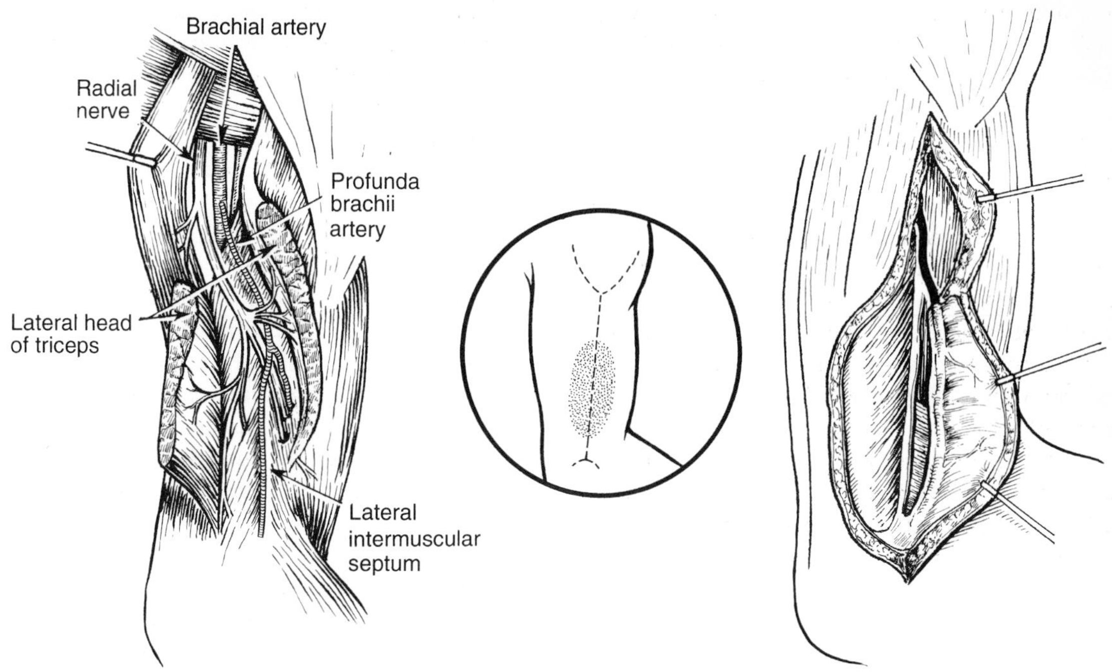

Fig. 4.54 The vascular basis of the lateral upper arm flap, the posterior terminal branch of the profunda brachii artery.

tum, is raised under tourniquet. Its breadth is limited to 6 cm because of the need to close the secondary defect directly; its average length is 10 cm. As a first step, the line joining the lateral epicondyle and the deltoid insertion, representing the line of the intermuscular septum, is marked out on the skin. Behind this line the flap contains no structures of note, and this makes it convenient to raise this segment first, and establish the plane between the investing layer of fascia and triceps at the outset, dissecting forward until the lateral intermuscular septum is reached. The muscle fibres can then be separated from the septum over its full depth and over the length of the flap, exposing the vessels and the nerves in the septum.

The skin incision is extended proximally to just behind the posterior border of deltoid, and this allows the vessels and nerves to be dissected out proximally, separated from the radial nerve, and traced back into the spiral groove. In carrying out this dissection triceps and deltoid are separated, and any fibres of triceps attached to the septum which are obscuring the groove are divided. With the vascular pedicle defined, the flap anterior to the septum can be freed from brachialis and brachioradialis, and its elevation completed. Throughout the dissection numerous small branches of the perfusing vessels supplying the surrounding muscles have to be divided.

When the transfer is as an osteofasciocutaneous flap, a strip of muscle is left attached to each side of the septum. These strips, carried down to the bone over the length to be raised, provide protection for the vessels in the septum which are perfusing the two elements of the composite transfer, skin and bone. As a preliminary to this part of the dissection the radial nerve should be retracted out of the way. A 1 cm broad, and up to 10 cm long, strip of the humeral shaft can be raised without compromising the strength of the bone.

Clinical usage

The skin element is thin and the underlying layer of fat is generally thin, the combination making for a flexible flap. The scar which represents the secondary defect, though in a site which may regularly be exposed, is not unduly obtrusive. The smallness of the diameters of its perfusing vessels is its major drawback, the trend generally being towards flaps with larger perfusing vessel diameters.

SCAPULAR FLAPS

These flaps (Fig. 4.55) are perfused by branches of the circumflex scapular artery and its associated veins. The artery is formed by division of its parent vessel, the subscapular, itself a branch of the axillary artery. The subscapular artery passes down on the posterior wall of the axilla for approximately 4 cm, where it divides into the thoracodorsal artery which continues down to reach the latissimus dorsi muscle, and the circumflex scapular artery, the latter the larger branch of the two.

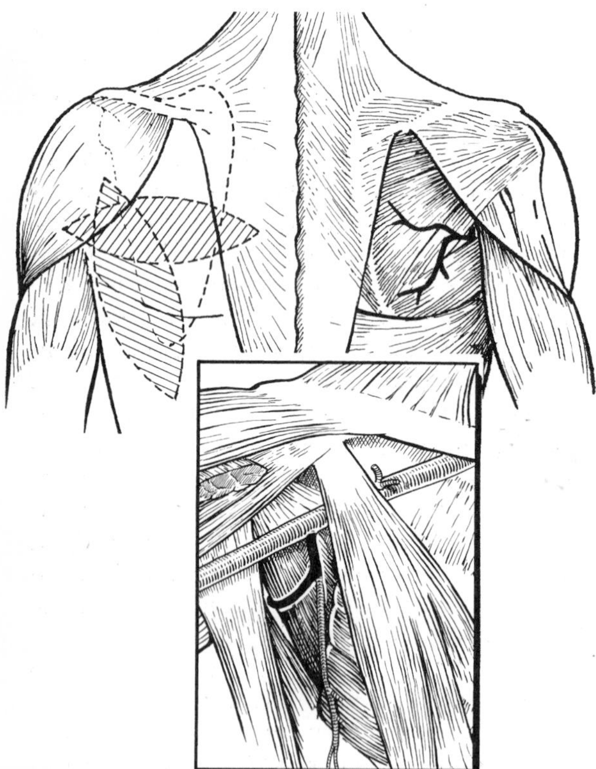

Fig. 4.55 Scapular flaps, showing the cutaneous branches of the circumflex scapular vessels as the vascular basis of the two flaps, one running horizontally towards the midline, and the other running along the line of the lateral border of the scapula. If a longer vascular pedicle is required, the circumflex scapular vessels may be traced back to the parent subscapular vessels in the axilla.

Almost immediately the artery passes into the triangular intermuscular space. This space is bounded above by subscapularis and teres minor, below by teres major, laterally by the long head of triceps, and the artery, while curving round the lateral border of the scapula inside the space, gives off musculo-skeletal branches. Emerging from between teres major and minor into the subcutaneous tissues overlying the scapula, it divides into a horizontal branch which runs towards the midline approximately 2 cm below the spine of the scapula, and a descending branch which runs obliquely downwards, parallel to the lateral border of the scapula. These terminal cutaneous branches have each been used as the basis of a fasciocutaneous free flap, one the **horizontal flap**, the other the **parascapular flap**.

The main musculoskeletal branch of the circumflex scapular artery is given off in the triangular space, and passes deep to infraspinatus into the infraspinous fossa. Before doing so, it gives off a branch which runs down parallel to the lateral border of the scapula as far as its inferior angle, where it anastomoses with the deep branch of the transverse cervical artery. In its course it gives off a series of small branches which provide a periosteal supply to the scapula along its lateral border, through its muscle attachments. These provide the perfusion source which allows a strip of the lateral border of the scapula to be transferred, usually as a vascularised composite along with one of the fasciocutaneous flaps.

The **horizontal flap** is designed approximately midway between the spine of the scapula and its inferior angle; the **parascapular flap** runs parallel to the lateral border of the scapula, both as ellipses. The two flaps share a common centre, the site where the cutaneous branch of the parent artery emerges from the intermuscular space, between the teres muscles. Identification of the space provides the point from which the central line of the ellipse is drawn on the skin, parallel to the spine of the scapula in the case of the horizontal flap, parallel to its lateral border in the case of the parascapular flap. The width of each flap is limited in practice by the need to be able to close the secondary defect directly, 24 cm × 12 cm being considered an absolute maximum.

Raising the flap

Both flaps are raised from their distant ends towards the point of entry of the vessels, the plane of elevation baring the underlying muscles to ensure that the flaps contain their axial vessels. As the vascular pedicle is approached the vessels become visible on the deep surface of the flap. It is a short pedicle, but it can be lengthened if the vessels are traced back to their subscapular origin in the axilla. Extension of the dissection in this way increases the length of the pedicle and the calibre of the vessels, both making for ease in transfer as a free flap. The degree of technical difficulty involved in the dissection is largely dependent on the amount of fat which surrounds the vessels, and in the obese patient this can be considerable.

When the transfer is as a fasciocutaneous flap, the musculo-skeletal branches of the circumflex scapular vessels are divided to allow the vessels to be mobilised, but when the transfer includes bone these vessels have to be carefully preserved. The segment of bone transferred, approximately 1.5 cm in width, is cut from the lateral border of the scapula from just below the origin of the long head of triceps, a length of up to 14 cm. This part of the scapula is perfused through its muscle attachments, and these must be preserved intact when the bone is being cut.

Clinical usage

The skin which both flaps transfer has the thickness and lack of flexibility typical of dorsal skin generally, and this may be a factor of importance when the method is being considered for use. The thickness of the subcutaneous fat is variable but can be substantial. The shortness of the pedicle and the small calibre of the vessels involved, unless extended to the origin of the circumflex scapular vessels, make for a degree of technical difficulty in the transfer, and the extension adds considerably to the difficulty of dissection. A further adverse factor is that both flaps involve turning the patient, unless the surgeon is willing to carry out the entire procedure, creation of the defect and elevation of the flap, in the lateral position, a position which for most surgeons lacks the virtue of familiarity. In its osteofasciocutaneous version a serious question mark concerning its use relates to the considerable disruption of the musculature of the shoulder girdle which it leaves in the scapular area. The potential it creates for frozen shoulder must be a major deterrent to its use, particularly in the older patient.

VASCULARISED FIBULAR TRANSFER

The fibula derives its blood supply from branches of the anterior tibial and the peroneal vessels, but when it is transferred as a vascularised bone graft, the peroneal vessels are the sole perfusion source. The peroneal artery is described as a branch of the posterior tibial artery, arising just below the division of the popliteal into the anterior and posterior tibial branches, but different arterial patterns exist, and when a fibular transfer is being considered it is essential to carry out preoperative arteriograms, anomalies and arteriosclerosis providing the two main contraindications to its use. The peroneal vessels run distally alongside the fibula, behind the interosseous membrane. In the upper half of the bone they are separated from the interosseous membrane by tibialis posterior, which there is taking origin from it, but in its lower half they lie directly behind the membrane. They provide the nutrient artery which enters the fibula a little above its mid-point, and also have branches which reach the surface of the bone. Septocutaneous perforators from the peroneal vessels also pass laterally behind the fibula in the intermuscular septum between the peroneal muscles and soleus, and perfuse the overlying skin. These allow the fibula to be transferred as an osteocutaneous free flap, as well as a vascularised bone graft.

The length of bone which can be harvested extends from just below the head to above the lower tibio-fibular joint, approximately 30 cm, and its segmental pattern of blood supply allows osteotomy to be carried out. The perforating branches are capable of supporting a skin island up to 10 cm × 20 cm.

Despite the loss of the shaft of the bone, the leg functions remarkably normally in the adult. In children and adolescents, where long bone growth is not complete, greater circumspection is required in its use, because of the risk of tibial bowing.

Raising the flap

The procedure (Fig. 4.56) is carried out under tourniquet, and the line joining the head of the fibula and the lateral malleolus is marked out on the skin.

When the transfer is of bone alone, a proximo-distal skin incision is made along the fibular skin marking, over a length to match that of the bone to be harvested, and the skin flaps are raised on each side to allow the septum which separates the posterior and peroneal muscle compartments to be identified. As a first step, the common peroneal nerve is identified, and care is taken to protect it. It represents the proximal limit of harvesting the bone, the ankle joint being the distal limit. The muscles on each side of the septum are separated from one another, and the lateral surface of the fibula reached.

When a skin island is being transferred with the bone as a composite, it is outlined on the skin as an oval placed symmetrically over the septum between soleus and peroneus longus, centred over the middle or the middle and lower third of the fibula. The skin incision is made, and extended proximally and distally as necessary, and the flap is elevated from its anterior and posterior borders, deep to the investing layer of fascia, as far as the intermuscular septum. The septum contains per-

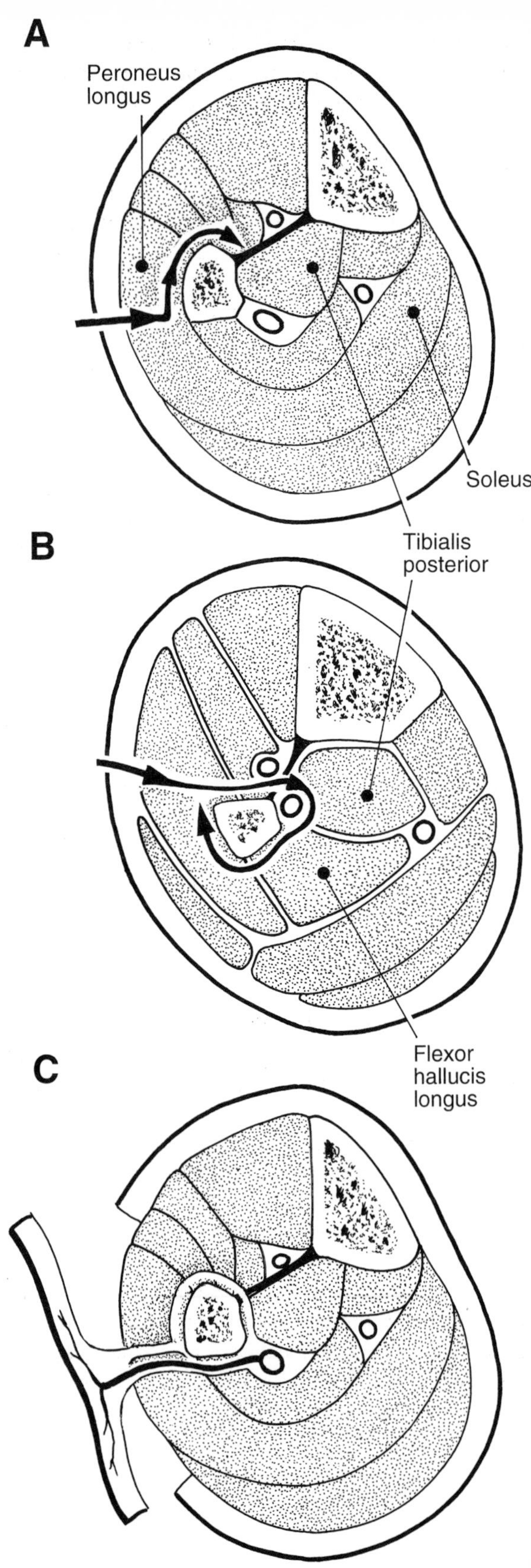

Fig. 4.56 Transfer of the fibula alone and with a skin flap. When the bone alone is being transferred, it is approached between the peroneal and posterior muscle compartments, and the mobilisation of the muscles from it is carried out anteriorly around the shaft of the bone. In the lower part of the dissection (**B**), the peroneal vessels lie directly behind the septum in direct contact with the bone, compared with the upper part of the dissection (**A**), where tibialis posterior, taking origin from the interosseous septum, separates it from the peroneal vessels.

When a composite of skin and bone is being transferred, (**C**) the skin flap is positioned symmetrically over the line of the septum between soleus and peroneus longus and elevated from both sides of it. The perforating vessels which pass to the surface from the peroneal vessels to perfuse it may emerge from the muscles, most often soleus, adjoining the septum, and they must be watched for so that, if necessary, some muscle can be included in the pedicle. This apart, the procedure is carried out as for the bone alone.

forating vessels, branches of the peroneal vessels, which provide the perfusion source for the skin island, but some of the vessels pass into the muscles on each side, and emerge from them near the septum. These should be looked for when the flap is being raised, and a cuff of muscle may have to be elevated with the flap to ensure that they are included in the pedicle. In the initial muscle dissection, separating them from the intermuscular septum, the perforating vessels have to be seen and preserved.

With the muscles on each side of the septum separated, the dissection proceeds in the same manner with both types of transfer. In mobilising the muscles scalpel dissection is used, the plane being extraperiosteal. The proximal and distal extent of the mobilisation depends on the length of fibula which is being transferred, but over that length they are mobilised completely.

Mobilisation is begun in the direction of the anterior surface of the bone, with division of the septum which separates the peroneal from the extensor compartment, and mobilisation of the extensor muscles, taking care to avoid damage to the anterior tibial vessels. Completion of the mobilisation of the extensors exposes the interosseous membrane from in front.

At this point, the fibula is sectioned proximally and distally at the levels required by the reconstruction, and the interosseous membrane is divided to expose the peroneal vessels which lie behind it. Section of the bone and division of the membrane, carried out in this order, allows traction to be applied to the membrane while it is being divided, and reduces the risk of injury to the peroneal vessels, in particular the venae comitantes, which are thin walled and easily damaged. It also allows traction to be applied to the bone, once the membrane has been divided, more effectively displaying the structures involved, and making dissection easier and safer.

Division of the interosseous membrane is best begun distally where the peroneal vessels lie directly behind the septum, and can be immediately identified, mobilised, and distally ligated. The vessels are traced upwards under direct vision, mobilising them and dividing branches directed away from the fibula, making sure at the same time that their attachments to the fibula are preserved. Proximally, where tibialis posterior is taking origin from the fibula, the vessels run between it and flexor hallucis longus, sometimes through the substance of the latter, from which they then have to be mobilised. Dissection and clearance of the vessels is continued up to their point of origin from the parent posterior tibial vessels, any residual muscle attachments being divided, and leaving the proximal vascular pedicle as the sole attachment.

The length of pedicle which is available for anastomosis is often less than ideal and, particularly when the transfer is as an osteocutaneous flap, lies in an awkward position. When the transfer is osteocutaneous, osteotomies can only be carried out with safety on the anterior or antero-lateral aspect of the bone. Transferred purely as bone, any of the surfaces can be used, other than the one from which the branches of the peroneal vessels are entering.

When bone alone has been transferred, skin suture with suction drainage is sufficient. When the flap is osteocutaneous the secondary defect is split skin grafted, preferably delayed. A splint is used for several weeks to support the lower leg and foot, and prevent the development of an equinus deformity, until the muscles heal and function normally. An ultimately normal gait is the rule.

Clinical usage

This transfer can be made either as one of bone alone, or as a composite with a flap of skin, its dimensions up to 20 cm × 10 cm. The characteristics of the bone, which determine its clinical role, are the length available, up to 30 cm, and its strength. Initially the bone is not strong enough to bear the body weight, but it has been demonstrated to be capable of hypertrophying to the extent of weightbearing successfully. It can safely be osteotomised, and should be able to accept osseo-integrated implants.

CHAPTER 5

Additional techniques

Several techniques have been developed which do not fit readily into a neat classification, either because they are not strictly surgical, though they are used in a surgical context, or have been taken from other surgical disciplines because they were found to be capable of solving, partially or completely, problems whose management by conventional plastic surgical methods was unsatisfactory.

TISSUE EXPANSION

In this technique, a silastic 'bag', not unlike an uninflated balloon, is placed under the skin and superficial fascia, and inflated at intervals by the injection of saline under pressure (Fig. 5.1). The saline is not injected directly into the 'bag', but into a small non-expansile reservoir placed at a distance from it, and connected to it by a fine-bore tube. The effect of the inflation is to produce an increasing bulge of the overlying tissue, and in so doing stretch the skin. In this way the skin is 'expanded', increased in area, and made available for reconstruction.

Expansion is exploited clinically in two ways. In one, as used in postmastectomy breast reconstruction, the expanded skin and the underlying cavity are both utilised, the cavity for permanent insertion of a silicone implant to recreate the breast mound, the expanded skin to provide an envelope for the implant.

The other way in which the principle is used is in the creation of an area of skin availability which, sited alongside a defect, allows it to be closed directly. The expanded area may be created beforehand, so that, when the defect is created, the expanded skin is already available to close it.

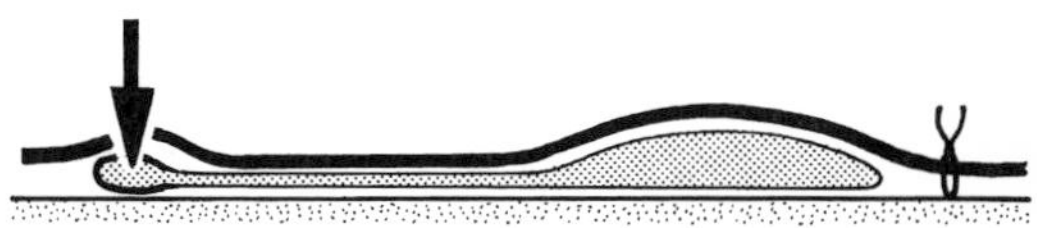

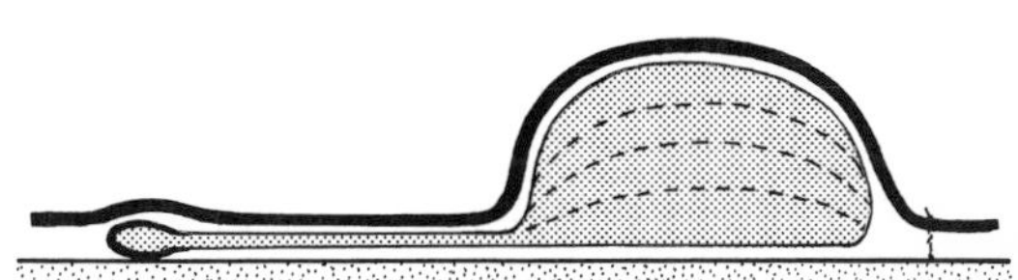

Fig. 5.1 The principle of tissue expansion. The 'expander', in an unexpanded state, in inserted in the area to be expanded, with the reservoir positioned at a distance from it. Saline is injected under pressure into the reservoir at intervals causing the 'expander' to increase in volume, stretching and 'expanding' the overlying skin.

Alternatively, it may be used to replace a skin graft, previously applied to cover the defect. The skin adjoining a defect is generally recognised to give the best result in reconstructing it, because they have similar characteristics, and this is a major virtue of the method, one which shows most strikingly when it is used to extend hair-bearing scalp in replacing an area of alopecia.

Various shapes of expanders are used, round, oval, and crescentic, with different sizes, depending on the amount of expansion desired. A skin incision is made, just long enough to allow the expander to be inserted without bending, and the pocket to accommodate it is dissected, generally at the deep level of the superficial fascia. A pocket is also made for the reservoir at a distance from the expander. The reservoir is sometimes positioned externally, making injection easier as well as painless, though it probably increases the risk of infection reaching the expander. A small volume of saline is injected immediately to smooth out the envelope of the expander, the incisions are closed, and the wounds left for 1–2 weeks to heal. Expansion is then begun, and repeated usually at weekly intervals. Whitening of the skin, indicative of local ischaemia, or a complaint of pain by the patient, are signs that expansion has gone far enough for the time being. Over the period of the expansion, a degree of capsule formation usually builds up and, depending on its severity, it is left, scored, or excised.

The technique has its strong advocates, but overall it has not achieved the popularity which seemed likely when it was first introduced. Adverse factors concern the time taken to achieve adequate expansion, 6–12 weeks, and the increasingly bizarre appearance of the patient as expansion proceeds. Even when circumstances are ideal, the complication rate is considerable, mainly the result of infection, haematoma or extrusion, and the nature of the technique means that any complication requires removal of the expander and spells failure of the method. The other substantial problem is that of designing the expansion, which involves three dimensions, to provide cover for a defect which, the breast and scalp apart, is usually two-dimensional.

The most effective applications of the method have been where the surface is convex with a bony base, as in the scalp and forehead, and in breast reconstruction.

LIPOSUCTION

Liposuction is a technique which permits 'blind' removal of subcutaneous fat through a small skin incision. Its most frequent clinical role is a cosmetic one, in the removal of unwanted subcutaneous fat as an element in 'body sculpturing', but it also has a small place in routine plastic surgical practice, in removing large lipomas and defatting unduly bulky skin flaps to make them conform to the surrounding contour after completion of their transfer.

It allows a large area to be defatted through a small skin incision, reducing scarring and simplifying postoperative care. Depending on whether the procedure is being carried out under local or general anaesthesia, the fat to be aspirated is infiltrated with a local anaesthetic agent or saline, containing adrenalin in low concentration. This facilitates aspiration and helps in achieving haemostasis.

A small skin incision is made, and the suction cannula is inserted into the subcutaneous layer in the area to be aspirated and attached to a high pressure suction pump. It is then moved to and fro like a piston, directed radially from the site of insertion through an arc. The cannula is blunt ended, and in its to and fro movements it disrupts the fat, which is sucked out into the suction pump reservoir, the blood vessels traversing the area largely escaping damage. It is important that the suction should not be applied, either superficially as far as the deep surface of the dermis which results in a lumpy skin surface, or deeply as far as the deep fascial layer which creates an area of adhesion of the skin. With suction completed, a pressure dressing is applied to the site. Local bruising can be considerable, but infective complications are infrequent.

Lipomas with little or no fibrous tissue are readily treated by this technique, but those with a more extensive fibrous stroma are difficult to remove, and may require formal excision. The flaps which benefit from debulking tend to be from the groin or hypogastrium, and although it is suggested that fat does not reaccumulate after removal, flaps from those sites are notorious for redeveloping subcutaneous fat if the patient puts on weight. When this occurs, the procedure may have to be repeated.

LASERS

In treating the port wine stain type of haemangioma, the use of cover by cosmetics, and surgical removal, have been the unavoidable mainstays despite their manifest inadequacy, but the development of laser technology has now added a third therapeutic possibility. Two main types of laser are currently used, **argon** and **tuneable dye** lasers.

Both instruments work on the principle that energy emitted by the laser is absorbed by the oxyhaemoglobin in erythrocytes within the ectatic vessels of the haemangioma. Diffusion of this energy damages the endothelial cells of the vessels and they undergo fibrosis. Circulation through the vessels ceases, and the port-wine appearance is lost. With both types of laser, the end result of treatment is largely the same, but they reach it in different ways.

The **argon laser** emits blue-green light, with most of the energy at 488 and 514 nm. Using a 1 mm laser beam spot, the dermis is penetrated to a depth of 0.75–1 mm. The energy of each pulse, though it is applied in very short pulses of 200 μs, tends to be dissipated beyond the blood vessels into surrounding tissues, giving rise on occasion to a degree of scarring. Focal alopecia can also occur. The area of staining is treated in such a way as to produce a confluent patch, but up to 2 months have to be allowed so that the tissues can recover before treatment of a skin area adjacent to a previously treated site can be carried out.

The **tuneable dye laser** uses a Rhodamine dye source, and emits light at 585 nm. Oxyhaemoglobin has an absorption peak at 577 nm, and the nearness of the two gives it the advantage over the argon laser of increased specificity, and penetration of the dermis to a greater depth, 1–1.5 mm. As a result, the risk of scarring is low. In contrast to the argon laser, non-contiguous areas are treated with a 5 mm laser spot. This initially produces a purpuric patch of skin, which reverts to a normal skin colour within a fortnight. Successive treatments are aimed at intervening residual areas of staining.

Regardless of which laser is used, multiple treatments are required at intervals of roughly 2 months to allow the tissues to recover. The comparative merits of the two types of laser are difficult to quantify. Clinical experience suggests that the argon laser produces better results in dark port-wine stains, while the tuneable dye laser is more effective in treating paler lesions, particularly in children.

In the older patient, the haemangioma tends to extend superficially, and in depth. Superficial extension has the effect of creating increasing irregularity of its surface; extension deeply usually brings the lesion beyond the limit of penetration, and as a result it does not respond well to laser therapy.

'Amateur' tattoos, produced with Indian ink, have been found to respond well to treatment using the Q-switched Ruby laser. With 3 J at 694 nm delivered in a 30 ms pulse, with a spot size of 5 mm, the effect is confined to the carbon pigment, which is converted to colourless oxides. Carried out under local anaesthesia, the vasoconstriction of added adrenaline has the effect of minimising any interaction between the blood and the laser beam. Improvement has also been found to occur in dark professional tattoos. The carbon component is removed, but unexpectedly significant fading of the red and green pigment has also occurred. This is felt to be the result of enhanced phagocytic activity, induced as part of the effect on the carbon component of the tattoo.

PART

2

Surgical applications

CHAPTER 6

Hypertrophic scars and keloids

When a scar, instead of becoming soft and pale in the usual manner, becomes red and thickened it is described as being either a *hypertrophic scar* or a *keloid*. These terms tend to be used rather indiscriminately, probably because it is difficult to define each with certainty.

The hypertrophic scar is raised above the level of the surrounding skin, rather red initially, but does not encroach on the surrounding normal skin, and shows an eventual tendency to regress spontaneously. The keloid is a much more florid lesion, grossly elevated, tending to spread and involve the surrounding normal skin. Itching of the involved area is common, its severity matching the degree of activity, sometimes with hyperaesthesia and tenderness to touch. The tendency to spontaneous regression is much less in evidence.

These are the extremes and as such easily recognised, but in reality there is a gradation from the completely quiescent scar through the very mildly hypertrophic scar to the most severe of keloids, and the point at which a hypertrophic scar becomes a keloid is a matter of opinion. The gradation rather suggests that the arbitrary division into keloid and hypertrophic scar is artificial and that the conditions are really a single entity of varying severity. The name is fortunately of subsidiary importance, for the treatment of both conditions is similar. Virtually nothing is known of the cause.

The clinical picture

A precise picture of the condition is difficult to draw, for clinical generalisations do not necessarily apply to the individual case and the condition itself is extremely variable and unpredictable. In the description which follows, the term keloid will be used to cover both conditions.

The tendency to develop keloids appears to diminish with age, but it is not possible in practice to forecast whether any particular patient will develop one. Nevertheless, any incision in a known 'keloid former' is more likely to develop into a keloid than a similar incision in a random patient, and recurrence following simple excision of a keloid is highly probable. Keloids are much more common in the black than in the white patient. The black also exhibits the condition in its most active form and the 'tumours' can on occasion reach quite grotesque proportions. In the white, on the other hand, even the frank keloid does eventually become less active, and takes on

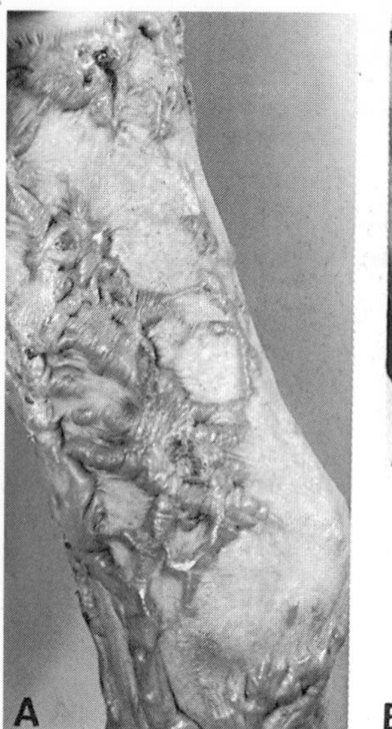

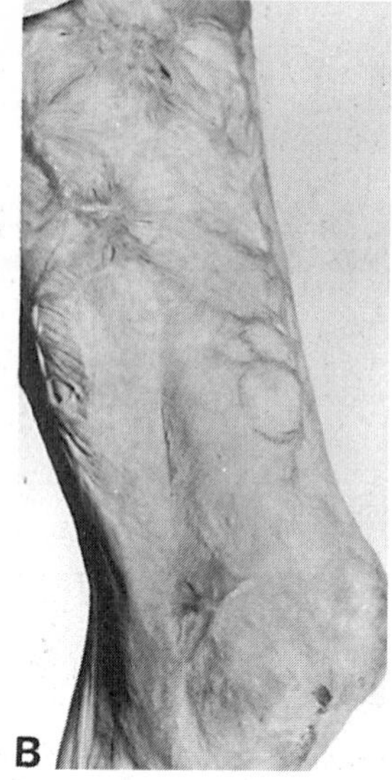

Fig. 6.1 Change from keloid to hypertrophic scarring over a period of two years. The area of most severe keloid was excised and grafted, but the settling of the areas left untouched is still clear-cut.

the characters and activity rather of a hypertrophic scar (Fig. 6.1).

Certain areas of the body have a particular tendency to produce keloids (Fig. 6.2); the presternal area is probably the most prone of all and here oddly enough the shape of the keloid often shows a sex difference — in the male it tends to be irregular in outline, in the female the pull of the breasts commonly gives it a butterfly outline. The deltoid area is another notorious site, most often following BCG inoculation. A scar may become keloid in only part of its length, a feature which shows particularly in the neck where the vertical scar is prone to keloid change while the horizontal scar is rarely affected. If a scar of neck is excised incorporating Z-plasties it is not uncommon for the horizontal scars to be completely flat and soft, while the vertical limbs of the Zs show keloid or at very least hypertrophic change. In general, scars in lines of election show less tendency to keloid than those which cross them.

Management

If a keloid is surgically excised, the probability that the resulting scar will develop into a fresh keloid is extremely high, and the more florid the keloid the greater the probability. For this reason surgery of keloids is generally to be avoided (Fig. 6.3). However, when the scar is hypertrophic rather than keloid and is bridging a flexure, so that contracture appears to have been a factor in its initiation, correction of the contractural element as part of the excisional treatment seems often to markedly reduce the likelihood of recurrence.

Prior to the introduction of pressure methods and injections of the highly active local steroid, triamcinolone, the mainstay of treatment was X-ray therapy. Whether the method had any real value or whether it was merely being given credit for the spontaneous tendency to regression is difficult to tell. Its use should never be countenanced in the young patient with a life-time ahead of him, and as the main problem in practice is the child with extensive postburn keloid, the undesirability of X-ray therapy needs no emphasis.

The circumscribed keloid might appear to be more of a candidate for X-ray therapy, but it is in this type of keloid that triamcinolone injected into its substance is most dramatically successful, with obvious flattening and softening in a matter of days. Nevertheless, it must be remembered always that triamcinolone is itself an extremely potent drug whose action is not fully understood. Caution in its use is essential. It must be injected into the substance of the keloid, and enough injected to make the whole keloid blanch. Injection can be repeated weekly. When the keloid has become flat with the surrounding skin, treatment should stop. Further injections will produce local skin and fat atrophy. Remarkably enough the drug is effective regardless of whether the keloid is red and ‘fresh’ or white and ‘mature’.

A recent additional form of treatment has come in the form of silicone gel. The gel is applied to the affected area and held in position by tape. The mode of action is unclear and the rate at which the activity of the keloid subsides varies. The method has the virtue of being non-invasive, which is particularly useful in children, and of having no side-effects. Although not effective in every case, experience has been that scars which fail to improve with silicone gel tend not to respond to injection of triamcinolone either.

The rate of change in the keloid appears to

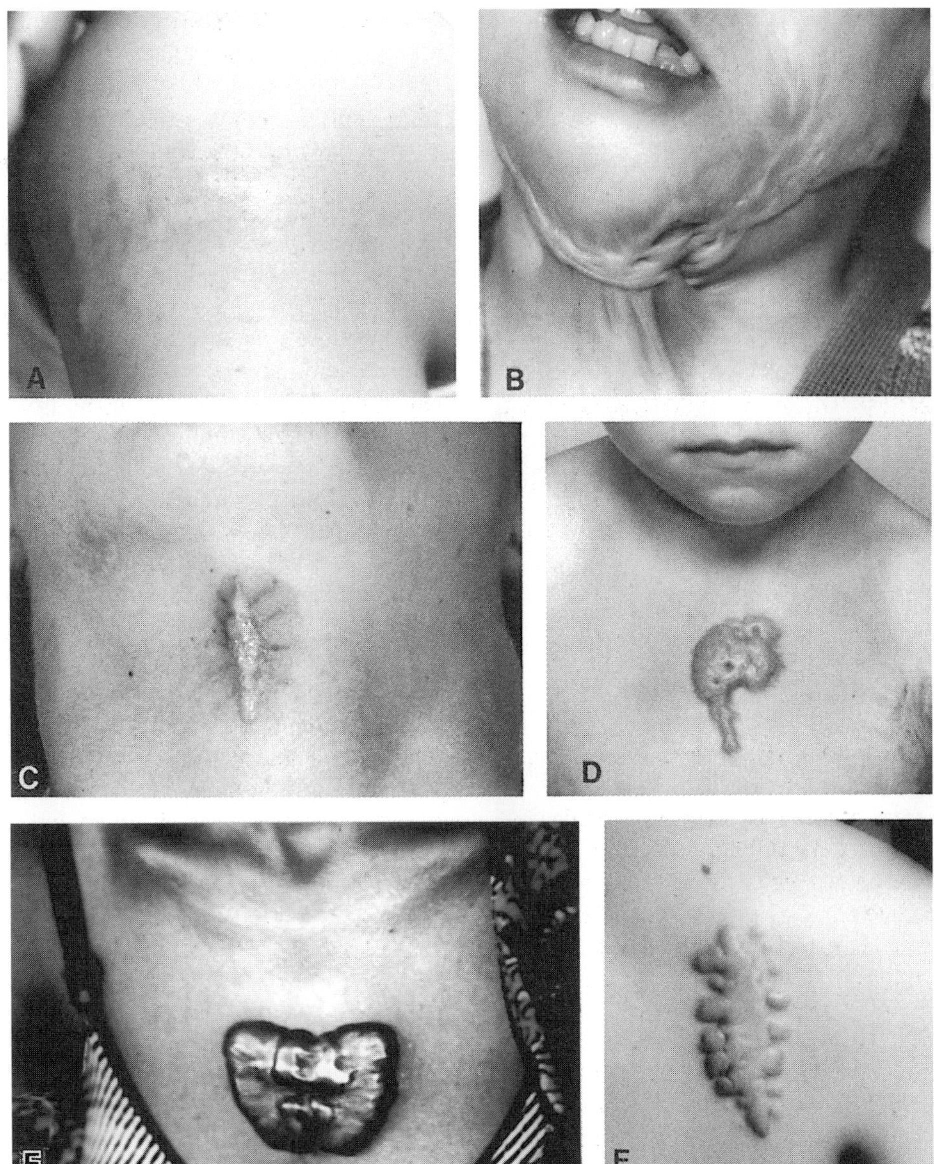

Fig. 6.2 Examples of hypertrophic scars and keloids.

A Mildly hypertrophic scar of the deltoid area.
B Severe post-burn hypertrophic scarring of the neck and chin.
C Hypertrophic scarring of the neck following the use of a vertical incision to excise a thyroglossal fistula.
D A pre-sternal keloid in the male.
E A pre-sternal keloid in the female black patient, showing the characteristic 'butterfly' outline. (Courtesy of Mr. Michael F. Green)
F A severe keloid of the scapular region.

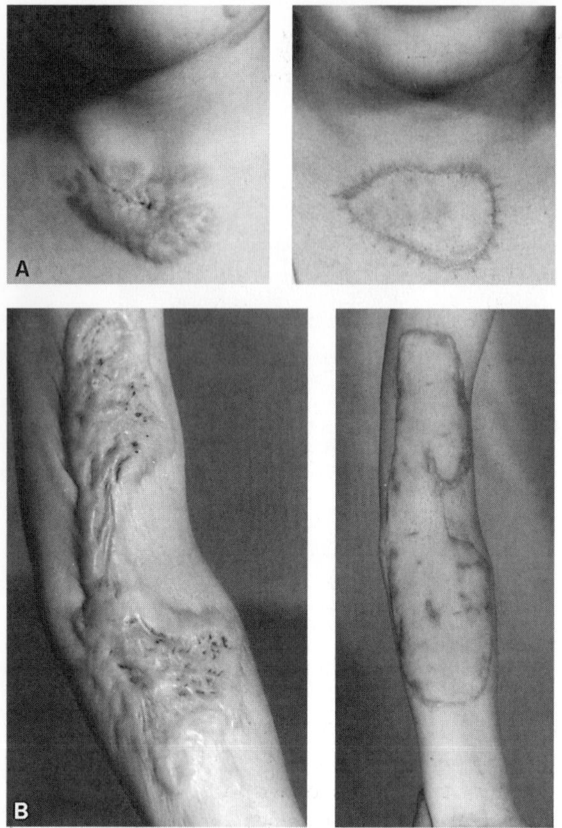

Fig. 6.3 Marginal recurrence of a keloid after excision and grafting.

depend on the length of time for which the gel is applied. Ideally it should be worn at all times other than when washing or bathing.

In clinical practice, the major problems arise when the condition complicates burns and degloving injuries, the extent of the keloid change precluding the use of steroids, and silicone gel. Quite apart from the appearance of the scarring and the contractural problems so frequently associated with it, the severity of the itch which usually accompanies it causes the patient to scratch the area, often to the extent of producing excoriation and exacerbating the problem generally. It is in this situation that the application of sustained pressure has had a dramatic effect both in mitigating the itch and in causing the condition to regress, with flattening and softening of the previously raised, indurated areas. The mode of action is not known, but its effectiveness has resulted in the development of garments custom-fitted to the individual patient, so that constant uniform pressure is applied to the areas involved. These garments are worn continuously until resolution is largely complete, and this may take a year and more.

CHAPTER 7

Radiation injury

The forms of radiation injury in which the plastic surgeon becomes involved are *radiodermatitis* and *radionecrosis* (Fig. 7.1), and the aspects which concern him are the ischaemia of the irradiated tissues and the association of radiation damage with neoplasia. Avascularity is stated to increase in severity up to 6 months postirradiation, plateauing thereafter, but the fact that both conditions manifest themselves clinically very much later than this would suggest that the ischaemic process may progress for a much longer period.

Radiodermatitis is most often seen today in the facial skin and scalp, and in skin sites which were used as portals in the process of irradiating deep structures, such as intra-abdominal tumours, thyroid tumours, or regional lymph nodes, usually in the neck. Radiotherapy was also at one time a standard method of treating such facial conditions as acne, sycosis barbae, or lupus vulgaris, and ringworm of the scalp. Although it may no longer be used in this way, patients are still seen with the problems which have resulted from its use. The type of radiation used did not penetrate deeply, and it is unusual to find the deeper tissues significantly involved. As a result, the excision required in treating an area of radiodermatitis does not often need to be carried deeply much beyond the skin and dermis. When there is doubt about how deeply the condition extends, the degree of mobility of the skin is a good guide, mobility indicating absence of deep involvement. The vascularity of the base left when the area of radiodermatitis has been excised will also give a good guide to the form that reconstruction should take, graft or flap. A free skin graft can generally be expected to take well, provided excision has been carried out to clinically normal well-vascularised tissue, though the defect left following excision of radiodermatitis of the scalp treated 40–50 years ago for ringworm is not usually successfully managed using a split skin graft.

Where the site has been used as a portal the situation is quite different. The entire block of tissue between the skin and the target site is involved. This form of radiodermatitis has much in common with radionecrosis, and in time frequently progresses to it.

Radionecrosis which involves the skin implies ulceration and is indicative of much more deeply extending ischaemia. In managing such an ulcer the first need is to establish whether or not the ulcer has a neoplastic component. Biopsy should be used as routine, and it should be both

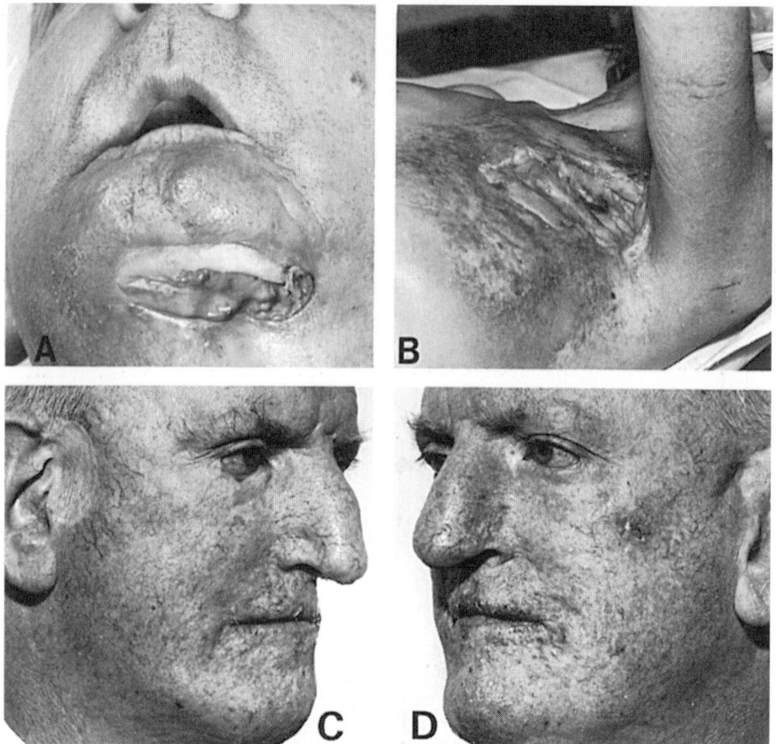

Fig. 7.1 Examples of radionecrosis and radiodermatitis.

A Radionecrosis of the chin, floor of mouth and mandible, with a salivary fistula, following irradiation of a squamous carcinoma of the anterior floor of mouth.

B Radionecrosis of the chest wall following radiotherapy used after radical mastectomy for carcinoma, showing central deep ulceration with exposure of ribs, and associated surrounding radiodermatitis.

C, D Radiodermatitis following radiotherapy for acne vulgaris. Over a period of years since this record was made, the patient has had excisions of multiple skin tumours, both basal cell and squamous cell carcinomas.

generous and representative. A diagnosis of radionecrosis made in the absence of pathological confirmation should not be accepted.

The surgical problems set by radionecrosis can be of considerable magnitude, both from the point of view of resection and of reconstruction. The tissues involved are woody hard, and when essential structures such as major vessels and nerves lie in the involved field the technical difficulties do not require stressing. Ideally the entire area of involvement should be excised both marginally and in depth as a preliminary to reconstruction, but this may not always be practicable, particularly in terms of depth clearance, because of the involvement of vital structures. Reconstruction of such a defect virtually always requires a flap with the blood supply which it brings with it. If it has not been possible to resect the radionecrotic area in its entirety, the pedicle of the flap used to reconstruct the defect, with its content of blood vessels, is best left undivided indefinitely. Division of the pedicle in such circumstances, even after a very prolonged period of time, is liable to be followed by necrosis of the flap, but if the zone of avascularity has been completely resected the problem does not arise. If a free flap has been used it is essential to use donor vessels outwith the area of radiation damage.

The association with neoplasia takes two forms, the tumour either arising *de novo* in the irradiated field, or occurring as continuing growth in a neoplasm treated by radiotherapy. The *de novo* tumour can appear as a late development in the tissues which were irradiated, even though the primary condition was neither malignant nor had malignant potential. The tumour can be a carcinoma or sarcoma, and often presents as an ulcer appearing in the area.

The extent of the resection required depends on the clinical problem for which the radiotherapy was used, and the type of radiation. Because of its effects on the local lymphatics, metastasis to the regional nodes is rare, and the local tumour tends to remain circumscribed both marginally and in depth, developing within the irradiated area. Unless the tumour has been grossly neglected, resection need be little more extensive than that required for the background of radiodermatitis or radionecrosis.

Tumour recurring following radiotherapy presents either as failure to respond to the radiation, or as recurrence after apparent cure. It tends to be clinically atypical, frequently masquerading as radionecrotic ulceration. Diagnosis is not made any easier when, as often happens, radionecrosis and recurrent tumour coexist in a single ulcer. As already emphasised, biopsy is essential. Detailed consideration of how post-irradiation recurrent tumour should be managed is beyond the scope of this book, except to comment that the pattern of behaviour associated with the particular tumour tends to be lost, and the destruction of lymphatic channels by the radiation may result in bizarre metastatic patterns.

CHAPTER

8 Pressure sore management

NON-PARAPLEGIC PRESSURE SORES

The usual sites of pressure sores in the non-paraplegic are the sacral area and heel, occasionally the iliac crest, and the background to their occurrence is immobility of the patient. Although immobility is ultimately responsible for the local pressure being prolonged for sufficiently long to produce the local ischaemia which leads to the sores, other factors are usually present which predispose to their occurrence. They occur most often as a complication of an emaciating illness. Loss of subcutaneous fat reduces the cushion it provides and, coupled with the reluctance of the patient to move as a consequence of the lassitude typical of such an illness, combines to create the conditions for their occurrence. When a pressure sore arises in a relatively young patient, a neurological factor, such as multiple sclerosis, is virtually always present.

Management of such a sore depends on the sites involved, how extensive each sore is and, most of all, to what extent the progress of the debilitating illness can be halted and, hopefully, reversed. In this respect the most important assessment of the plastic surgeon is whether the sore is extending in extent or depth, is static, or is showing signs of healing with marginal epithelialisation.

While the sore is extending the plastic surgeon has no active role to play. The problem is essentially a nursing and medical one. Once the sore has become static and, even more, shows signs of healing, the question becomes one of deciding whether meeting the conditions needed for successful reconstruction of the ulcer, whether by graft or flap, might halt or even reverse the improvement in the patient's medical state. A most important element in making the decision is to appreciate that the change from the bedridden to an ambulant state is likely to allow the healing process to progress, even although healing may be by marginal epithelialisation, and will be a slow process.

The patient at very least must be able to keep pressure off the site of the sore before active surgery can even be contemplated. This aspect of the problem has to be emphasised very strongly, and the need to observe it is paramount, even if it precludes surgery in the majority of patients. If it is not strictly observed, failure is virtually certain, to achieve healing in the short term, and to maintain healing in the long term.

In practice, the number of patients suitable for an aggressive surgical approach to the problem is very small. The solution lies more often in getting the patient ambulant. Ambulation immediately relieves pressure on the typical ulcer sites, allowing spontaneous healing to begin. A striking example of this is seen in the pressure sore of the heel, typically sited posteriorly over the tendo Achillis and the adjoining os calcis, which begins to heal as soon as the patient begins to walk and pressure is transferred to the normally weight-bearing part of the heel. Certainly one should not rush into surgical treatment of such sores.

Management is most difficult when it is apparent that the patient is likely to be permanently bedridden. Considerable judgment is required in managing such a situation, and sympathy for the unfortunate patient must not be allowed to override a realistic assessment of the problem. The decision is usually in the direction of saying that surgery is contraindicated.

The dilemma is seen in its most acute form in the patient, frequently young, who is suffering from multiple sclerosis, and who has developed a pressure sore. The harsh fact is that the development of a pressure sore is often the first step in the downward course of the patient with multiple sclerosis, and the question the surgeon must ask himself is whether his surgery will not have the effect of accelerating the downward course. Such a patient virtually always requires a flap to reconstruct the defect and the position which has to be maintained for a successful result all too often results in a fresh pressure sore elsewhere.

When a decision has been made that the defect should be treated surgically the choice lies between a graft and a flap and the selection depends on the character of the defect. The defect with little or no undermining is likely to be suitable for grafting; the defect with significant undermining is rarely suitable for grafting, and requires a flap. The flaps suitable for the various sites are largely similar to those used in the paraplegic patient.

The sore involving the heel is best left to heal spontaneously no matter how long it takes. The alternative reconstructions make demands on the patient which are not acceptable in the age group typically involved.

PARAPLEGIC PRESSURE SORES

Although discussion of pressure sores in the paraplegic patient is confined to the problems of reconstruction, it cannot be emphasised too strongly that *the procedures to be described for the various types of decubitus ulceration are only a small facet in the overall care of the paraplegic, and they must be regarded as merely providing the ulcerated area with a fresh start in the best conditions.*

The sites in the paraplegic which are particularly liable to develop pressure sores lie over the pressure-bearing bony prominences. Compared with the sores which develop in the non-paraplegic, the ulcers tend to have an 'iceberg' quality, with extensive undermining, and osteitis of the underlying bone, or even pyoarthrosis in severe cases. Surgical treatment consists of the covering of the completely excised ulcer with a movable pad of healthy skin and subcutaneous tissue, and simultaneous reduction of any underlying bony prominence which appears to be acting as a focal pressure point. This latter procedure is generally essential, since such prominences left untouched reproduce the mechanical pressure which was responsible for the original ulcer.

During the acute phase of the spinal injury, the common sites are over the sacrum and femoral trochanter; after recovery, prolonged sitting in a wheelchair makes the ischial area the most frequent site. Sacral ulcers tend to be large and flat with minimal undermining; ulcers of the trochanter and ischium usually have a small opening, leading into a large slough-lined cavity into the base of which the bony prominence projects.

The anaesthetic tissues of the paraplegic heal poorly, and with the slightest provocation the wound will fail to heal following surgery. Tension on suture lines must be avoided, haemostasis must be even more meticulous than usual, cavities and dead space must be positively eliminated — failure in any one aspect will result in failure as a whole. If skin loss is minimal, excision and direct closure may suffice, but in most instances a flap is needed. The secondary defect created by transfer of the flap has often to be grafted and, as discussed on p. 88, the graft need not necessarily be applied at the time of the flap transfer. The collection of a haematoma under the flap is particularly undesirable in the paraplegic patient, and leaving the secondary defect ungrafted in this way is a valuable way of ensuring that a large area is available through which any haematoma can

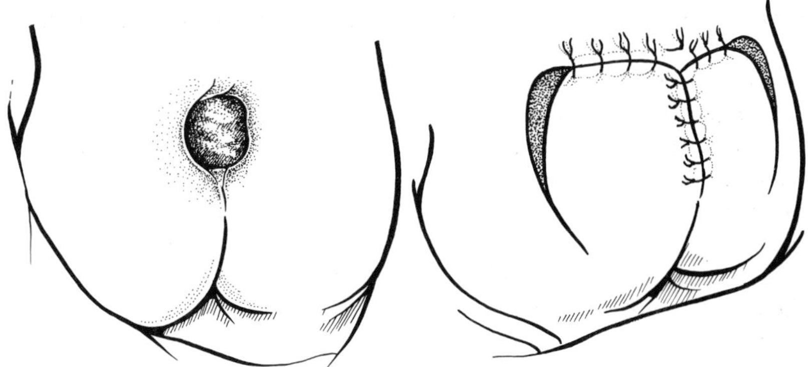

Fig. 8.1 Sacral pressure sore in a non-paraplegic patient, repaired using bilateral rotation-transposition flaps of buttock skin.

drain instead of collecting under the flap to cause tension, infection and necrosis. The graft can be applied 7–10 days later.

Sacral sores

The appropriate type of flap depends on the shape of the ulcer. Frequently suitable is the bilateral flap of buttock skin based on the inferior gluteal fold (Fig. 8.1), and this double flap is especially useful in the sacral pressure sore in the non-paraplegic patient. If the shape and extent of the ulcer make this flap unsuitable, alternatives are the transposed or rotation flap using buttock skin, extending on to the lumbar region (Fig. 8.2). Gluteus maximus has been incorporated into these flaps to add to their safety and effectiveness, and more recently flaps have been designed to use the gluteus maximus muscle in a more formal way (Fig. 8.3). Each muscle, together with a triangle of the overlying buttock skin, is detached from its sacral insertion and mobilised, preserving the inferior gluteal nerve and the gluteal vessels, and advanced to meet its fellow in the midline to reconstruct the postexcisional defect of the sacral ulcer, providing skin cover along with an underlying pad of muscle.

In using the glutei in this way there are several considerations which need to be taken into account, and which are not immediately apparent. One concerns the fact that gluteus maximus is not an expendable muscle, and if the transfer will result in denervation it can only be used in the paraplegic patient. The advancement myo-

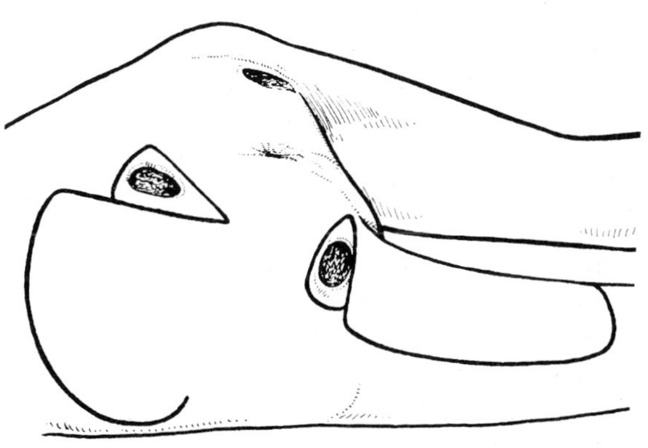

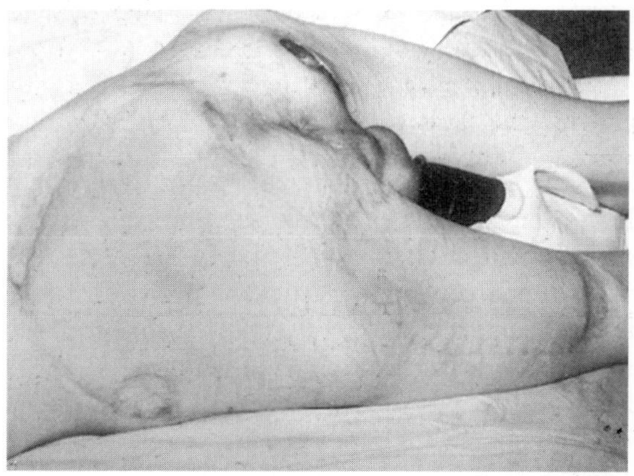

Fig. 8.2 Sacral and bilateral ischial ulcers in a paraplegic patient, the sacral ulcer repaired using a rotation flap of buttock skin, and the left ischial ulcer using a transposition flap of posterior thigh skin as shown in Figure 8.5.

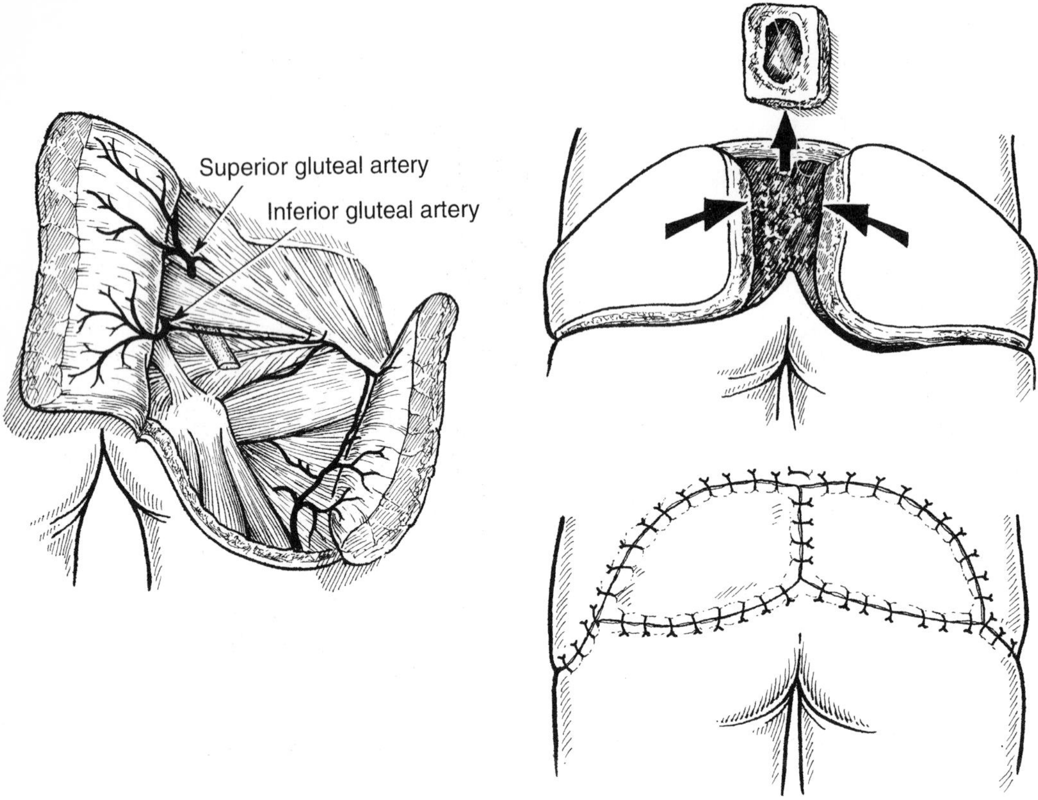

Fig. 8.3 The vascular basis of the gluteus maximus myocutaneous flap, and its incorporation in a bilateral advancement flap to cover a sacral ulcer.

cutaneous flap as described should retain the nerve supply and can thus be used in the non-paraplegic. The entire area is also extremely vascular, and dissection involving gluteus maximus, indeed dissection generally in this area, both in the paraplegic and non-paraplegic patient, involves considerable blood loss.

Trochanteric sores

The greater trochanter is the projection which determines the site of the trochanteric ulcer. Initially, the main cavity of the ulcer is the trochanteric bursa which overlies the projection and, if this alone is involved, permanent closure may be achieved without interfering with the bone. As the condition progresses the trochanter and neck of femur increasingly project into the cavity, and excision of trochanter and appropriate cortex of the shaft is required to let the soft tissues collapse and obliterate the cavity. In the most severe instances a pyoarthrosis of the hip joint may develop and, once present, this complication is virtually impossible to eradicate without amputation of the limb.

The ulcer is so undermined in most cases that free skin grafting is seldom practicable. Cover by a flap is necessary. When this takes the form of a skin flap a transposed flap is used; its precise situation and shape will depend on the size and shape of the ulcer, with the proviso always that the secondary defect should be on an area free from subsequent weight-bearing. Added safety can be provided by incorporating the iliotibial tract in the flap, in the form of a tensor fasciae latae myocutaneous flap (Figs 8.4 and 8.7).

Tensor fasciae latae flap

In the lateral aspect of the thigh the fascia lata is markedly thickened to form the iliotibial tract, receiving into its upper part the insertions of

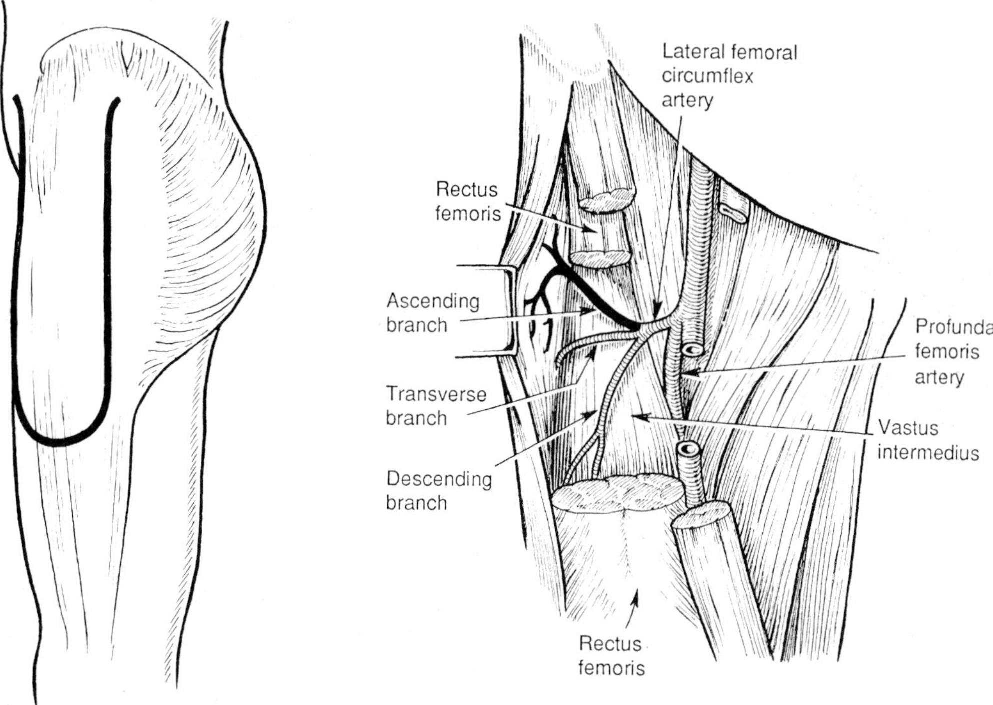

Fig. 8.4 The vascular basis and the typical dimensions of the tensor fasciae latae myocutaneous flap.

gluteus maximus behind and tensor fasciae latae further forward. As the tract passes distally it overlies vastus lateralis but there is no attachment between the two structures. Although the fascia lata encircles the thigh the thickening which constitutes the iliotibial tract virtually ceases along a line dropped vertically from the anterior superior iliac spine.

The tensor fasciae latae muscle is perfused in its lowest part from the ascending branches of the lateral femoral circumflex vessels which reach it about the level of the pubic tubercle. This supply appears to extend into the upper two-thirds of the iliotibial tract.

The tensor fasciae latae myocutaneous flap is designed on the lateral aspect of the thigh with its base superior, and makes use of the iliotibial tract as its 'muscular' element. Its anterior border runs vertically along a line brought just lateral to the anterior superior iliac spine in order to avoid the lateral cutaneous nerve of thigh. Its posterior border approximates to the line running down from the greater trochanter. The length of the flap is determined by the geometry of the transfer but it can safely extend to the junction between the upper two-thirds and the lower third of the thigh. The flap is technically easy to raise because the plane between the tract and vastus lateralis is so well defined and avascular. It can be raised proximally to the level of the pubic tubercle. Its usual use is as a transposed flap, moved posteriorly to cover a defect of trochanter and/or ischium. The secondary defect is split skin grafted as a rule.

Ischial sores

The cavity of the ulcer consists of the ischial bursa but, as the condition progresses and extends, the ischial tuberosity increasingly projects into the cavity and becomes the seat of chronic osteitis. An advance in the treatment of this type of ulcer has been reduction of the prominence of the ischial tuberosity jointly with the appropriate soft tissue surgery. Even where the bone is not pathologically involved it is still the main cause of the ulceration.

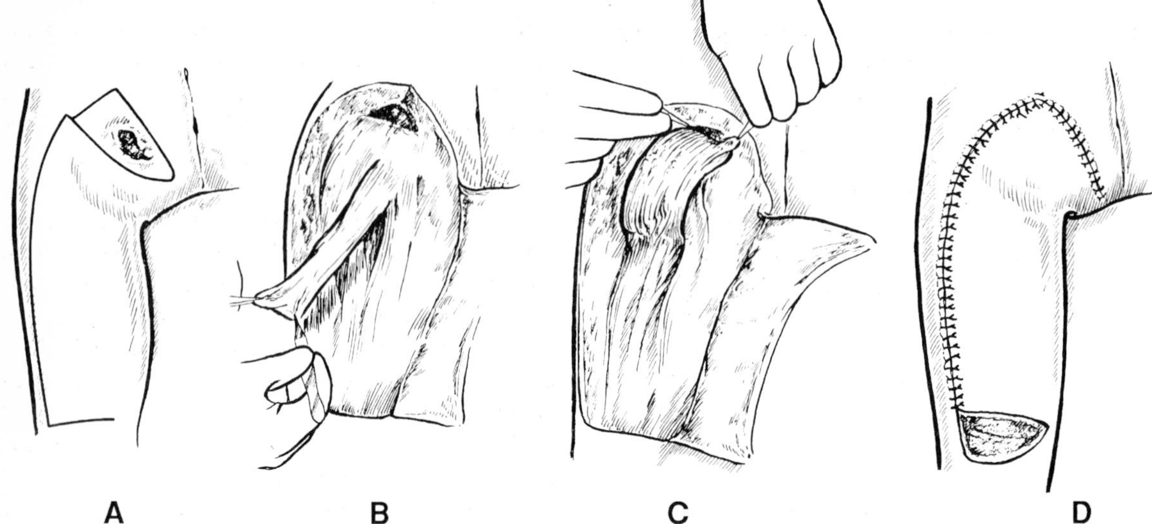

Fig. 8.5 A transposition flap of posterior thigh skin used to repair the defect left following excision of the ischial ulcer, and reduction of the projection of the ischial tuberosity, the cavity of the ischial area filled by detaching near its lower end and mobilising such biceps femoris muscle as is available.

When planning the appropriate flap the patient should have the hip flexed to imitate the sitting posture to ensure that residual scars do not overlie the tuberosity. A useful flap is very broadly based medially along the greater part of the thigh and moved upwards (Fig. 8.5). A virtue in this situation is its generous dimensions which, on the one hand make it extremely safe, and on the other permit further rotation (Fig. 8.6) should the ulcer

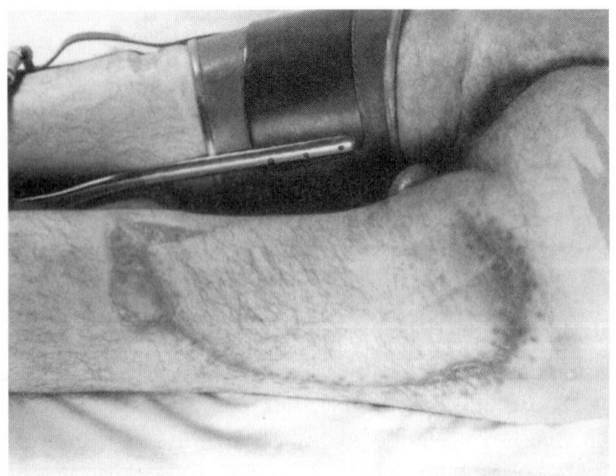

Fig. 8.6 Rotation of a previously used posterior thigh flap to repair a recurrent ischial pressure sore in a paraplegic patient. The segment of the flap beyond the line of the scar of the previous flap was delayed prior to rotation of the flap.

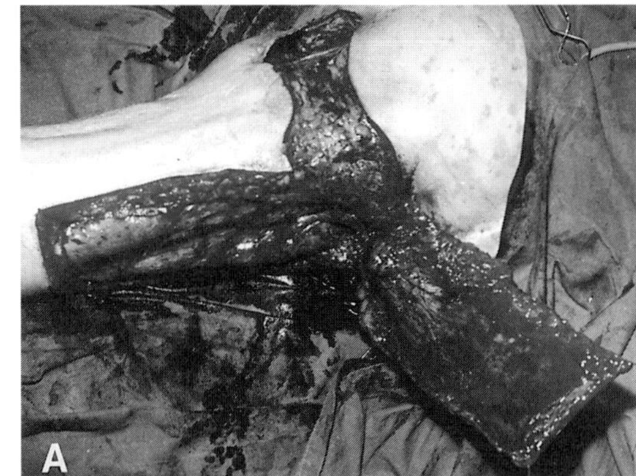

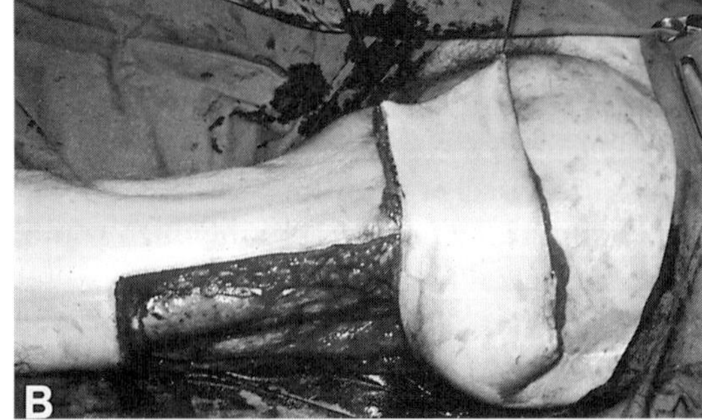

Fig. 8.7 A tensor fasciae latae flap used to provide simultaneous cover for a trochanteric and an ischial pressure sore in a paraplegic patient, showing (**A**) the defect, and (**B**) the flap raised and transposed, ready for suture.

recur. An added advantage is that it provides simultaneous access to the hamstring muscles, and the atrophic remnant of the biceps muscle can be detached at its lower end and mobilised by dividing approximately half of the perforating vessels. The muscle can then be rolled up and tucked into the dead space left by the ischiectomy.

An alternative possibility is the tensor fasciae latae flap. Used for this purpose the length of the flap required is rather greater than for the trochanteric ulcer, a flap of 30 cm or even more being needed. Where trochanteric and ischial ulcers coexist, the single flap may be able to cover both simultaneously (Fig. 8.7).

Total obliteration of the pressure point by ischiectomy, used in conjunction with an appropriate flap for skin cover, appeared to be a promising advance when it was first introduced. The late results have shown up its deficiencies. The major defect as in all procedures in the paraplegic is the tendency to recurrent or fresh ulceration. The body weight has to be supported somewhere, and the effect of surgical procedures is merely to transfer the pressure to a new area where a fresh sore is liable to develop. Following the use of ischiectomy, sores tend to develop on the posterior aspect of the thigh at trochanteric level and also towards the perineum and scrotum. Ulcers in these areas, particularly the perineoscrotal, are extremely intractable, and with flaps already used for ischial sores are very difficult to deal with surgically.

With the ischial ulcer it is better to compromise and, instead of carrying out a formal ischiectomy, to restrict bony excision to the obvious area of projection.

CHAPTER 9

Limb trauma

Limb trauma predominantly involves skin, muscle and bone. Infection does not loom large as a hazard if the skin is not involved, but it has to be added to the list of possible complications when there is a break in the skin barrier, and this can be particularly serious when a fracture is part of the injury. It is for this reason that the effective provision of skin cover becomes a matter of urgency, though its provision has to be coordinated with the management of the other damaged structures, each of which carries its own imperative.

When skin loss is a major element in a limb injury, whether in isolation or as part of combined skin-bone trauma, it usually takes the form of **degloving**.

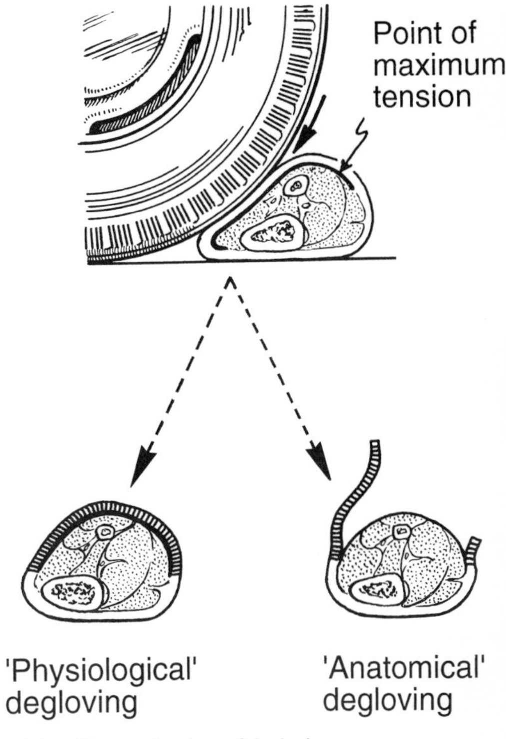

Fig. 9.1 The mechanism of degloving.

DEGLOVING INJURIES

The distinguishing feature of a degloving injury is the flaying of the skin, the result of a severe shearing strain, as for example in the 'running over' of the limb by a pneumatic tyre (Fig. 9.1). The plane through which the skin is detached is sometimes superficial, sometimes deep to the investing layer of deep fascia, and the skin may tear, creating a flap. Alternatively, the skin may remain intact, though detached deeply. The effect of detachment is to disrupt the perfusion pattern of the skin and superficial fascia. The vessels which reach the investing layer of deep fascia and through it perfuse the superficial fascia and skin, described on p. 67, are avulsed. The sudden extreme tension set up by the shearing strain also disrupts the vascular network in the superficial fascia and skin, the combined effect being to produce ischaemic necrosis of the skin which is detached. Depending on the mechanism of the injury there may also be friction burning of part or all of the degloved skin.

At first sight, the severity and extent of the damage to the skin circulation may not be particularly striking, but there is failure of the skin to blanch when pressure is applied, with return of colour when the pressure is released and, when a skin edge is present, no dermal bleeding, both indicating absence of circulation. The skin area demonstrated to be devoid of circulation, although its epidermis at that point in time may be viable, progresses to ischaemic necrosis.

Accurate assessment of the extent of the area lacking circulation is desirable, and fluorescein, administered intravenously, 15 mg/kg in 200 ml of saline, over a period of 10 min has been used as a visual aid to estimating this. Viewed under ultraviolet light, normally perfused skin clearly fluoresces while avascular skin does not. Unfortunately, difficulty is liable to arise in the areas where help is most needed, where damage is partial. Such areas show a mottled pattern of fluorescence. Towards the margin of a degloved flap they are likely to go on at least to superficial necrosis, and are probably better managed as part of the frankly ischaemic skin area.

The principle of management in such an injury is that the non-viable skin area should be excised, and the defect split skin grafted with the minimum of delay. The patient's general condition may overshadow the local and dictate at least temporary delay, but a local assessment should be made as soon as possible, and the excision carried out. It is positive evidence of perfusion which decides viability, and in its absence the skin should be excised.

It is not essential that the graft should be applied immediately following excision. There may be advantage in waiting for a few days to allow for further excision if any dubious areas remain, either of the degloved skin or the surface exposed by the degloving. Grafting with a minimum of delay is nonetheless desirable (Fig. 9.2). As much skin as possible should be applied, with priority to the flexures and areas with underlying tendons.

Damage to muscle may also be present, recognisable by the darkening of the muscle fibres, and failure of the fibres to contract when pinched. Excision to healthy muscle is then required, since it is only on a healthy base that a graft will take. Residual necrotic muscle will mean local graft failure.

The fact that the skin after the injury, though without a blood supply, remains viable makes it possible to use it on occasion as a free skin graft to resurface the area at least in part. If it appears largely undamaged, it is worth considering its reapplication to the debrided surface as a full thickness skin graft after its subcutaneous fat has been carefully excised. Successful use of the skin in this way gives a better ultimate result than a split skin graft cut from elsewhere.

It is important that the nature of the injury and its vascular significance should be recognised, so that the situation is not allowed to drift until a slough forms and separates slowly and spontaneously. If the injury has not been recognised primarily, and only becomes obvious when a slough forms, it should be excised as soon as it has demarcated, and the area immediately grafted.

SKIN-BONE INJURIES

The fractures most often associated with skin loss involve the long bones, tibia and, much less frequently, ulna. Before the management of such an injury can usefully be discussed, it is necessary to have an understanding of the principles which underlie its treatment, for the detailed handling of the injury is the expression in practical terms of these principles. A primary objective in treating such a combined injury is to prevent infection, and this is achieved by **fixing the fracture**

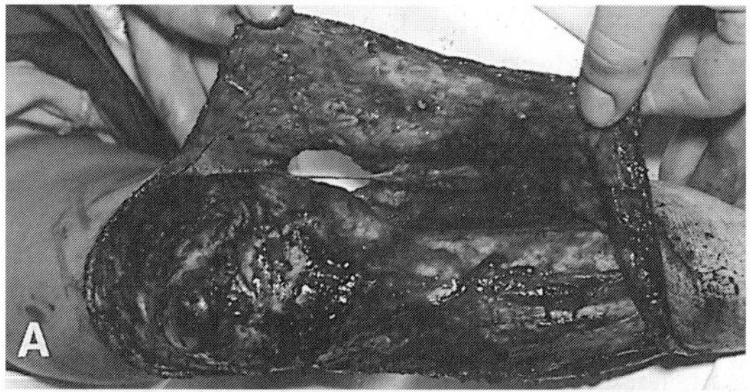

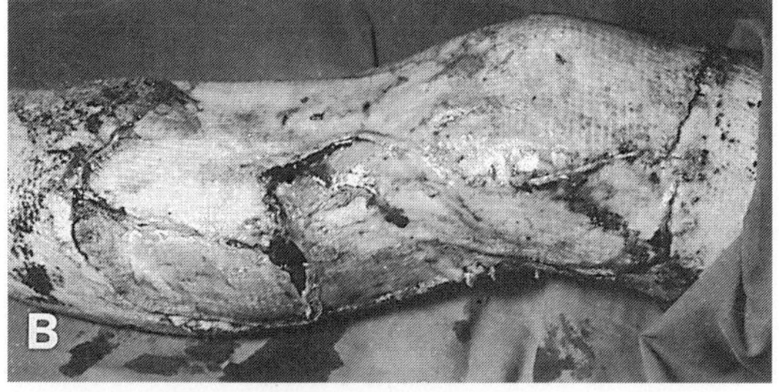

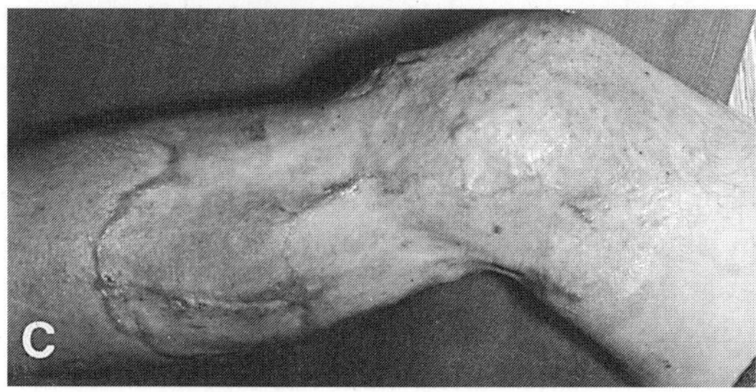

Fig. 9.2 A degloving injury of the leg resurfaced primarily with split skin grafts.

The extent of the injury (**A**), the appearance 7 days later (**B**), following the application of sheet split skin grafts immediately following debridement of the wound, and the healed appearance (**C**), with full function.

and by **providing skin cover** to isolate it from the surface.

An X-ray of a fracture gives an incomplete picture of the total injury in the way that it ignores the soft tissue element. The severity of this latter element and the form it takes are of major importance when the soft tissues around the fracture site, muscle, fascia and skin, are being assessed for damage, and even viability, or as potential sources to provide cover for the bone, fractured or merely bared by the injury.

The **injury to muscle** can take the form of obvious tearing of muscle fibres, but damage at a less gross level can also occur, resulting in swelling of the muscle belly. Even so, muscle is unexpectedly resilient in practice, and has been successfully transferred in the form of a flap shortly after the original injury, though its use in this way is not without risk.

The **injury to skin** takes a different form, seen most strikingly when part of the injury involves degloving of the skin and superficial fascia. Degloving as an isolated injury has already been described, but when it is associated with bony trauma it has to be considered also in relation to the extent to which it might be possible to use degloved skin and its underlying layer of fascia as a local flap to cover the surface defect. Before the use of such skin could be considered, there would have to be clear evidence of circulation in the skin area, and even when this criterion has been fulfilled it has not proved a reliable flap source.

The various elements of a mixed skin–bone injury can vary widely in their severity, and the plastic surgeon is liable to have a biased view of the situation. He is likely to see only the injuries at the most severe end of the spectrum, and assume that they are the norm, whereas in fact the less severe injuries are being successfully managed by the orthopaedic surgeon on his own. Nonetheless, if a harmonious and effective relationship is to be built up, the plastic surgeon is best invited to see the patient at the acute stage if the orthopaedic surgeon considers that there is even a remote possibility that he may have to be involved in treatment later.

Role of the periosteum

The periosteum plays a crucial role both in the management of the fracture and in the provision of skin cover. In addition to providing an effective barrier to infection, a significant proportion of the blood supply to the superficial cortex of the bone reaches it through the periosteum. This explains why avascular necrosis of the superficial cortex and surface sequestration regularly occur where bone is left denuded of periosteum by the injury, and also provides the reason why nothing should be done in manipulating and fixing the fracture which might denude more bone or add to the periosteum already damaged. If plates and screws are being used they should be applied on top of the periosteum even though this may add to the technical problems of fixation. The surgeon has to accept the therapeutic problems posed by the cortical bone denuded by the injury, but he should not add to them by surgically stripping periosteum.

In relation to the role of the periosteum in the provision of skin cover, cortical bone which is covered with periosteum will accept a split skin graft; cortical bone denuded of periosteum cannot be expected to accept a split skin graft.

Fixation of the fracture

Fixation of the fracture is the responsibility of the orthopaedic surgeon, but in choosing the method he has also to ensure that his choice does not conflict with the needs of the soft tissue injury. The essence of the method used is that it should provide rigid fixation of the fracture, and the potential alternatives are **plaster of Paris**, with or without a window, **internal fixation** using plate and screws, **intramedullary nail fixation**, and **external fixation frame**.

With **plaster of Paris fixation** there is no access to the area of skin loss unless a large window is cut. A window of adequate size is likely to affect fixation of the fracture adversely, and on these grounds is undesirable. However, if a window is to be avoided, the skin cover used at the time of primary treatment has to be restricted to split skin grafting at the very most, and it is therefore not an option where skin damage is a significant part of the total injury. Even without a window, plaster of Paris fixation alone may not be considered capable of providing the rigid fixation regarded as essential when the fracture is unstable.

Internal fixation using plates and screws may be an effective method in the closed tibial fracture but in the compound fracture with skin loss its role is more dubious. The site of skin loss nearly always overlies the subcutaneous surface of the tibia, and addition of the incisions and dissection required to expose the bone to insert an anteriorly applied plate extends the area of soft tissue damage to an undesirable degree, in the surface where the tibia is most vulnerable from the point of view of overlying skin necrosis. Application of the plate to the posterior surface is an alternative, but the posterior approach has not become standard practice in this context.

In the comminuted fracture particularly, the method is unlikely to be the one of choice, and even in the absence of comminution it has the serious disadvantage of adding considerably to the amount of bone exposed and soft tissue dissected.

Intramedullary nail fixation might appear to have adverse factors. It might well be felt that the exposure of the entire medullary cavity to the surface, which the insertion of such a nail entails, would invite the spread of infection from end to end of the bone. The fact that it is being successfully used, admittedly in conjunction with the provision of well-vascularised flap cover, would indicate that this fear is largely groundless. Viewed in relation to the provision of skin cover it has the considerable virtue that its use does not place any restraints on the method of providing skin cover selected by the plastic surgeon.

The **external fixation frame** also has the virtue of leaving the fracture site unimpeded from the point of view of providing skin cover. The transfixion pins inserted into the bone at a distance from the fracture provide virtually absolute stability without interfering with the fracture site once the frame has been set up. The absence of interference with the soft tissues, damaged or undamaged, at or around the fracture site, allows the two components of the injury, bone and soft tissue, to be managed with minimal reference one to the other. Almost the only aspect of the bony fixation which may affect soft tissue management is the site of insertion of the pins. This determines the line of the interconnecting bar, and thought should be given to this aspect to ensure that it does not make the reconstruction which the plastic surgeon wishes to use less easy technically, or even impossible. With this proviso, it leaves the entire range of reconstructive techniques available for use.

Provision of skin cover

In the combined injury of skin and skeleton, skin damage can vary from minimal up to extensive degloving.

Where skin loss has been minor, but closure

by direct suture can only be achieved under tension, a 'relaxation incision' is often recommended. The idea is that by making such an incision tension will be reduced, and skin closure will be easier. The method sounds safe enough in theory, but it is less so in practice. A 'relaxing' incision really creates a bipedicled flap which moves across to allow closure of the original wound. It is a well-recognised fact that even in optimal circumstances a bipedicled flap transferred in this way is an unsafe procedure and is liable to necrose. Used in a mixed skin and skeletal injury it is even more hazardous, for soft tissue damage and degloving have so often added their quota to the local devitalisation of skin. The presence of degloving is a virtual contraindication to its use, and even in the absence of degloving the method should be used with the greatest of care. It is likely to be safest and most effective when closure is difficult because of local swelling of the limb from oedema and haemorrhage, rather than because of skin loss. The incision itself should be straight, placed at a considerable distance from the wound, and run in the long axis of the limb. Undermining of the skin should be avoided.

When skin loss is more extensive, the replacement methods available are: **free skin graft**, **skin or fasciocutaneous flap**, **muscle or myocutaneous flap**, and **free flap** — usually used individually, occasionally in combination.

Despite the alternative reconstructive methods available today, **split skin grafting** should be the first choice if the raw surface is suitable. In determining which surfaces are suitable for grafting, the key role of the periosteum has already been stressed. Excision of avascular tissue, fixation of the fracture, conservation of periosteum, closure of joint by suture of the capsule when possible, or cover with a muscle flap to create a graftable surface — all combine to give a graft the best chance to take. The split skin graft has the great virtue also of being able on occasion to stabilise a clinical situation at minimal cost to the patient. It gives the surgeon a breathing space, and even if the graft is unsuitable as definitive cover it is possible to replace it at leisure once the patient's condition has become stable.

Split skin grafting can be used in conjunction with other techniques. A muscle flap, for example, may be needed to cover the bare bone element of a composite injury, but the graft can still be applied all around the area covered by the muscle as well as providing cover for the muscle itself.

Skin and fasciocutaneous flaps, rotation or transposed, raised locally, have little if any place in acute injuries of this sort. Although safer when they include the fascial layer, they have not been assessed objectively in the context of acute skin–bone trauma. Before contemplating the use of a flap of this type, it would be essential to gauge the damage to the overall vascularity of the skin which it is proposed to use as the flap, particularly when an element of degloving is involved. In any case the size and shape of the typical defect and the state of the surrounding skin would preclude its use.

The cross-leg flap may have been increased in safety by incorporating the fascial layer, but for the surgeon with little experience in its use (and such experience is becoming rarer as the method is losing popularity in other contexts) it must be regarded as distinctly hazardous. Such flaps have also to be used with particular circumspection, even as elective procedures in older patients because of peripheral vascular problems in the ageing limb, and problems of joint stiffness. These considerations would apply with redoubled force in an emergency situation, especially in the lower limb where the problem really arises. In a lower limb injury a cross-leg fasciocutaneous flap can be contemplated only by an experienced operator, in the young patient with unimpaired peripheral circulation and joints capable of tolerating the immobilisation, a combination of limitations likely to restrict its usage to near zero.

Local fasciocutaneous flaps being generally unsuitable for use at the acute stage of a combined skin–bone injury, the question arises whether the skin–fascia combination is capable of recovering sufficiently to be safe to use at a later date, and if so when. It is difficult to believe that degloved skin can recover to total circulatory normality, though it has been reported as being successfully used for subsequent reconstruction, which would suggest that at least a degree of recovery can take place. The cautious surgeon is unlikely to accept this as a blanket finding. Reasoning from other clinical contexts, such observations as the amount of superficial scarring of the skin, its degree of comparative mobility, and the thickness of the layer of superficial fascia, would all play a part in decision making.

The use of **muscle and myocutaneous flaps** raised locally would be confined to defects of the knee and upper half of the anterior tibia. The medial head of gastrocnemius is capable of covering the medial aspect of the knee joint and the upper third of the tibia.

Transfer is probably better carried out as a muscle flap rather than as a myocutaneous flap when the option is present. Even used in late reconstruction the virtues of a muscle flap with grafting of its exposed surface, as compared with grafting of the secondary defect left by the transfer of the corresponding myocutaneous flap, have been recognised. The potential hazard of the presence of muscle damage in assessing its usage in muscle transfer has already been discussed, and its unexpected tolerance of transfer as a flap even when showing signs of injury.

Where the necessary facilities and microvascular expertise have been available, **free flaps**, fasciocutaneous, muscle and myocutaneous, have been increasingly used in managing the more severe mixed injuries of skin and bone. The techniques involved may be demanding, but the results, judged in terms of healing time, time to fracture union and time in hospital, are all better. Muscle, transferred as a flap, appears also to bring with it a degree of vascularity which, used to cover a surface which shows damage, prevents the damage progressing to necrosis, and it seems to retain these virtues even when it is part of a free flap. In a situation where periosteal stripping and continuing exposure of bare cortical bone is so often followed by sequestration of its outer layer, this is a particularly valuable attribute. The muscle is also able to fill any bony defect which may have resulted from the removal of comminuted bony fragments judged to be avascular, and in this way eliminate dead space.

A free flap frequently used is the latissimus dorsi flap. Its long pedicle and reliable vessels of a good calibre make it among the less technically demanding transfers. The large area of muscle which can be transferred also makes it possible to cope with the more extensive defects successfully so that, even if part of the area of skin loss is graftable, it may still be convenient to cover the entire area with the flap. The rectus abdominis flap has become a popular, and equally suitable, alternative. Both flaps tend to be used as muscle rather than as myocutaneous flaps, leaving skin cover to be provided by grafting.

For the smaller defect, alternatives are the radial forearm, the lateral upper arm flap, and the scapular flap. The comparative virtues of the three are discussed in Chapter 4.

The vessels at the fracture site chosen for anastomosis will depend on the site of injury and the extent of vascular involvement. They must be examined with extreme care for signs of damage, and interpositional vein grafts may be needed if it proves necessary to reach a healthy vessel wall which can be used for anastomosis. Immediately post-traumatic, reliable criteria of total normality of the vessel wall present a problem. Seven to 10 days later, signs of damage to vessels are more obvious, with oedema and thickening of the wall.

The state of the other main arteries of the limb may also need to be assessed to ascertain to what extent the artery chosen for anastomosis is sustaining the limb alone or with minimal assistance from the other main arteries. The findings may preclude the use of end-to-end anastomosis to the flap artery, and even in the absence of damage to other vessels end-to-side anastomosis may be preferable. The information provided by arteriography is, as already stressed (p. 102), only partial and must be matched against the findings at operation.

Clinical management

Once the fracture has been reduced and fixed, it becomes possible to make a proper assessment of the soft tissue component of the injury, and carry out an initial excision of irreparably damaged tissue, skin, fascia and muscle. The criteria for assessing viability of skin have already been described, and the excision of damaged fascia can safely be radical, since the muscle surface exposed will accept a graft. Excision of fascia may also have the beneficial effect of decompressing muscle swollen and oedematous as a result of the injury. The only structure, vessels and nerves apart, which should be managed conservatively throughout is, as already stressed, periosteum. Even at this early stage, some idea of the reconstruction likely to be required is usually possible, and a provisional strategy can be drawn up.

If skin grafting is considered feasible, it is not obligatory to apply the graft there and then. There is much to be said for a 'second look', with a further debridement in order to improve the surface. Carried out 4–6 days later, the further debridement should leave only viable soft tissue exposed, and definitive decisions regarding reconstruction can be made. When a skin graft is used after such a delay, the ultimate healing time may actually be reduced, take of the graft becoming 100%, rather than patchy.

The decision regarding the best form of skin cover will depend very much on the site of the injury, the state of the bone, and the surface it presents. This, in turn, may well depend on the type of fracture, whether it is comminuted or not, and the estimated viability of any detached fragments. The site most often involved by such a mixed injury is the lower half of the tibia, and in that site, if a reconstruction requires more than merely a free skin graft, the most effective alternative is likely to be a free flap, and the greater the deficiency in depth the more valuable will be the muscle component of the free flap. This aspect might determine whether or not a latissimus dorsi or rectus abdominis muscle flap is chosen.

The timing of free flap reconstructions remains controversial, whether they should be carried out at the acute stage or postponed for a few days. The advocates of definitive free flap reconstruction at the acute stage tend to be enthusiasts for the method, but for most plastic surgeons the more severe forms of these mixed injuries are infrequent, and the results claimed for 'acute' free flap transfers are not necessarily repeatable by the occasional operator, who perhaps should be more cautious. What can be stated with certainty is that, if the decision is made to use an immediate or even a delayed primary free flap, the debridement which immediately precedes the application of the flap should be more than usually thorough, making sure that no non-viable tissue is left to provide a focus of potential infection.

In managing these injuries, the question must arise at some stage whether or not a damaged lower leg and foot is salvageable. The question is not whether the limb can be preserved viable, but whether the result will be a useful functioning limb. Severely injured lower limbs are salvaged today in a manner which would have been inconceivable until comparatively recently, and this is extremely satisfactory. As with many advances, however, the pendulum may have swung further than is ultimately desirable, with limbs being preserved which are never likely to function effectively. Such results represent a triumph of enthusiasm for a technique over realism concerning its results. The injury which is likely to be most crippling in the long term is one where there is anaesthesia of the weightbearing surface of the foot. Experience in other contexts has shown that such a foot does not do well. It would be wrong to deprive a patient of the chance to save his lower limb entire but it should also be recognised that on occasion conservation can be carried too far. With the currently available prostheses, a below-knee amputation need not be a significant disability, and the surgeon needs to compare the alternatives both in terms of final function and in terms of time spent in hospital. Without suggesting that a decision should be made at the acute stage, the possibility that amputation may be required, if the possibility is a real one, should be put to the patient early on, and a decision, if it has to be made, should not be delayed. As time goes on the patient is likely to become increasingly unrealistic, and unwilling to face an unpleasant truth and, having already spent time, may wish to continue in the forlorn hope of ultimate success.

A further aspect of the management of tibial fractures associated with skin loss which is often neglected concerns the ankle and foot. In the absence of positive steps taken to prevent its occurrence, one regularly sees clawing of the toes being allowed to develop, often with a degree of foot-drop as well. This becomes increasingly difficult to correct, and left uncorrected, the patient ends up unable to walk properly, even after the fracture is united and the soft tissues are stable.

OSTEITIS AND INFECTED FRACTURES

When the plastic surgeon is asked to help in

managing a problem arising from infection occurring in a bone, the bone involved is nearly always the tibia. The pathology is usually one of periodic flare-ups of chronic osteitis, with the background either an old infected fracture or the residuum of acute osteitis, the latter less frequently today with more effective control of the initial episode, possibly with the background of a sequestrum. The problem relates either to the skin overlying the subcutaneous border of the bone and/or the bone itself.

There are several reasons why the tibia should be the bone so often involved. Apart from being the long bone whose shaft is probably most frequently fractured, it has a larger subcutaneous surface than any of the others. Less obviously significant, but probably just as important, a much smaller area of its total surface is covered with attached muscle. The cover provided by the extensive muscle attachments to the other long bones distances them from the surface, and eliminates to a large extent the problem of providing effective skin cover after surgery. In this they provide a sharp contrast to the problems created by the long subcutaneous surface of the tibia, particularly if the injury has involved skin damage, or there is the deep skin fixation which so often follows previous surgery in the area.

The muscles attached to a bone are also important providers of blood supply to the cortex to which they are attached. The lower half of the tibia, the segment of the shaft most at risk from fracture, has virtually no muscles attached to it, and this leaves perfusion of the bone largely reliant on its nutrient artery. In a comminuted fracture, bony fragments which appear on X-ray to be detached from the main tibial shaft cannot rely on the perfusion source which the presence of a muscle attachment would provide, increasing the likelihood of sequestration.

This explanation of the reasons why the problems exist provides at the same time some clues to their solution. At a clinical level one of the problems concerns the most effective way of replacing the scarred and deeply adherent skin overlying the tibial shaft. When chronic infection of the bone with periodic flare-ups is an additional problem, avascularity and sclerosis are added to the pattern. The objectives then become ones of providing stable skin cover for the subcutaneous surface, trying to add to the blood supply of the sclerotic bone, and filling any defect in the bone which may result from the activities of the orthopaedic surgeon, if he has to carry out a sequestrectomy or remove sclerotic bone.

In managing the acute combined skin–bone injury, vascularised muscle used to cover the defect and fill any gaps in bony continuity has been found to have a beneficial effect in salvaging damaged tissues, and it has proved equally useful in these subsequent problems.

The form which soft tissue replacement should take, whether by fasciocutaneous or myocutaneous flap, will depend on the local circumstances, but it should be generous in area, and planned with enough reserve to cope with any minor infection which might arise from the bone subsequently. At which precise point the bony problem should be tackled in relation to the timing of the flap transfer is a matter for discussion with the orthopaedic surgeon but, in general, operation on the diseased bone should be undertaken only when it can be immediately and completely covered by the flap.

The extent of the typical area of pretibial scarring is likely to make the possibility of using local tissues to reconstruct the defect a remote one. The use of a distant flap is unavoidable, and the demands of time and patient comfort and convenience are strong arguments in favour of a free flap. The form it should take will depend on the details of the local problem. If skin replacement alone is required a fasciocutaneous flap would be adequate. If surgery of the bone will be required, and particularly if there is the possibility of dead space after its completion, or surgery of sclerotic, relatively avascular bone is involved, a flap which includes muscle is likely to be preferable, bringing a more effective blood supply to the site, and capable of filling dead space.

Safe use of a free flap in this context requires as much knowledge as possible of any changes in the major vessels which may have resulted from the original injury. Caveats regarding the use of vessels which are already damaged, and the use of end-to-side rather than end-to-end anastomosis, have already been discussed in relation to the acute skin–bone injury.

TENDON AND NERVE INJURIES

When a nerve and/or tendon is injured in association with extensive loss of skin, and it is apparent at the outset that their repair or reconstruction will be required, the management of that aspect of the overall defect has generally to be subordinated to the provision of skin cover.

In order to function properly in the case of a tendon, or for axon regeneration in the case of a nerve, a covering of subcutaneous tissue as well as skin is necessary, and this carries the implication that cover by a flap will be required.

When the skin defect is being reconstructed primarily using a flap, the possibility of carrying out the tendon and/or nerve reconstruction simultaneously theoretically exists, but the decision may well depend on the degree of experience of the surgeon(s) involved. The considerations which would determine such a decision concern the degree of tissue damage and wound contamination present, and whether an adequate primary debridement is possible, whether failure to reconstruct primarily is likely to result in much poorer final function, and whether the posture which may be required of the tendon/nerve reconstruction will preclude the use of the method of providing skin cover considered otherwise appropriate. The cautious approach is to provide primary flap cover and carry out the tendon/nerve reconstruction as a secondary procedure.

When the initial skin cover has been provided by a free skin graft, tendon/nerve reconstruction has to await replacement of the graft by a flap. Here again the considerations are essentially the same as those involved in decision making at the acute stage, except that tissue damage and potential contamination are not part of the equation. A single-stage reconstruction, with the opportunity present for preoperative planning, simultaneous tendon/nerve reconstruction may be a reasonable approach; multi-staged, it is safer to wait until the flap transfer is complete and the flap well settled before carrying out the tendon/nerve reconstruction.

Sometimes disease or previous injury makes it necessary to replace the overlying skin to allow surgery of bone, joint or tendon to be carried out. A flap is then usually required, and the considerations involved are similar to those described for the combined skin–tendon/nerve injury.

PLANTAR DEFECTS

The plantar aspect of the foot has two distinct types of skin surfaces, weightbearing and non-weightbearing. The major weightbearing areas are the heel, a strip corresponding to the line of the metatarsal heads, and a strip which joins the two, running along the lateral border of the foot. Subsidiary areas of weightbearing are present on the pulp areas of the toes, that of the great toe being much the largest. In static situations the heel carries the bulk of the body weight; activity increasingly transfers the weight to the skin overlying the metatarsal heads and the pulp areas of the toes, the great toe particularly.

The distinction between the two areas is matched by differences in their skin. Non-weightbearing skin is soft and barely more keratinised than skin in other sites; weightbearing skin is heavily keratinised, to a degree which depends on the demands which are put on it. The heel has a thicker keratin layer than elsewhere, and the foot of the barefoot individual shows a much greater degree of keratinisation of the weightbearing areas overall than the individual who habitually wears footwear.

Other adaptations to functional demands are also seen with the strong fibrous attachments which bind the skin deeply, countering the shearing strains to which the weightbearing skin is subject.

The literature on reconstruction of defects of the foot has demonstrated a general unwillingness to assess the long term results of the reconstruction being described, and a failure to separate the defects according to whether the site involved is an obligatory weightbearing area or not. The few publications which have examined results critically from this point of view have demonstrated clearly that reconstructions of defects of the weightbearing areas have been successful in the long term only when the patient has been able, by altering posture or footwear, to convert the site involved into one which is virtually non-weightbearing.

When one considers the degree of structural specialisation of such areas, the keratinisation of the epidermis and the deep fixation by fibrous septa to counter shearing stresses in the obligatory weightbearing areas, and the fact that these cannot be reproduced by any technique currently available, this lack of success is not surprising. Nonetheless it is a fact which has to be kept in the forefront when options are being discussed with a patient.

The defects which arise in practice vary in the site involved, in extent and in depth, all factors which influence the likely result. Factors which may also be relevant are the state of the patient's peripheral circulation, and his tobacco smoking habits. This latter factor may preclude reconstruction altogether.

When the area is non-weightbearing, the problem of reconstruction will depend on whether the surface exposed is graftable or not. If the defect is small in area a full thickness skin graft has certain advantages, experience being that such a graft develops better sensation than a split skin graft. A split skin graft may be unavoidable when the defect is more extensive though the dermal cushion of a thick graft is then desirable. A problem which arises regularly following the grafting of such a defect is the subsequent development of a line of callosity with fissuring of the skin along the line of the skin adjoining such a graft, and there is no way of preventing its occurrence.

When the surface is unsuitable for grafting the type of flap used will depend on the extent and site involved. Defects confined to the non-weightbearing areas are typically small and a local flap may be possible. Transfer of such a flap is likely to leave a secondary defect, and in planning this, a weightbearing area should be avoided. The instep area, and the medial border of the foot extending on to the adjoining dorsum, may be potential areas on which the flap can be designed. The larger defect will require the use of a distant flap, and then its long-term success is likely to depend on whether it is confined to a non-weightbearing area or strays on to one which bears weight.

When the area is weightbearing, the problems of reconstruction are greatly increased, and much depends on the size of the defect. The small defect can often be grafted, and the whole skin graft has the advantage of being more likely to develop sensation. It may also function adequately, even in an obligatory weightbearing area, because its thickness compared with the depth of the defect leaves it forming a local depression, so that the weight is borne by the surrounding normal skin, though the development of an area of callus around may require regular paring.

The large defect is almost invariably the result of traumatic degloving, and the plane usually leaves virtually no soft tissue covering the bone, particularly over the calcaneum. This is the kind of injury which, despite being successfully covered with a flap, even one where a degree of sensation is provided, is unlikely to remain healed unless the patient is prepared to permanently subordinate his lifestyle to its demands, or is able to convert the posture of the foot into one which leaves the heel non-weightbearing. Few patients walk on soft tissue reconstructions of the heel, altering their gait to walk on the forefoot.

One recognises that, in the initial assessment of such an injury, to consider amputation of a foot which, apart from its weightbearing surface, is normal, seems an outrageous thought, unlikely to be mentioned to the patient and, if it is discussed, understandably likely to be rejected out of hand. Nonetheless, personal experience has been that patients, after experiencing years of recurring ulceration, have welcomed amputation, and found it an effective solution to their problems. When the outlook is being discussed with the patient with a severe degloving injury, involving the heel particularly, and a realistic prospect is being presented, amputation should perhaps be mentioned as the bottom line.

CHAPTER 10 Neoplastic conditions

CARCINOMA OF THE BREAST

The problems of reconstruction which follow mastectomy have changed as the pattern of the mastectomy has changed. With movement away from radical mastectomy, through simple mastectomy, to 'lumpectomy', the need for skin grafting of the postexcisional defect has diminished greatly, but it has been replaced by an increased demand for postmastectomy reconstruction. The first reconstructions which were used took the form of replacing the resected breast tissue with a latissimus dorsi myocutaneous flap (p. 96), augmented where necessary with a silicone implant. More recently the rectus abdominis myocutaneous flap (p. 99) has been used as an alternative. This latter method is particularly appropriate when, as regularly happens in such circumstances, the patient has a redundancy of her lower abdominal skin, the island of skin normally discarded in carrying out an 'apronectomy' being transferred to reconstruct the breast. Depending on its bulk, this flap may obviate the need for a subsequent implant.

The principle of tissue expansion (p. 121) has also been applied to the problem of the postmastectomy defect, and the method has proved effective in creating a space which is then filled with a silicone implant. The use of such an implant creates its own problems, particularly those of capsule formation, and such a reconstruction seldom results in an appearance which matches the normal breast alongside it.

A controversial aspect of reconstruction after mastectomy, and one which has not been completely resolved, concerns whether the reconstruction should be carried out immediately postmastectomy or as a secondary procedure. There is a general feeling among plastic surgeons that secondary reconstruction is preferable. The patient undergoing reconstruction secondarily has seen her postmastectomy appearance and this makes her more ready to accept the fact that, while the reconstruction will never match the original, it will still be a marked improvement. Tissue expansion requires that the area should be healed, and it is therefore unsuitable for use immediately postmastectomy.

TUMOURS OF THE SKIN

The specific problems of neoplasia of the head and neck apart, the policy of skin replacement following excision of a malignant tumour of skin might be expected to be a straightforward one, with the cosmetic aspect of subsidiary importance, and the split skin graft as the routine method employed because it does not obscure the field when recurrence is being watched for. One of the few situations which would require cover by a flap is a surface left following excision which is unsuitable for grafting, for example bare cortical bone or tendon. The virtues of a flap would then have to be weighed against the degree of certainty of adequate excision, particularly in depth, this being the part most likely to be hidden by the flap.

In many clinical situations and with many patients this is the standard approach, but it is not one which commends itself to every patient. Some patients are extremely concerned about the appearance of the graft. The concern is likely to be greatest in the female patient where the defect is of the lower limb, generally because of the hollow resulting from resection to deep fascia, and replacement with the thinness of a graft. The surgeon may take the view that the skin graft, even with the hollow, is an acceptable price to pay for the greater certainty of early recognition of recurrence, but an important factor in this equation is the type of tumour and its pattern of spread.

The problem arises in its most acute form when the tumour is a malignant melanoma. In reconstructing the post-excision defect, the use of a free flap has been advocated, in the lower leg, for example. An added complication is the current trend to more conservative marginal excision when the Breslow thickness is at the lower end of the spectrum. With the strongly adverse effect that local recurrence of melanoma has on prognosis, neither approach can currently be regarded as definitive. The problem remains an aspect of management where the decision should be shared with a patient who has been adequately informed on the issues involved.

CARCINOMA OF HEAD AND NECK SKIN

This section is primarily concerned with the techniques used in reconstructing the defects resulting from the resection of neoplasms which involve the skin of the head and neck, but *it should be stressed that, although the techniques are discussed in the context of neoplasia, comparable defects arise in these sites for other reasons, and the reconstructions described are equally effective in those circumstances. Also, to avoid repetition, the text, and the captions of the figures used to illustrate it, have been coordinated to give an overall view of the reconstructions discussed, their background, indications, and limitations, as well as an account of the surgical technique involved in carrying out each.*

The reconstruction used when a neoplasm of the skin of the head and neck is excised is determined by a variety of factors, predominantly pathological and anatomical, but tempered by those of cosmesis. To explore all of these aspects in depth is beyond the scope of this book, but there are certain principles which need to be discussed if the techniques pertaining to reconstruction of soft tissue defects in these sites are to be used effectively.

Excision and direct closure is used whenever possible, but when a defect cannot be closed directly the decision has to be made concerning the form that its reconstruction should take, whether a free skin graft or flap. The problem of deciding between the two arises because the demands of effective tumour treatment and those of cosmesis can conflict, and the surgeon has then to decide on the relative priority to give to each.

Pathological aspects

These concern the influence that the tumour type, its speed of growth and pattern of infiltration, are likely to have on certainty of tumour clearance, this being an important determining factor in whether a graft or a flap should be chosen to reconstruct the defect. When grafts and flaps are compared in relation to ease of recognising marginal recurrence, the difference in thickness between the two is not of great importance, since marginal recurrence is likely to show equally quickly with either. It is in relation to the certainty of clearance in depth that the comparative thickness of graft and flap becomes important, to the extent that it may be a major determinant as to which should be used. The thin graft is less likely to hide recurrence, compared with the thicker flap which may conceal recurrence until it is disastrously extensive.

In assessing the adequacy of depth clearance, whether it has proved possible to make use of a 'tumour barrier' may also determine suitability for use of a flap. Cartilage, and to a lesser extent bone also, are effective barriers to tumour spreading through them, and the act of removing them as part of the overall resection may convert the probability of clearance in depth into certainty, making the use of a flap, if preferable on cosmetic grounds, acceptable on pathological grounds.

Important also is the state of the surrounding skin. Skin tumours arise either in skin which has a normal appearance, or as the most neoplastically advanced focus in a skin which is diffusely dysplastic, most often as a result of sunlight damage. Such skin is seldom suitable for transfer as a local flap. Essentially pre-malignant, it is unsuitable on pathological grounds. Frequently atrophic, it is less than ideal for use as a local flap on technical grounds.

The infiltrative characteristics of the particular tumour type, whether it tends to remain superficial or infiltrate deeply, may also influence the type of reconstruction. At the opposite ends of the spectrum are the localised basal cell carcinoma with its typically lateral spread, and the 'single' squamous cell carcinoma with its pattern of deep as well as marginal spread. The skin tumours arising on sun damaged skin are also generally slow growing, and remain superficial unless neglected over a long period.

In judging the certainty of clearance at a clinical level, the degree of experience of the surgeon becomes important, the accuracy of his judgment in assessing the clearances appropriate to the various tumour types, and his skill in making use of tumour barriers. A further factor in the equation is whether there will be any increase in the lethal potential of the tumour should it recur locally. This in turn may depend on the anatomical site involved, and whether the pattern of growth and infiltration has been altered by the previous ineffective use of radiotherapy.

Problems of cosmesis

Skin grafts from certain donor areas give outstandingly good results in specific sites, but these apart, a well-chosen local flap will give a much better cosmetic result. Despite this, pathological factors cannot be ignored in making the choice. Skill in achieving the proper compromise between the two is generally a measure of experience. The less experienced surgeon should probably be using grafts more frequently, but most surgeons gradually move to an increasing use of flaps as their experience widens and their clinical judgment improves.

When the demands of the pathological situation and those of cosmesis appear to be incompatible, as for example when depth clearance is doubtful but a flap is cosmetically desirable, a compromise may be reached where, with the patient's agreement, a graft is used as a temporary measure despite its poor appearance. This allows the site to be watched until cure can be regarded as virtually certain, say after 12–18 months, depending on the tumour type, at which time the graft can be replaced with the definitive and cosmetically satisfactory flap.

Sometimes the characteristics of the defect make the use of a prosthesis appropriate during the period of observation, Further, when the age of the patient and the complexity of the reconstruction envisaged are considered, and the appearance likely ultimately to be achieved is compared with the appearance wearing the prosthesis, it may be that the latter should be used as the permanent 'reconstruction'. This situation arises most often when the pinna, and to a lesser extent the nose, are the organs involved (Fig. 10.1).

Local flaps are generally preferable to distant flaps, from the point of view both of convenience and the cosmetic result. A distant flap almost invariably gives a poorer colour and texture match, and though it may weather with time, the improvement is seldom enough to make it comparable with a local flap. The most frequent reason for using a distant flap in preference to a local flap is the size of the defect.

Distant flaps can be pedicled or free, and which is chosen may depend on whether the surgeon has the facilities and expertise which allow him to make the choice. For the surgeon confined to the use of pedicled flaps, the deltopectoral flap waltzed to its destination is probably the most

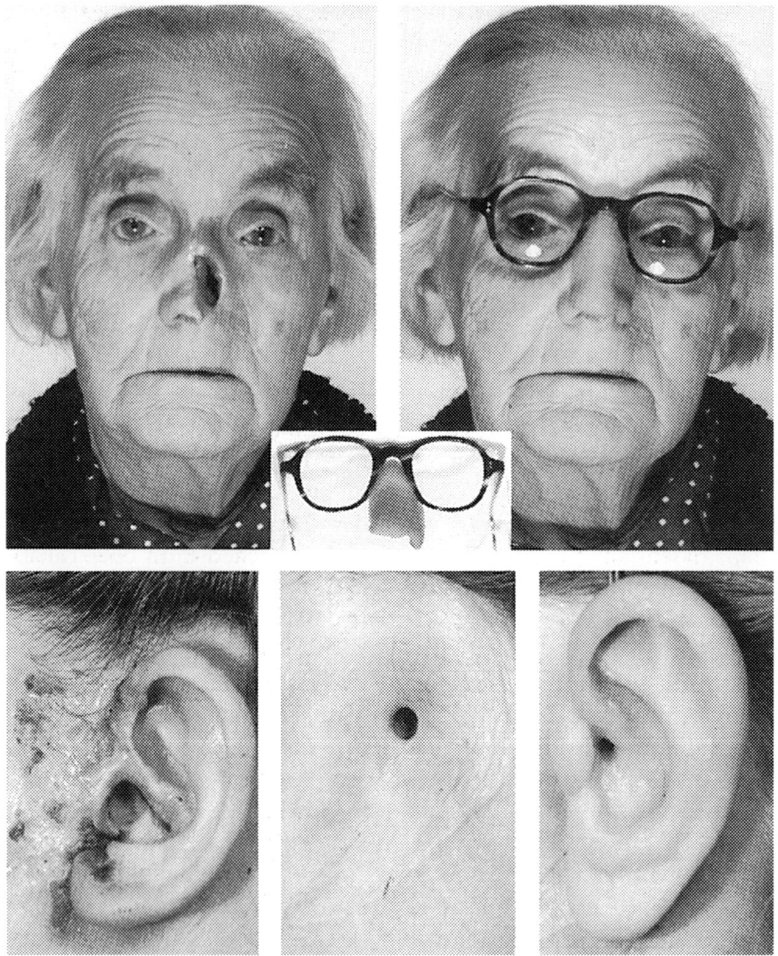

Fig. 10.1 The use of prostheses in the management of postexcisional defects, of the nose and of the pinna.
In both instances the prosthesis was used as the permanent 'reconstruction'. The age and general condition of the patient was considered to preclude definitive reconstruction of the nasal defect using the patient's own tissues. The defect of the pinna resulted from excision of a basal cell carcinoma of the pre-auricular skin, involving the pinna and the outer part of the external acoustic meatus. The defect was resurfaced with a split skin graft.

generally useful, though the restriction of its reach to the level of the zygomatic arch is a limiting factor. Even for the surgeon who has the liberty to choose, the deltopectoral flap is still worthy of consideration for defects within its reach.

Occasional overriding circumstances dictate departure from these general principles, and examples of these are:

1. Where a salivary fistula will be produced by the excision, it is preferable to carry out a primary definitive flap repair. Patients in general, and older patients in particular, do not tolerate such a fistula well. In any case such excisions usually involve the full thickness of the cheek or lip, and marginal recurrence alone need be watched for.

2. Where the tumour is inoperable in depth, the use of a flap is likely to make the use of radiotherapy easier and more effective.

RECONSTRUCTIVE TECHNIQUES

The use that can be made of **direct suture** in closing a post-excisional defect is dependent on the local availability of the facial skin. This parallels the presence of a wrinkle pattern, so often part of the ageing process, and how deeply it is etched in the skin. As already stressed (p. 3), the most obvious wrinkle patterns run at right angles to the underlying muscles of facial expression, and are concentrated around the mouth, eyelids and forehead, creating the vertical striations around the mouth, the nasolabial fold, the glabellar pattern, the 'crow's foot' pattern radiating from the lateral canthus, and the forehead wrinkles. These, and their magnitude at different sites, are indicative of the habitual facial expression of each individual. The occasional adult is met in whom there is a virtual absence of wrinkling, usually in association with a degree of facial rotundity. In such an individual, skin availability is minimal.

The wrinkle pattern indicates laxity of tissue on each side of the wrinkle, and it indicates also the line along which, or parallel to which, skin ellipses should be placed to give the best cosmetic result (Fig. 10.2).

An exception to this generalisation is provided by the forehead. The predominant wrinkle pattern in the forehead is horizontal, but in making use of excision and direct suture an overriding consideration is maintenance of the symmetry of the eyebrows. The anatomy of the galea–frontalis complex, fixed above and mobile below, means that a horizontal ellipse, excised and closed directly, is liable to raise the level of the eyebrow and create asymmetry. Because of this, unless the excision is a narrow one, vertical excisions are to be preferred. Unexpectedly, they result in remarkably inconspicuous scars if the wrinkle lines are matched on both sides.

The design of **local flaps** depends on the effective use of the areas of availability present in most adult facial skin. Elsewhere in the body the secondary defect left by the transfer of a local flap is covered with a split skin graft, but in the face the flaps are designed to leave the secondary defect in a site of skin laxity, allowing direct suture to be used.

The more obvious sites of such laxity are in the *mandibulomasseteric area*, the *nasolabial area*, the *temple*, and the *glabellar area* (Fig. 10.3). The amount of available skin varies greatly in different

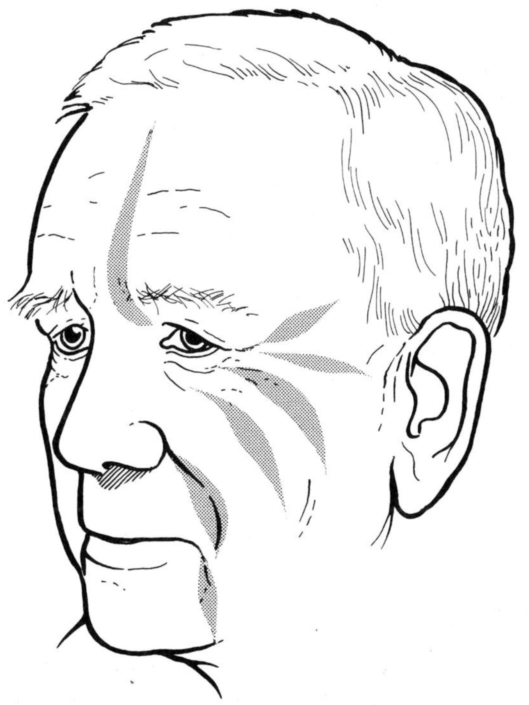

Fig. 10.2 Examples of elliptical excisions making use of the wrinkle pattern of the face.

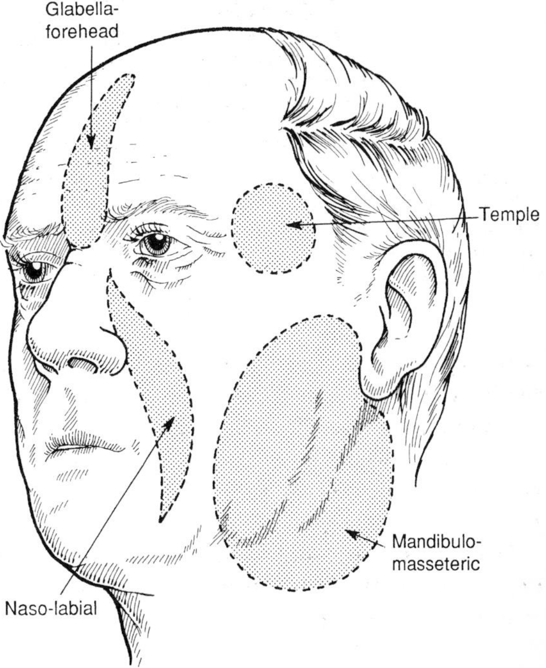

Fig. 10.3 The areas of skin availability which are exploited most frequently in local flap transfer – the mandibulomasseteric, nasolabial, glabellar and forehead areas, and the temple.

individuals, and parallels the presence of wrinkle lines. As already stressed in discussing the use of direct suture, the face which is free of wrinkles has little skin available, and this lack makes it also unsuitable for designing local flaps.

Many local flaps have been described, and each surgeon has his favourites, but the most useful, and the most frequently used, are those which fill a regularly recurring therapeutic need, and at the same time exploit the areas of availability most effectively. As part of the process of assessing suitability for the use of a flap, and designing it, it is essential to work out which area of availability is being made use of, and ascertain whether it is available. If it is not present, the flap is unlikely to be the appropriate one to use.

Flaps raised in the head and neck have certain distinctive qualities. They possess a richness of vascularity (Fig. 4.2), which permits a degree of laxity in design requirements unacceptable elsewhere. Below the level of the zygomatic arch, this is due to the richness of the dermal and subdermal circulation; above the arch, it is due to the wealth of vessels of a sizeable calibre which form an anastomotic pattern running horizontally between the skin and the galea, without deep connections, derived from vessels reaching the area from its periphery. The absence of deep connections means that delay of a scalp flap need never include elevation, and flaps with no overt axial pattern are raised both in the scalp and forehead which behave in transfer as though they did have such a system. In the face, the standard plane for elevating a flap is subdermal, superficial to the facial muscles; in the neck, it is deep to platysma, and designed to include as much of the superficial venous system as possible; in the forehead, it is deep to frontalis; in the scalp, it is deep to the galea.

The smaller flaps raised in the face also have a rich enough blood supply to allow the precise thickness of the defect often to be duplicated in the segment of the flap to be inset, though it may be wise to thicken the flap to the standard plane in passing from the segment to be inset to the pedicle.

The copious blood supply of flaps raised in the face and scalp also permits their bridge segment to be left raw without any danger of infection, for tubing is rarely technically possible. During the 3 weeks between initial transfer and division, the bridge segment tends to tube itself by fibrotic contraction of the raw surface and by marginal epithelialisation. If the bridge segment is being

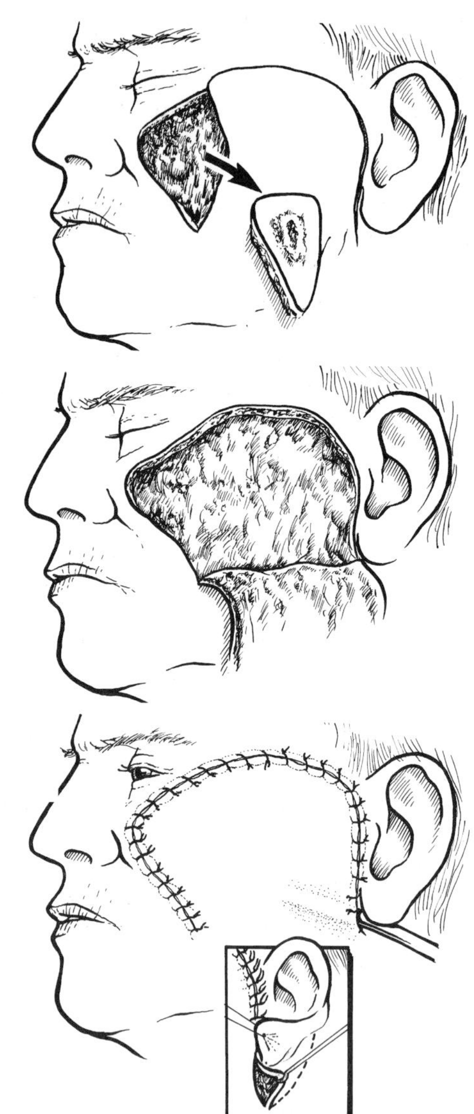

Fig. 10.4 Inferiorly based rotation flap used to reconstruct a defect of the cheek following excision of a basal cell carcinoma.

The skin excess adjoining the ear lobule, created by transfer of the flap, was managed using the method shown in Figure 4.32, with the scar resulting from the triangular skin excision concealed in the postauricular sulcus.

The anterior margin of the flap is designed to be slightly longer than the defect, and in passing back from the defect the curve of the flap initially rises. Both of these steps are designed to ensure that no downwards traction on the lower eyelid which might produce ectropion results from transfer of the flap.

discarded after division, this is of no moment, but if it is being returned to the donor site, untubing requires complete excision of the fibrous tissue, and the marginal spread epithelium is also best removed. Even so, the flap usually remains a little narrower than it was when first raised, and the margins of the donor site may have to be mobilised to allow easy suture.

Following division of the bridge segment, it is usually safe to inset the flap straightaway and, as with the direct flap (Fig. 4.22), a little thinning of its margin may be necessary to allow it to sit neatly into the defect.

CHEEKS AND SUBMANDIBULAR AREA

Defects of these sites may result from excision of tumours arising in the skin itself or tumours which have arisen in deeper structures, such as the parotid gland, and have spread to involve the skin, and they vary greatly in site and size. Full-thickness cheek defects can also result from deeply invasive tumours of the buccal mucosa, but their reconstruction is beyond the scope of this book.

Defects in the region of the nasolabial fold which are too broad for direct suture, are sufficiently close to a flat skin surface often to allow effective use of the rotation flap principle. The site and shape of the typical defect which is appropriate for the method most often suits an inferiorly based flap (Fig. 10.4), and it can give an excellent result. With the site of the defect a little higher, the superiorly based rotation flap (Fig. 10.5) can be equally effective, though the occasions to use it arise less frequently. Defects

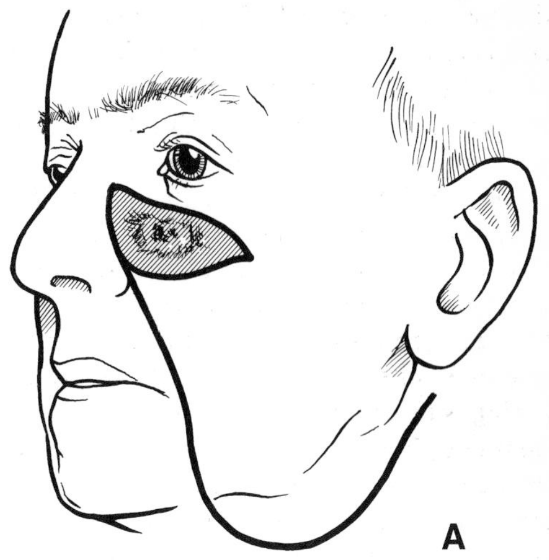

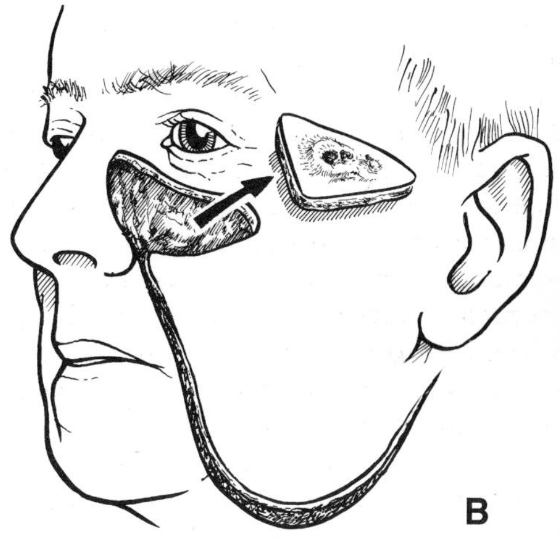

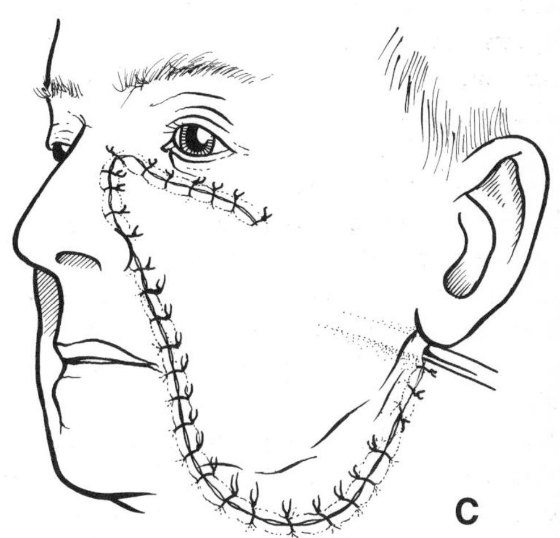

Fig. 10.5 Superiorly based rotation flap, used to reconstruct a defect of the cheek following excision of a basal cell carcinoma.

It was possible to transfer this flap without a back-cut because of the degree of general facial skin laxity, indicated by a marked nasolabial skin crease continued down beyond the angle of the mouth, and a submandibular skin crease with mandibulomasseteric skin redundancy, resulting in vagueness of the pivot point, as referred to in Figure 4.30. The use of the skin creases as the line of the flap helped to conceal the final scars. The junction line between the nose and the cheek was used as one of the resection margins, with the resection carried up towards the glabellar area beyond the medial extent of the medial canthus. This allowed the deep anchorage of the nasal skin to be used to counter the effect of gravity on the transferred flap, maintain it in its elevated position, and ensure that ectropion did not result.

over the parotid and the submandibular area are managed effectively by a free flap or a delto-pectoral flap, the latter capable of reaching almost as far as the zygomatic arch (Fig. 4.34). The initial pallor of both flaps makes them somewhat conspicuous, but their appearance improves appreciably as they weather with time.

FOREHEAD, TEMPLE AND SCALP

In these sites, there are anatomical differences in the constituents of the soft tissues, which influence both the resections and the reconstructions carried out. In the *scalp*, the skin, superficial fascia and galea are firmly attached to one another and are managed as a single structure. The tissue layer separating the galea from the pericranium provides the surgical plane, both in resection and reconstruction. Tumours superficial to the galea are resected to that plane, regardless of how superficial they may be, and flaps are also raised in that plane.

In the *temporal area*, the temporalis muscle, with its covering of temporal fascia, intervenes between the galea, thinner in this area, and the skull, and the surgical plane changes to one between the galea and the temporal fascia.

In the *forehead*, the galea is replaced by the frontalis muscle, and its presence makes it possible to raise flaps superficial as well as deep to it. The plane superficial to it is not a natural one, and has to be created by scalpel dissection. Its usage is generally confined to small flaps.

The use of these surgical planes leaves a graftable surface, whether pericranial or fascial.

In planning reconstructions in these areas, a major consideration is the mixture of sites, some hair bearing, some hairless, with the need to retain each in its proper position. A further complicating factor may be the pattern of baldness, both the one already present and the one likely to develop.

Forehead defects can be primary, the result of a local tumour excision, or secondary to the transfer of a flap. In both instances their management depends on the width of the defect. When direct suture is possible, vertical closure is generally best, with care to match wrinkle lines. When a defect is too large for direct closure, it usually has to be split skin grafted, though the use of tissue expansion (p. 121) may allow the graft to be excised subsequently.

The *temple* is a regular site for small tumours, and their excision provides the problem of devising a reconstruction which will allow the position of the anterior hairline and the eyebrow to be maintained, and the distance between them. An effective solution makes use of the **rhomboid flap** (Fig. 10.6). Around the lesion, with adequate local clearance, a rhomboid is drawn on the skin, with a short diagonal which equals the lengths of the sides, giving the appearance of two equilateral triangles placed side by side. The diagonal is extended for a distance equal to its original length and, from the extremity, a back cutting line is drawn parallel to one of the sides of the rhomboid. The rhomboid of tissue which contains the lesion is excised, and the rhomboid-shaped flap, outlined by the extended diagonal and the backcut, is raised and transferred into the defect, which it fills neatly. The resulting secondary defect is closed directly.

Although the dimensions and shape of both defect and flap are precise, there are variables in planning, namely which of the four potential flaps should be used, and the axis around which the excisional rhomboid can be drawn. It is possible to manipulate these variables in such a way that closure of the secondary defect makes use of the laxity of skin present in the temple area, as indicated by the wrinkle pattern extending back from the outer canthus. With completion of the transfer, the rhomboid flap has filled the rhomboid defect, and the relevant distances and positions of the eyebrow and the hairline have been maintained.

Management of defects of the *scalp* is dominated by its physical characteristics, its rigidity and inextensibility. Direct suture can only be used for small defects. It is generally stated that 'scoring' of the galea will act as relaxing incisions, but the amount of advancement achieved in practice is virtually nil. Fortunately, scalp is more tolerant of suture under tension than most tissues. The strength and inextensibility of the galea appear to prevent tension from being significantly transmitted to its vascular system.

The majority of defects which are too large for

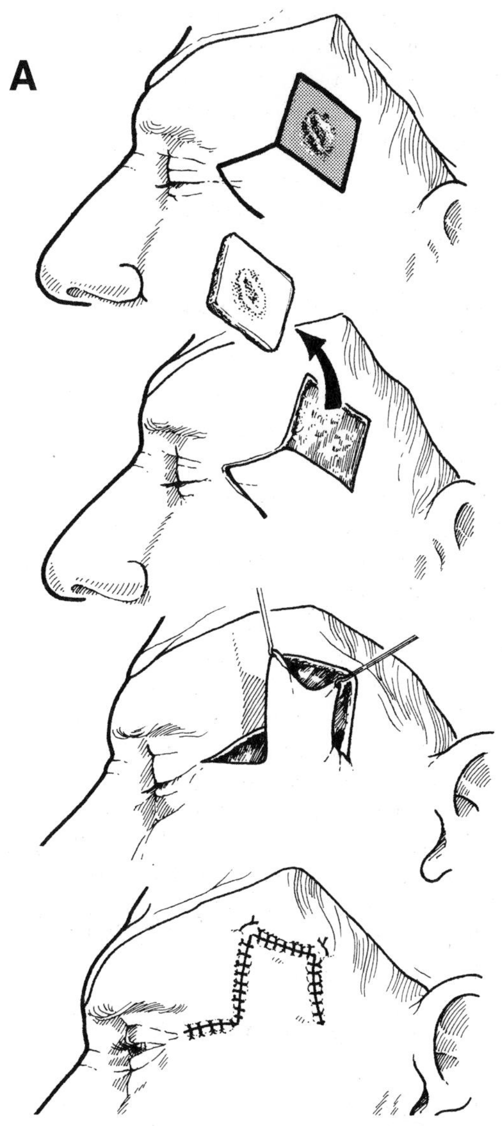

direct suture are split skin grafted. In their subsequent management, the tissue expander has an obvious role in eliminating the hairless area, should the patient be concerned about it.

Flaps are used mainly when the tumour has extended into or beyond the pericranium, and its resection has left an area of bare skull. The area of hairbearing scalp without anatomical features around such defects makes it possible as a rule to design both transposition and rotation flaps. When a transposition flap is used, the excellence of the local blood supply makes it safe for a flap to be designed which is narrower than it is long (Fig. 4.25). In the case of a rotation flap, the rigidity of the scalp and its inextensibility set very strict limits on design. The flap should be made as large as possible, since that reduces the relative amount of rotation involved, and a back-cut is almost invariably required. The secondary defect it leaves has to be split skin grafted.

When the defect is of a size or in a site which precludes the design of a satisfactory local flap, the appropriate reconstruction today is probably a free flap.

LIPS

The orbicularis oris muscle acts as a sphincter, functioning in conjunction with dilator muscle groups in normal activity. In reconstructions of the lip the surgeon aims for continence of the oral cavity, and the maintenance of sphincteric function is his primary concern. An important contribution to the blood supply of the area is made by the labial arteries which run across each lip at the level of the skin–vermilion border between the mucosa and the muscles of the lip, meeting in the mid-line. These vessels make possible the safe transfer of the large segments of lip tissue used in several of the standard lip reconstructions.

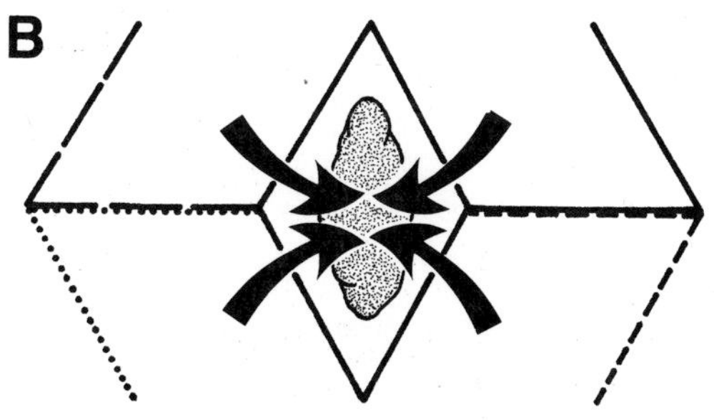

Fig. 10.6 The rhomboid flap used to reconstruct a defect of the temple, leaving the relationship between the eyebrow and the hairline undisturbed, and the scar of closure of the secondary defect in a line of election. The steps of the transfer are shown (**A**), and the possible four flaps which are theoretically available to reconstruct the rhomboid defect (**B**). The flap selected in practice depends on the local availability of skin, and whether there is enough 'slack' present locally to allow the secondary defect to be closed directly.

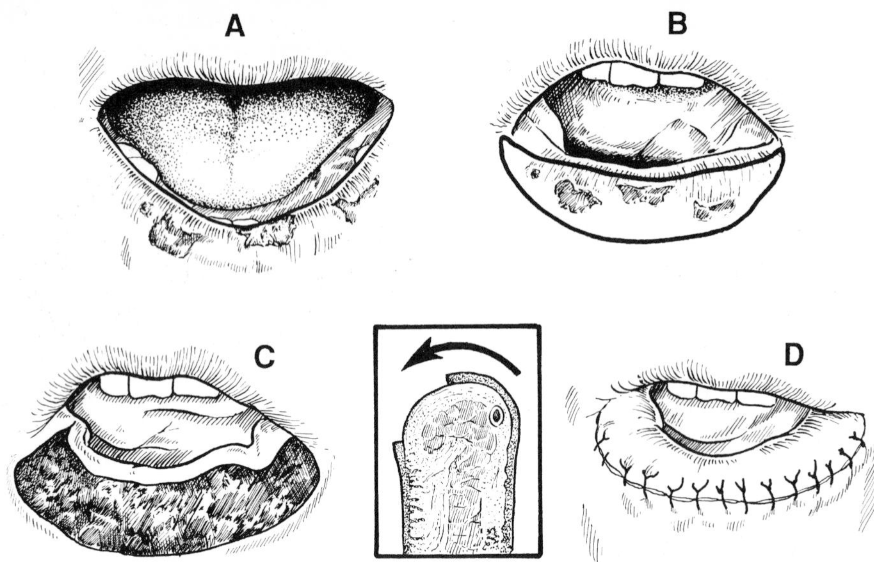

Fig. 10.7 The lip-shave with mucosal advancement.

A Shows the lesion, multifocal premalignancy of the vermilion, suitable for such resurfacing.
B The extent of the area of vermilion, angle-to-angle, to be excised.
C The defect following the lip-shave.
Inset shows the extent and depth of the vermilionectomy.
D Closure of the defect of the vermilion by advancing the mucosa.
Undermining of the mucosa to permit advancement is not necessary, and its use can result in mucosal necrosis.

The commonest tumour involving the lips is actinically induced squamous cell carcinoma, and the commonest site is the vermilion of the lower lip. It may arise as a single lesion, or as the most neoplastically advanced area in a diffusely premalignant vermilion, and the premalignant state can also occur on its own. Such actinically induced neoplasms generally progress slowly.

The vermilion which shows premalignant change is treated by a **lip-shave** (Fig. 10.7). The exposed vermilion is stripped from angle to angle, and the mucosa lining the lip is advanced to close the defect and resurface the lip margin.

When there is also a focal area of greater induration suggestive of early invasion, and requiring greater clearance in depth, more of the substance of the vermilion needs to be removed. The roundness of the margin can then be restored by using a **tongue flap** (Fig. 10.8) to replace the resected tissue. This involves the raising of a mucomuscular flap along the anterior margin of the dorsum of the tongue, and suturing it to the skin resection margin of the lip, the flap being divided when it has settled in its new site, usually by the 10th day. The method is also used to provide a vermilion substitute in certain of the more elaborate reconstructions of the lower lip, described below.

A focus of frankly invasive squamous cell carcinoma is treated by excising a full thickness segment of the lip. *The extent of the resection depends on the size of the tumour but, because the reconstructions used in practice require the creation of suitably shaped defects, a certain amount of normal tissue is also excised as part of the total resection, beyond the excision necessary to clear the tumour, in*

Fig. 10.8 *(opposite page)* The 'deep' lip-shave resurfaced with a tongue flap.
1 Shows the lesion of the lip, a squamous carcinoma showing very early invasion, with diffuse premalignancy of the remaining vermilion, and **2** the defect following excision. **3** Shows the line of the incision along the anterior margin of the tongue with the incision begun, **4** completed, and **5** the tongue flap raised. **6** Shows the depth of the excision, and how the tongue flap covers the defect, **7** the flap sutured in position, and **8** the result after the division of the flap two weeks after the initial transfer.

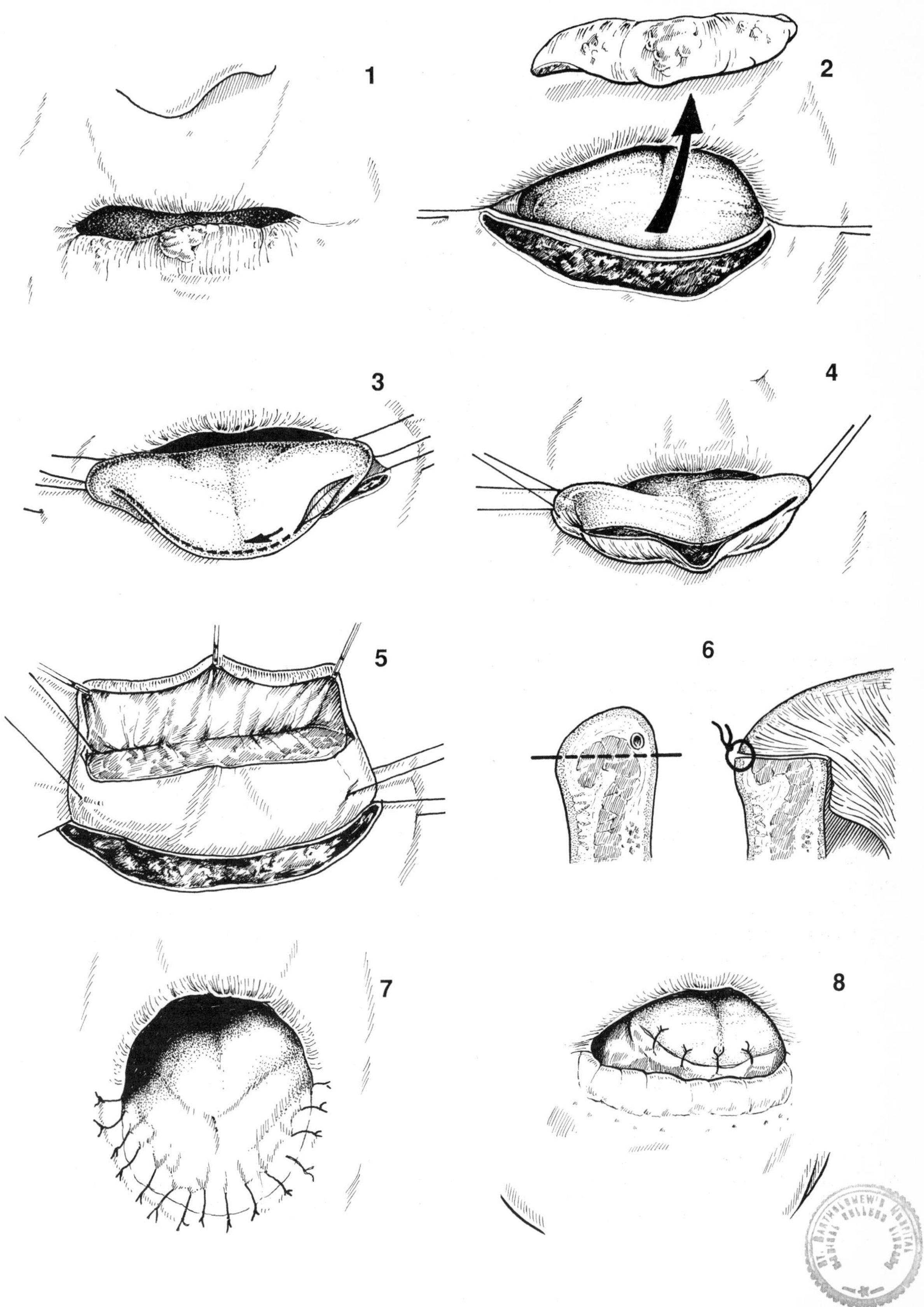
1
2
3
4
5
6
7
8

order to create the desired shape. This principle applies also in many of the resection/reconstructions described in this Chapter.

When the focus of invasive tumour coexists with diffuse premalignancy of the vermilion, the techniques of managing each element are used in combination, with a full thickness excision of the main focus of squamous cell carcinoma, and a lip-shave of the remaining premalignant vermilion.

Wedge excision and direct suture (Fig. 10.9) is used when the defect measures less than one-third of the lip, this being the breadth of lip which can be excised as a V, and closed directly without unduly constricting the opening. The defect is closed in two layers. Undermining of the skin for 2–3 mm defines a mucomuscular layer on each side of the V, and the two are approximated with vertical absorbable mucomuscular mattress sutures. These take the strain of the repair

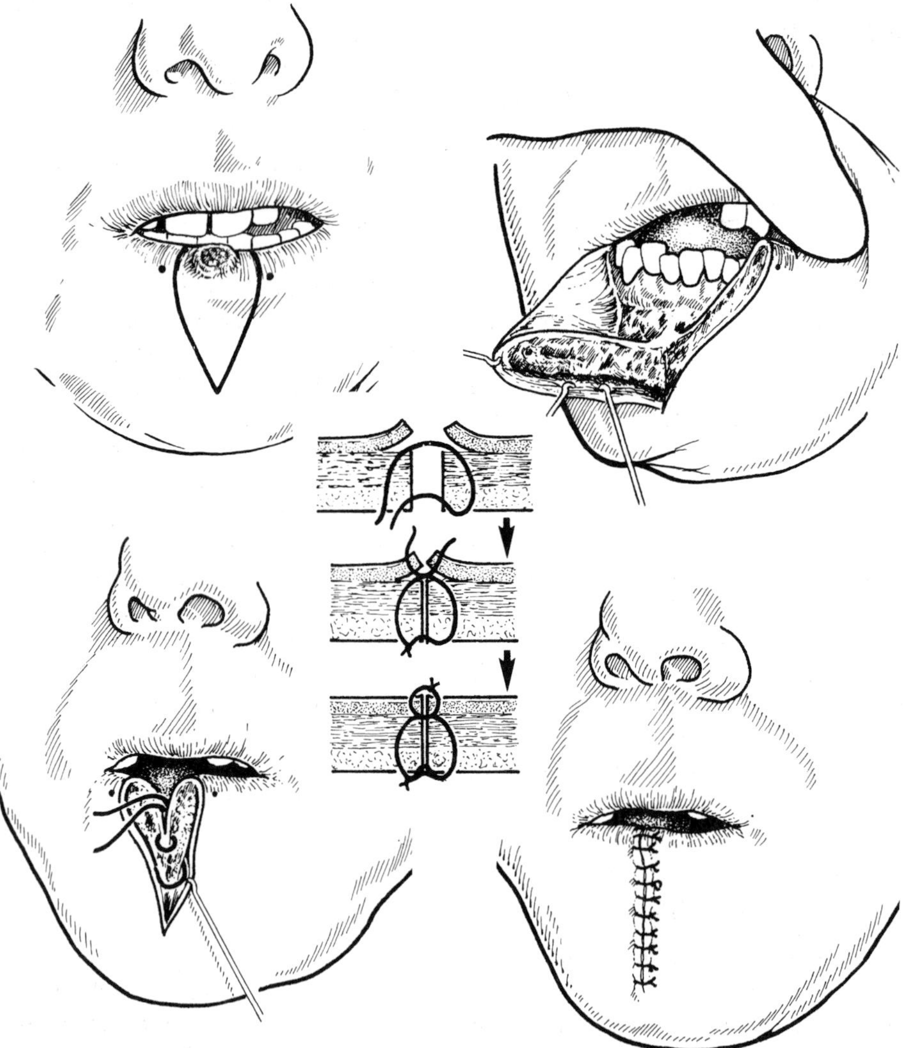

Fig. 10.9 Wedge excision of the lower lip and direct closure.
The skin and subcutaneous layer is mobilised from the mucomuscular layer for 2–3 mm from the cut edge of the lip. A two-layer closure is used, muscle and mucosa joined with a single mucomuscular mattress absorbable suture which takes the strain of the closure, followed by skin closure.
Preoperative tattooing with Bonney's Blue is used to mark the junction of the skin and the red margin on each side of the excision to facilitate subsequent matching. This technique is used in lip reconstructions where such matching is required.

and allow the skin edges to be closed without tension or tendency to invert. This suturing method is also used in the reconstructions described below.

In repairing cleft lip defects it is common practice to incorporate a Z-plasty of the vermilion to give a smoother margin to the lip, but in cancer surgery it is preferable to retain the straight suture line so that a single line only has to be watched for recurrence of tumour.

When resection results in loss of more than one-third of the lip, a formal reconstruction of the resected segment is required and, for the reason explained above, the excision is generally carried out in the form of a rectangle. When the defect is of one-half of the lower lip and extends to one angle reconstruction can make use of the **fan flap** (Fig. 10.10A). In this an approximately circular flap of the full thickness of the cheek is raised lateral to the angle of the mouth and centred on it, with a final back-cut which reaches almost to the vermilion at the angle leaving a narrow pedicle, but one which contains the superior labial vessels. The flap is rotated to fill the lower lip defect and sutured in position. The effect is to leave the angle at its original site and maintain the width of the mouth. The secondary defect in the nasolabial area is closed directly, taking up the slack which is present in that area of availability. The reconstructed lip segment lacks a vermilion, and this is best provided by incorporating a tongue flap. When a combined resection and lip-shave of the remaining pre-malignant vermilion is required, a tongue flap is used to reconstruct the vermilion, angle to angle.

On the rare occasions when the entire lip is excised this fan flap technique can be duplicated, the flap raised on each side being rotated to meet its fellow on the opposite side (Fig. 10.10B), with a tongue flap to reconstruct the vermilion. The fan flap, single or double, designed in this way, is totally denervated, but sensation returns gradually, although usually effectively. Motor activity is also restored, but more slowly.

When the lip defect involves up to two-thirds of its width, but preferably does not reach either angle, the reconstruction which produces the best result is the **neurovascular (Karapandzic) fan flap** (Fig. 10.11). On each side of the rectangular defect, a circular line with radius equal to the vertical height of the lip defect is drawn on the skin around the angle, stopping just short of the alar base. Along the two lines the skin is incised, and deepened to, but not through, the mucosa, its proximity recognised by the presence of the grape-like clusters of minor salivary glands. In the process, the dilator muscles which are part of the orbicularis complex are divided, but the nerves, motor and sensory, and the blood vessels which cross the incision lines are carefully preserved. From each side of the defect the mucosa also is divided laterally for 1 cm. This allows the excision margins to be approximated and sutured vertically, in the process rotating the fan flaps of skin and muscle on each side. The skin incisions on both sides are sutured together in their new position, taking up the disproportion all the way along. With preservation of the nerves, the reconstructed lip retains both motor power and sensation from the outset.

The upper lip is a much less frequent site of tumour, but when excision leaves a full thickness defect it is usually filled with a **lip-switch (Abbe) flap** (Fig. 10.12). This is a flap of the entire thickness of the lower lip, generally constructed in the form of a V, with a narrow pedicle containing the inferior labial vessels. It is rotated into the upper lip to reconstruct the defect, and the defect of the lower lip is closed directly. The presence of the pedicle tethers the lips together at its site until it is divided 2 weeks later. The lower lip is able to provide a flap up to one-third of its width, and the reconstruction can be used for defects at any site on the upper lip of a suitable size and shape. When the defect extends to the angle of the mouth, the same method can still be used, in the form of the **Abbe–Estlander flap**, the pedicle becoming the new angle (Fig. 10.13).

EYELIDS

The tarsal plates form the skeletal basis of both eyelids, held against the eyeball by the attachment of the palpebral ligaments, medial and lateral, to the margin of the orbit. Their strength is not great and, in the lower eyelid particularly, they are very susceptible to tightness of the skin, resulting in ectropion.

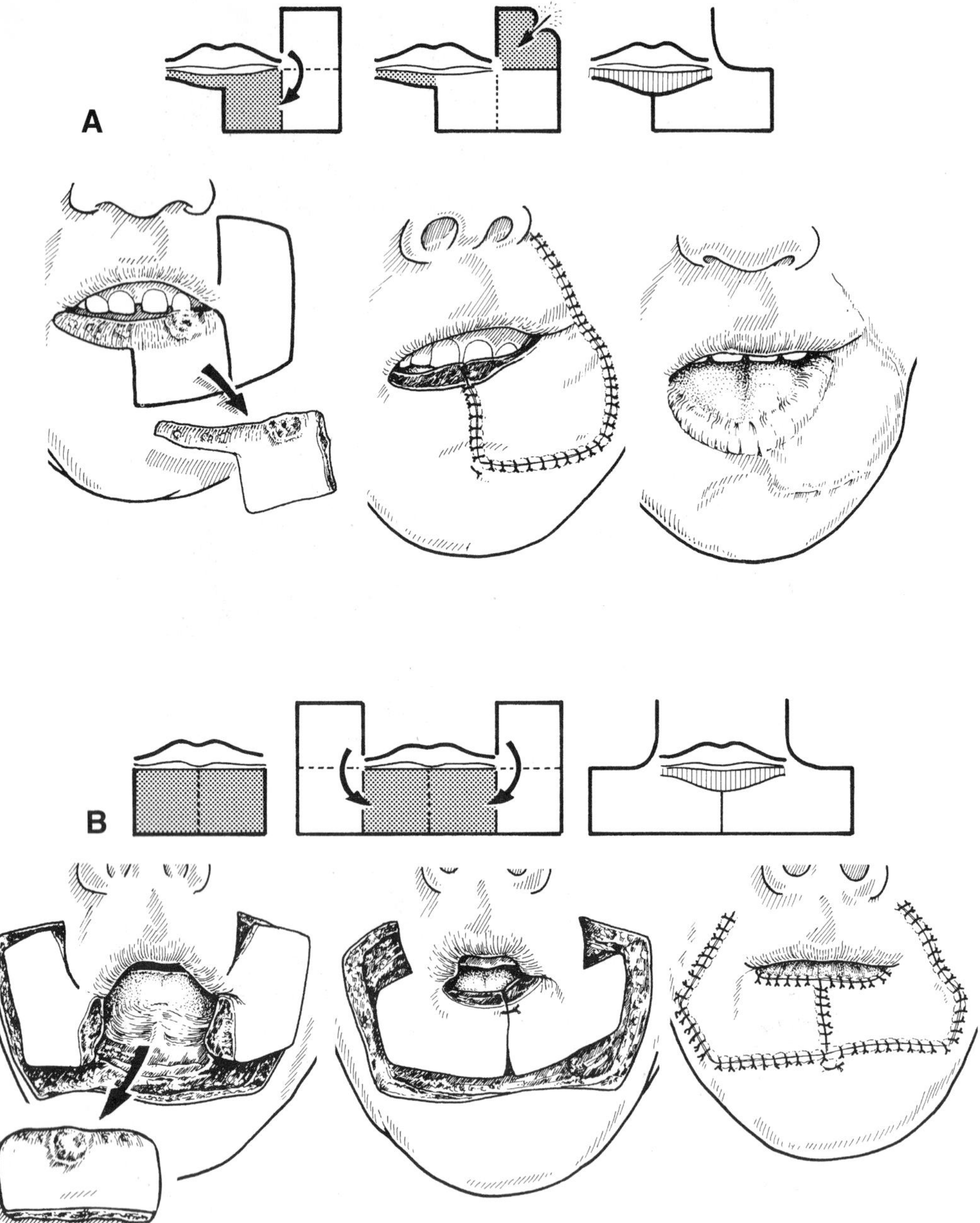

Fig. 10.10 The fan flap, used in combination with a tongue flap, to reconstruct full thickness defects of the lower lip.

A The method used following resection of half of the lip. The extent of the resection of the lesion, a squamous carcinoma with associated diffuse premalignancy of the adjoining vermilion, is outlined and the flap used to reconstruct it. The flap, which includes the full thickness of the cheek, is rotated into the lip defect, leaving a nasolabial defect which is closed by advancing the nasolabial tissues. The vermilion is restored with a tongue flap, using the method shown in Figure 10.8.

B The fan flap used bilaterally in combination with a tongue flap following resection of the entire lip. The steps are similar to those shown in **A**, but with a fan flap raised on each cheek, each flap rotating to form half of the reconstructed lip.

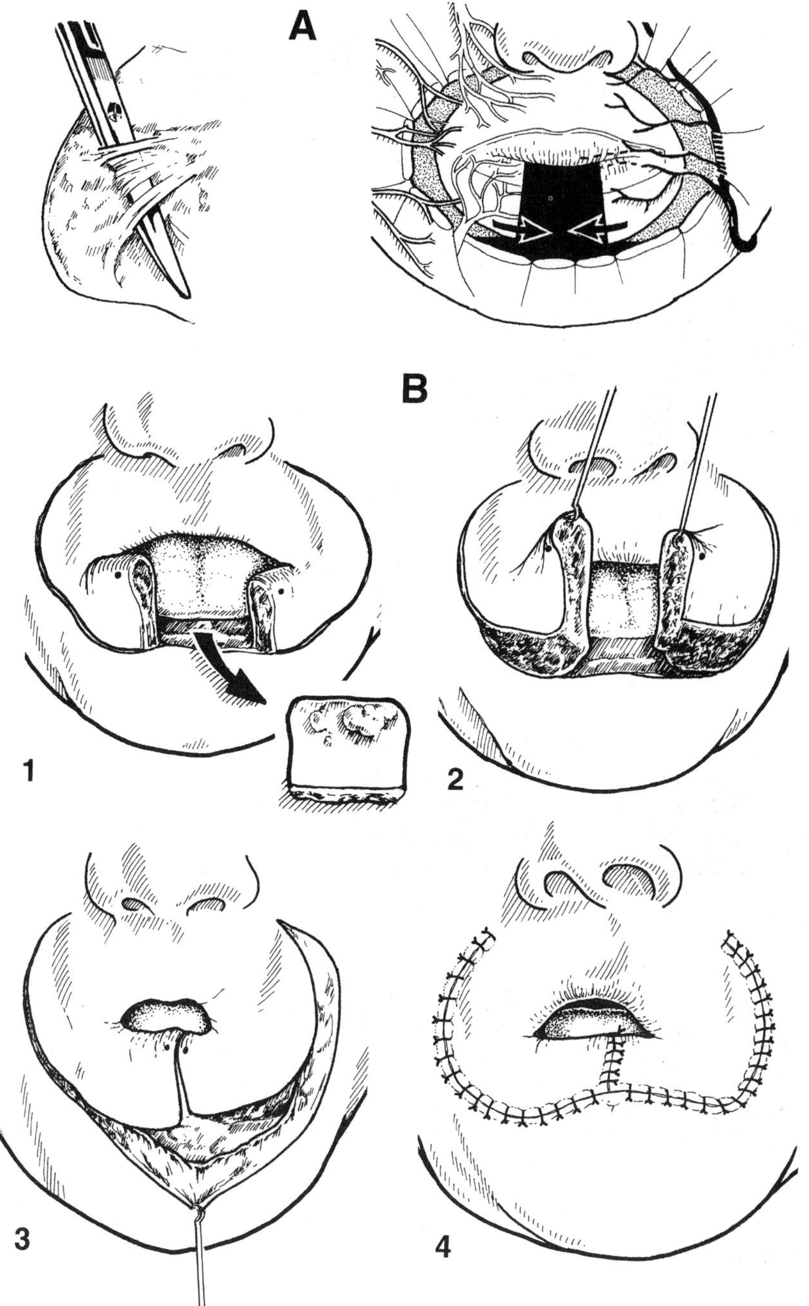

Fig. 10.11 The neurovascular fan flap, used to reconstruct the defect left following full thickness resection of the central two-thirds of the lower lip.

A shows the principle of the method, reconstructing the defect while preserving the neurovascular supply of the lip.

B The steps of the reconstruction. Following the full thickness lip resection, a semicircular incision, centred on the angle of the mouth, is made on each side (**1**), from the resection margin round to the alar base. Except at its commencement, where the incision is made through the full thickness of the lip, skin and muscle only are divided (**2**), the nerves and blood vessels crossing the line of the incision being carefully preserved. The flaps which this creates on each side are advanced to the midline (**3**) and sutured to one another, the skin incisions being then closed (**4**).

The very considerable virtue of this method lies in the maintenance of an intact nerve supply, motor and sensory, to the reconstructed lip.

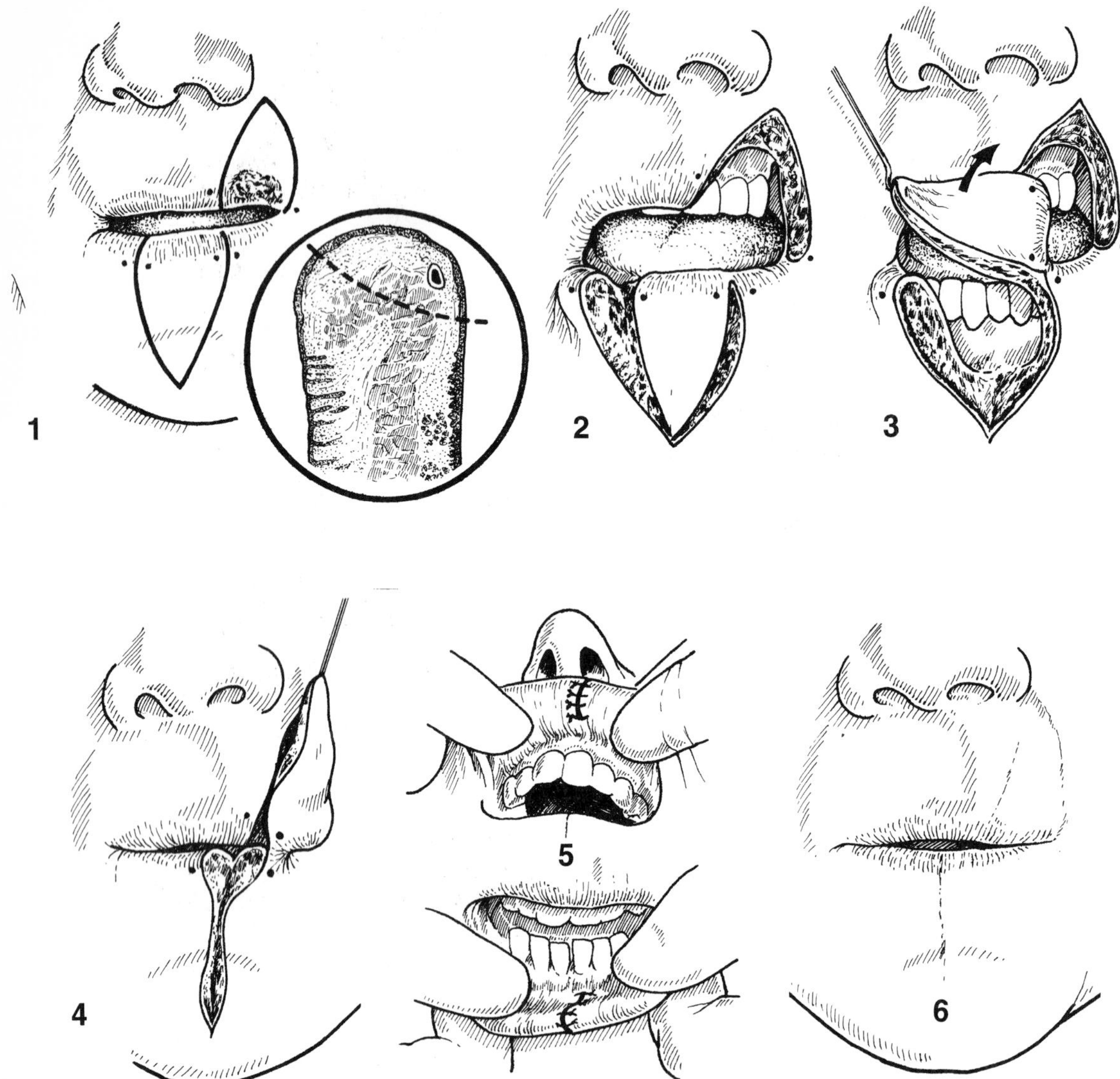

Fig. 10.12 The lip-switch (Abbe) flap, used to reconstruct a full thickness wedge excision of the upper lip.

The flap is outlined on the lower lip as a wedge to fill the defect of the full thickness of the upper lip resulting from the resection of the tumour involving the vermilion (**1**). **Inset**, the pedicle of the flap with its content of inferior labial artery. With the upper lip defect and the Abbe flap raised (**2**), its pedicle, as shown in the inset, is confined within the vermilion. The flap is rotated upwards on its pedicle (**3**), and filling the upper lip defect, is sutured in position (**4**) using the layered closure shown in Figure 10.9, with the lower lip defect closed in the same way. Two weeks later the pedicle is divided (**5**), and sutured following division, with (**6**) the final result.

The construction of the pedicle completely within the red margin allows the various skin-vermilion borders to be matched at the stage of the initial transfer so that no adjustment is required when the pedicle is divided.

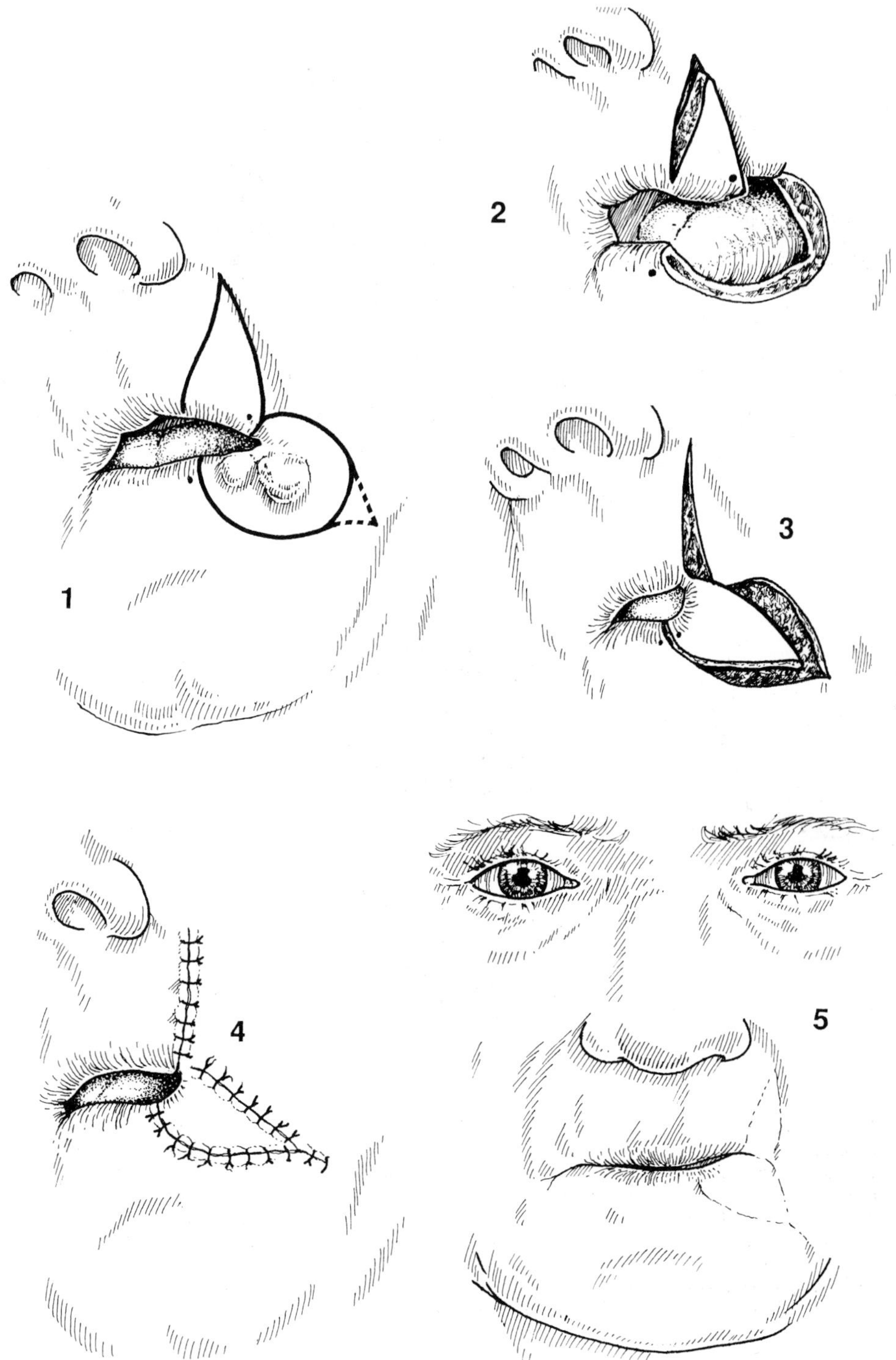

Fig. 10.13 The modified lip-switch (Abbe–Estlander) flap. This flap is used when the defect of the lip is at the angle of the mouth, and the pedicle of the flap becomes the angle of the reconstructed mouth.

The lesion is of the lower lip directly adjoining the angle of the mouth, shown with the resection outlined (**1**), and the flap marked out on the upper lip. The resection is carried out (**2**), and the flap raised, its pedicle similar to that shown in Figure 10.12. The flap is rotated into the defect (**3**), and sutured in position, using the two layer closure shown in Figure 10.9, suture of the skin (**4**), completing the reconstruction, with (**5**) the final result.

In the upper eyelid, an element of skin laxity is almost invariably present in the age group usually involved by neoplasia. In the lower eyelid, there is never the same degree of skin laxity and, with gravity working against the surgeon, direct suture of a post-resection defect is rarely an option if ectropion is to be avoided.

Ideally, skin grafted to an eyelid defect should be as thin and flexible as normal eyelid skin, but in practice the need for mobility varies at different sites, greatest at the upper palpebral furrow, less on the lower eyelid below the tarsal plate, least over the tarsal plates, lower and upper, and the canthi. In managing postresection defects the full thickness graft of postauricular skin has proved in practice to have sufficient mobility to make it entirely acceptable, with an excellent colour and texture match, and no tendency to contract secondarily. The technical aspects of its use in this site are illustrated in Figures 3.7 and 3.17.

The skin of the upper eyelid is made use of for reconstructive purposes in the so-called **Tripier flap** (Fig. 10.14). This flap, raised together with the underlying orbicularis muscle, extends across the entire width of the eyelid and is swung on its two pedicles, in the form of a 'bucket handle', to fill a lower lid defect. The secondary defect is closed directly, and this, together with the degree of skin redundancy present in the lid, determines the limit of its width. Despite its remarkable length:breadth ratio, necrosis of a Tripier flap is virtually unknown. The explanation may lie in the fact that in the age group involved the flap is extremely thin, despite its content of orbicularis muscle, and its thinness probably allows it to 'take' partly as a graft. The dusky colour which it frequently develops during its elevation and transfer can be ignored. In providing cover, it has the virtues associated with upper eyelid skin used as a free skin graft.

With the postauricular full thickness graft and the Tripier flap both available to reconstruct lower lid defects, and each capable of giving an excellent result, cosmetic and functional, a problem of choice arises. The posterior surface of the ear is capable of providing enough skin to resurface any potential eyelid defect, and to that extent it has the greater versatility. The width of the Tripier flap is restricted by the need to be able to close the secondary defect of the upper eyelid, and this limits its potential.

The Tripier flap is used to provide the skin element in reconstructing full thickness defects of the lower lid where extension of the tumour has been predominantly horizontal, and it has been its effectiveness in that role which has led to its use in partial thickness defects. Within its limitations of breadth, and these can be established at the planning stage, the flap can be used for defects of the lower lid where tumour extension has been predominantly horizontal, within the extremes of medial to lateral canthus.

Depending on the site of the defect on the eyelid, the transferred flap may have a bridge segment. This segment tubes itself extremely rapidly, and even the segment of the flap which is inset into the defect has a marked tendency to tube itself. This is prevented by using a lightly applied tie-over dressing to positively untube it. The mild pressure which such a dressing exerts may also help the flap to attach deeply and vascularise quickly. When a bridge segment is present, division and insetting is required to complete the reconstruction, although patients often express a reluctance to have it carried out, since the intact bridge segment is barely noticeable and gives them no trouble.

Where the resection is near one or other canthus, and extends only as far as the centre of the eyelid, the design can be modified, to use only half of the flap, with a single pedicle.

Many of the tumours which involve the lower eyelid are small enough to be suitable for a Tripier flap reconstruction, particularly when they are near one or other canthus, and the flap itself is thin enough not to obscure any tumour recurring deep to it.

The regular sites of basal cell carcinoma, the tumour which involves the eyelids most often, are the medial canthal area and the lower lid. The upper eyelid in the skin overlying the tarsal plate is an occasional site.

When the tumour arises in the *medial canthal area*, the eyelid, upper and/or lower, becomes involved by marginal extension, and resection generally leaves a surface, both in the nasal bridge and the eyelid/s, which accepts a free skin graft. Resection of the entire lid thickness is only

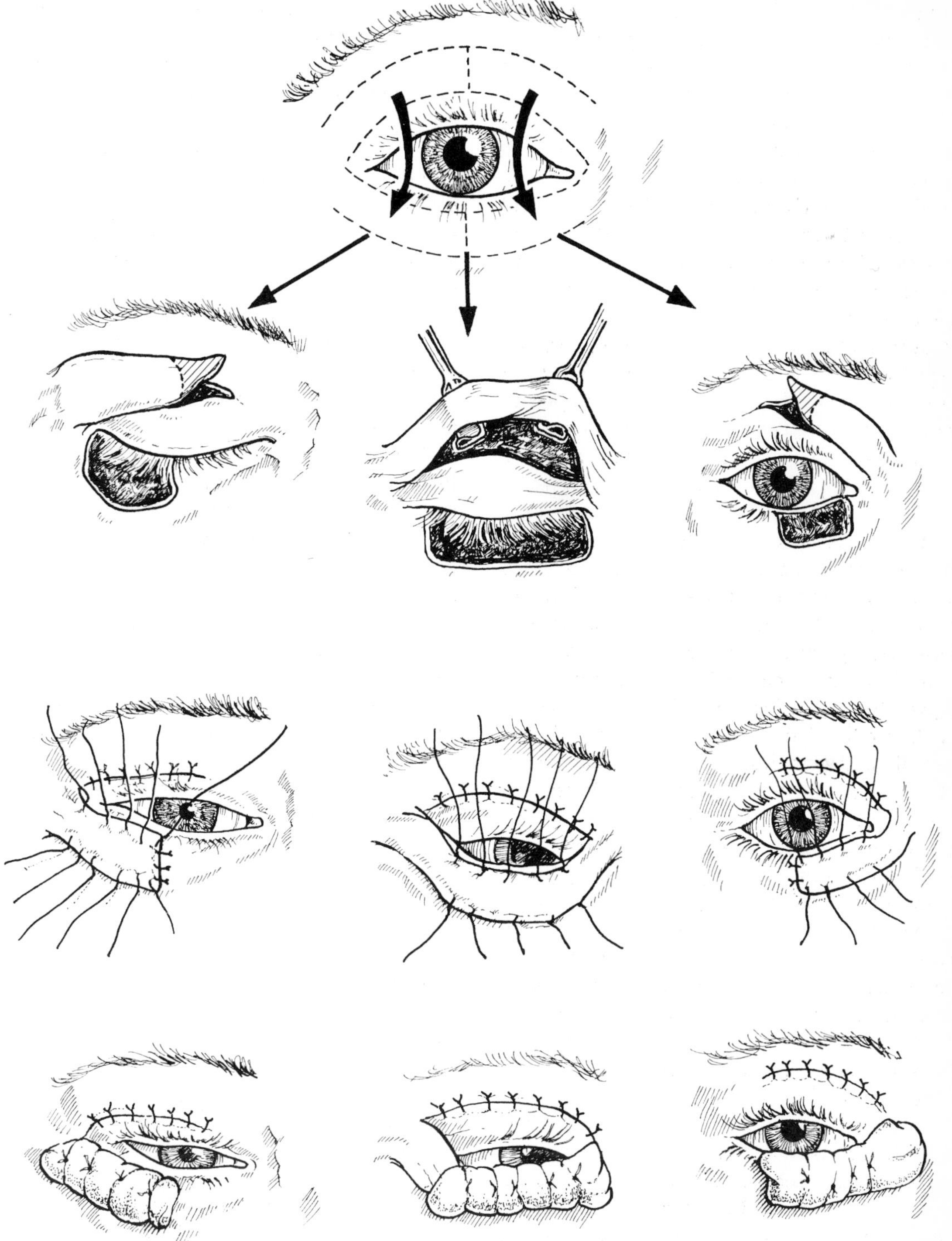

Fig. 10.14 The Tripier flap, as used to provide the skin component of lower eyelid defects.

The flap, raised on the redundant skin usually present in the upper eyelid of the older patient, and including the underlying orbicularis muscle, is extremely versatile, capable of being used with a single pedicle to reconstruct defects near the canthi, medial or lateral, and as a 'bucket handle' bipedicled flap, to reconstruct defects of the central segment of the eyelid.

The Tripier flap has a marked tendency to tube itself, and to prevent this from happening it is usual to use a light tie-over dressing to hold the flap in a positively untubed position during the healing phase.

required when such a tumour is deeply invasive over the whole area, and the management of such an advanced tumour is beyond the scope of this book.

When the primary site is the *lower eyelid*, resection leaves a defect which can vary from one of skin alone up to the full thickness of the lid. The degree of mobility of the tumour on the orbicularis muscle and tarsal plate is an excellent indicator of whether a partial thickness resection of the lid will be adequate, or whether a full thickness resection is needed. The majority of the tumours seen in clinical practice are superficial, and only require resection of skin and part thickness of orbicularis muscle, though the closer the lesion to the lid margin the more likely it is to be found that a full thickness resection is required. The presence of distortion of the lid is virtually diagnostic of the need for a full thickness excision.

The management of a tumour involving the upper eyelid depends very much on its site and extent. The skin laxity of the eyelid in the age group generally involved is maximal in the region of the palpebral furrow, and allows direct closure of a larger defect in that site than one might expect. The degree of laxity there also allows the skin to be advanced downwards over the tarsal plate to close a defect in that site directly. The postauricular full thickness graft also gives an excellent result when a superficial tumour overlying the tarsal plate is excised (Fig. 10.15). It is most often when the lid margin is involved that a full thickness excision becomes unavoidable, and the reconstruction of such a defect is beyond the scope of this book.

When the extent of a lower eyelid tumour and its shape requires excision of a V-shaped wedge of the eyelid, the defect is closed by approximating the two limbs of the V. Making the V-defect involves dividing the full thickness of the eyelid–conjunctiva, tarsal plate and skin at the same level, and this is best achieved using sharp pointed scissors, rather than a scalpel, with the lid on each side of the cut supported with skin hooks (Fig. 10.16). The skin is so mobile on the

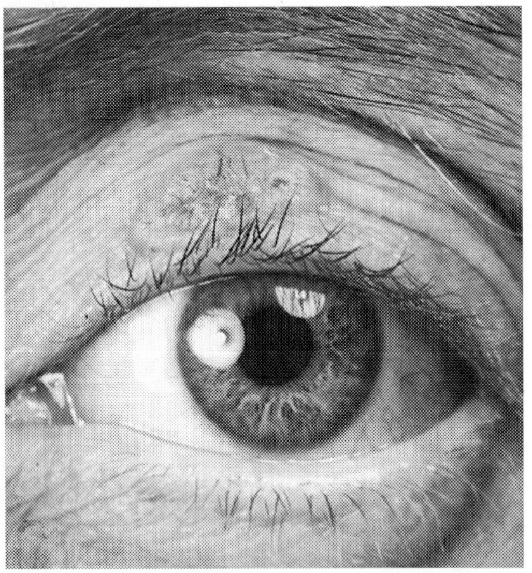

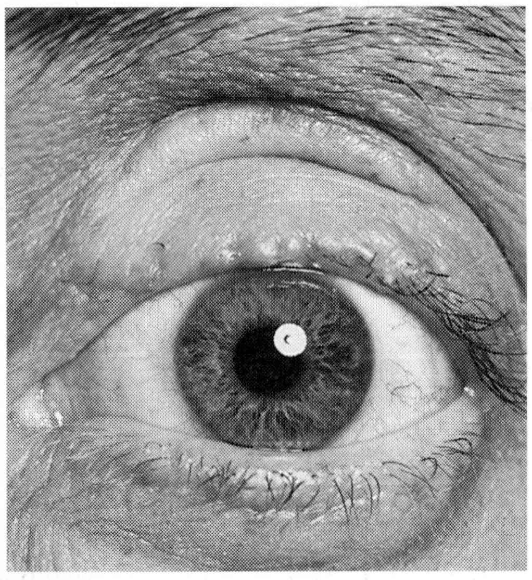

Fig. 10.15 A full thickness skin graft used to reconstruct a defect overlying the tarsal plate of the upper eyelid following excision of a basal cell carcinoma.

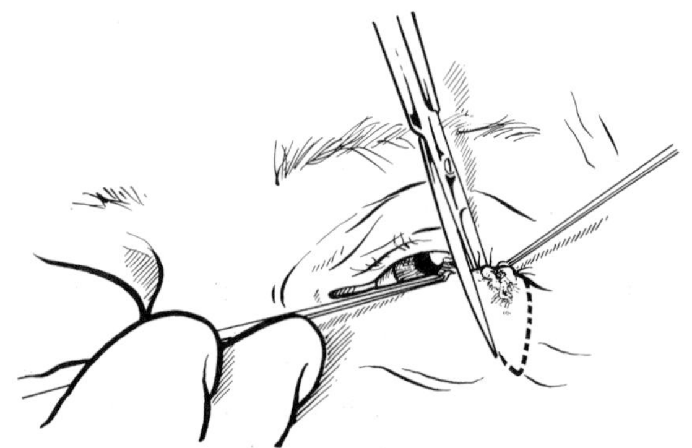

Fig. 10.16 The use of sharp pointed scissors to section the eyelid. The lid margin on each side of the proposed line of cut is steadied with skin hooks.

tarsal plates that cutting with a scalpel tends to result in a less tidy cut.

V-excision and direct suture (Fig. 10.17) is used when the V is narrow, and the landmarks of the lid margin – eyelashes, the grey line, the junction of conjunctiva and skin – are used in matching the two sides of the V. The method of suture used to close the defect is designed to avoid suture material being exposed in the conjunctival sac, since it causes irritation of the cornea where the two come into contact. The tarsal plate is closely adherent to the conjunctiva, and the two behave as a single structure, making it possible, by matching the tarsal plates, to approximate the margins of the associated conjunctiva, which then heals very rapidly. The defect can be closed in two layers, a tarso-conjunctival and a skin–muscle. Using 6–0 catgut on an atraumatic needle, the margins of the tarsal plate are approximated using interrupted sutures with the knot placed on the skin side. The skin and orbicularis muscle are then closed as a single layer. To use 6–0 catgut successfully in this way, tension across the tarsal plate suture line must be minimal, and this limits the width of the V which can be closed directly to a little less than one-quarter of the eyelid width.

When it is apparent that tension across the suture line is likely to be unacceptable, it can be reduced by dividing the limb of the lateral canthal ligament to the eyelid, approaching it through the conjunctiva at the lateral canthus, **V-excision and lateral canthotomy** (Fig. 10.17).

When tension is still too great despite this manoeuvre, a formal reconstruction of the defect becomes necessary, medially advancing the eyelid skin lateral to the defect, and the skin beyond the lateral canthal region, in the form of a transposed flap, **V-excision and transposed flap** (Fig. 10.17). The flap is outlined by continuing the upward curve of the eyelid margin on to the temple almost as far as the hairline, with a downward back-cut, equal in length and parallel to, the lateral limb of the V. The flap is elevated, dividing the lower limb of the canthal ligament, and the flap is transposed medially. It may be necessary in addition to divide the orbital septum and any other lid attachments deep to the skin which are felt to be limiting movement of the flap medially. There is ample slack in the conjunctiva present in the lateral fornix to be taken up as the flap is drawn medially, and provide lining for the part of the flap which is forming the reconstructed eyelid segment. The two limbs of the V are approximated and sutured together, and the free edge of the reconstructed eyelid segment is sutured to the conjunctiva which it has drawn medially with it. The effect of transposing the skin flap medially in this way is to leave a triangular secondary defect laterally, corresponding to the wedge initially resected from the eyelid. This is closed by rotating a small triangular flap, outlined at the planning stage of the procedure, at the lateral extremity of the transposed flap, and giving the appearance locally of a Z. Rotation of the flap downwards to fill the lateral triangular defect completes the reconstruction.

The method works best when the defect does not extend to one or other canthus, and there is sufficient tarsal plate on each side to provide good material for suturing. It can be applied to defects which extend a little beyond half of the eyelid, and this makes it applicable to the majority of tumours whose excision can be encompassed by a V-shaped wedge.

NOSE

Considered from the point of view of tumour resection and reconstruction, the nose has an outer layer of skin and a lining largely of mucous membrane, the two separated by the nasal bones and the nasal cartilages, lateral and alar. Over the bones and lateral cartilages, the normal mobility of the skin makes it a reliable clinical test of depth of tumour involvement. Over the alar cartilages the skin is fixed deeply, and the test is not reliable.

The degree of activity of the sebaceous glands in some patients can create problems in the use of the various reconstructive techniques. Sebaceous activity normally increases from the bridge of the nose to the tip and, when it is marked, the thickness of the involved skin, its lack of flexibility, and its proneness to infection and bad scars, make it unsuitable as surgical material.

Closure by *direct suture* is only suitable for defects which are strictly limited in size, and the potential usage of the method diminishes with

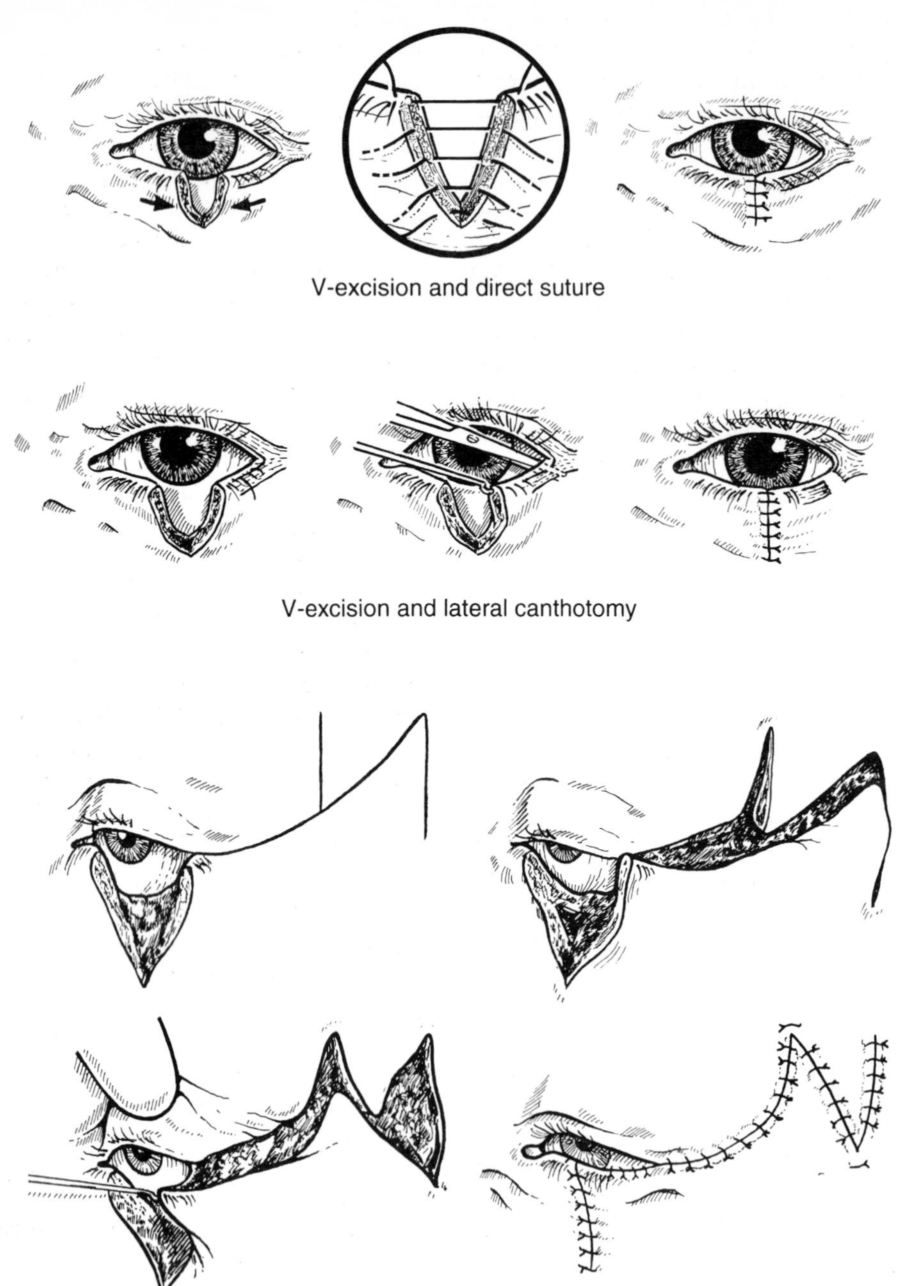

Fig.10.17 The management of a full thickness V-excision of the eyelid, showing the changes in the methods used to allow closure of the defect to be achieved without tension as the V increases in width.

The narrow V is closed by **direct suture**, the inset showing the two layer closure used, with fine catgut used to approximate the margins of the tarsal plate, while avoiding any exposure of suture material in the conjunctival sac. When the tension of closing the wider V is considered to be too great, **excision and lateral canthotomy** is used, in which the limb of the lateral canthal ligament to the eyelid is divided, allowing the V to be closed without tension. When the V is still wider, and it is considered that canthotomy will be inadequate, tissue is advanced medially from the malar area and temple as a **transposed flap, closing the secondary defect with a Z-plasty**.

passage towards the nasal tip. Because of the virtually total attachment of the skin to the alar cartilage, direct suture used in that site generally results in asymmetry of the nostrils because of the distortion it produces, and the presence of sebaceous activity in the area is a virtually absolute contraindication to its use.

Free skin grafts have a useful, if limited, reconstructive role, particularly over the nasal bones and lateral cartilages, where a deep plane of resection which leaves a readily graftable surface is easy to achieve. The full thickness post-auricular graft gives an excellent cosmetic result in those sites, though when the resection has been carried to the periosteum of the nasal bone, or the perichondrium of the lateral cartilage, the thinness of the graft often fails to match the depth of the defect, and a hollow results.

Local flaps are thicker, and are liable instead to create a bulge. They are also subject to the problem that their thickness makes early recognition of deep recurrence more difficult. The use of 'tumour barriers', as discussed on p. 155, can provide a solution to both problems. By removing the nasal bone and/or cartilage as part of the resection, deep clearance can be assured, and the increase in the depth of the defect makes it also able to accommodate the flap without creating a local bulge.

The local flaps most often used make use of the nasolabial or the glabellar areas of availability. The glabellar area provides the **glabellar flap**, the **finger forehead flap**, and the **glabellar advancement flap**, and the nasolabial area of availability provides the **nasolabial flap**. The reconstruction of larger defects, and defects which involve the full thickness of the nose are beyond the scope of this book.

The **glabellar flap** (Fig. 10.18) is used to reconstruct defects of the side of the nose in the glabellar area. It has a limited reach, but the area is a common site of basal cell carcinoma, and it is regularly required.

When a defect beyond its range requires flap cover, a variant in the form of a vertical **finger flap** (Fig. 10.19) can be designed, still based on the glabellar area, but extending vertically upwards over the forehead. Its additional length, limited by the height of the forehead, makes it possible to reconstruct defects at a greater distance. In many patients it can reach as far as the nasal tip and, in addition to being available to resurface the nose, it can be used to reconstruct defects of the cheek close by the side of the nose within the limits of its length (Fig. 10.20). Its breadth is restricted by the need to be able to close the secondary defect directly. The transfer has generally to be carried out in two stages, the entire flap not being inset at the outset. At the second stage the pedicle is divided, insetting is completed, and the bridge segment is discarded.

The **glabellar advancement flap** (Fig. 10.21) is designed for the specific purpose of resurfacing the midline defect of the upper third of the dorsum of the nose, a problem which does not arise often, but one for which there is no easy alternative solution.

The **nasolabial flap** (Fig. 10.22) exploits the nasolabial area of availability, and it provides a versatile method for reconstructing nasal defects, predominantly of the lower third, and mainly of one or other side. The flap is usually based superiorly, occasionally inferiorly, and unless it abuts directly on the defect, the transfer requires a second stage, with division of the pedicle, and completion of insetting.

In planning the flap, the intention of the surgeon may be to approach the nasal defect from a particular direction with the breadth of the flap cut to match, but it is often found that the planned approach is not the eventual approach, and if the breadth of the flap proves to be insufficient for that approach, the result can be disastrous. Such an embarrassment can be avoided by creating the defect as far as possible in the shape of a circle. The direction from which the flap then reaches the defect becomes immaterial, and the only important flap dimension, other than making it long enough, is to give it adequate width.

The siting of the flap in relation to the nasolabial fold is dependent on the sex of the patient, and whether the defect is in a hairless area. In the female the flap can be positioned astride the nasolabial fold, but when the defect is in a hairless area in the male, the flap has to be positioned lateral to the beard area, usually just beyond the line of the fold.

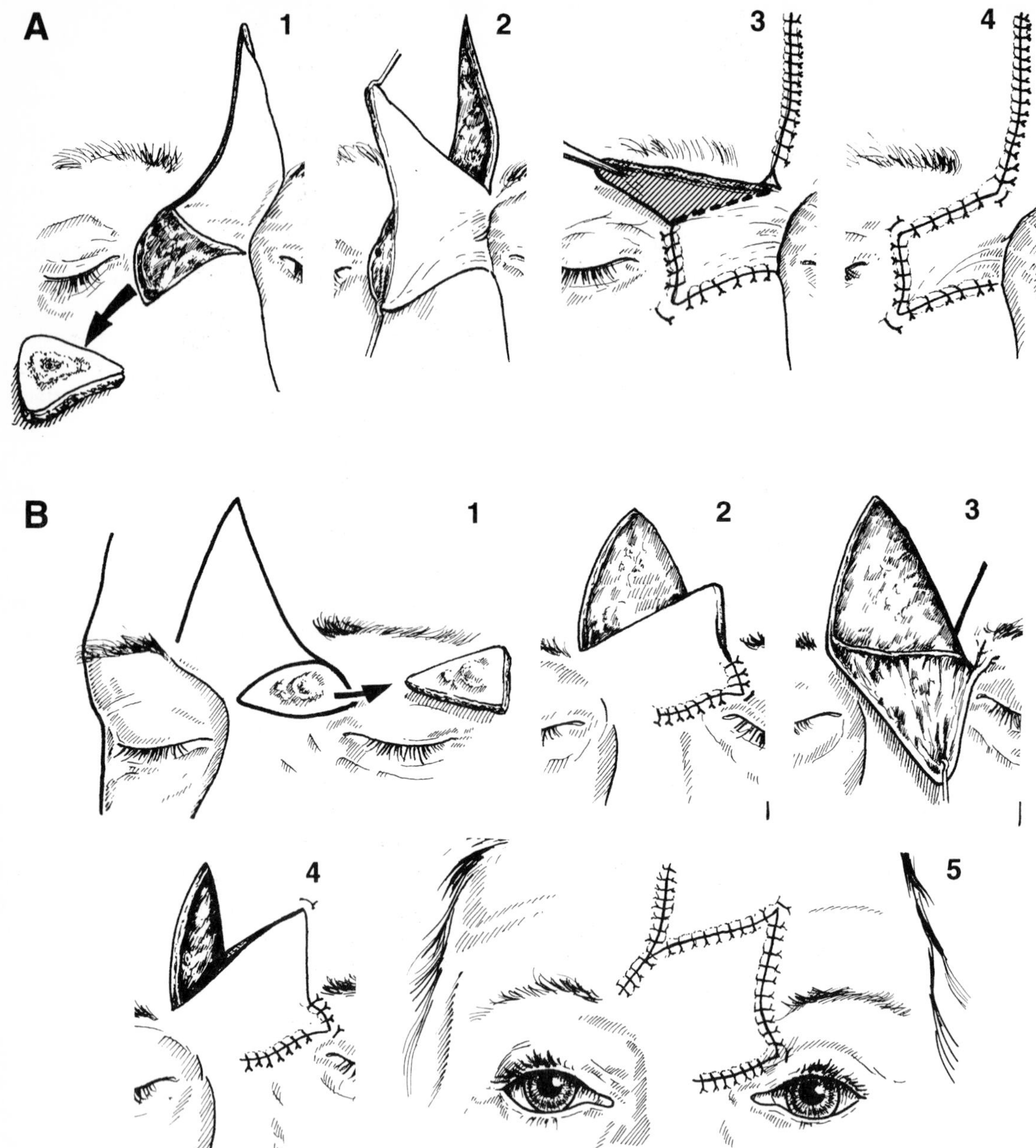

Fig. 10.18 The glabellar flap, used to reconstruct defects in the area between the bridge of the nose and the canthus, showing the two possible designs. The design selected in practice is usually determined by the estimated ease of closing the secondary defect. When closure is easy, the method shown in **A** is used, when it is likely to be difficult the method shown in **B** is used.

A The defect and the flap outlined, is shown in (**1**), and (**2**) shows the flap elevated and moved into the defect. The secondary defect is closed (**3**), and suturing of the flap carried out until the triangle of excess skin is delineated, and excised, allowing suturing to be completed (**4**).

B The lesion, with the defect and the flap outlined, is shown in **1**. In **2** the flap has been raised, moved into the defect, and sutured in position. At this stage it is apparent that it will not be possible to close the glabellar defect directly. An incision is made as shown in **3**, and the triangular flap which results is moved medially (**4**), reducing the tension of closure, and allowing suturing to be completed (**5**).

The flap is usually made as broad as the distance between the eyebrows and this determines the breadth of the secondary defect, and the ease or difficulty of closure.

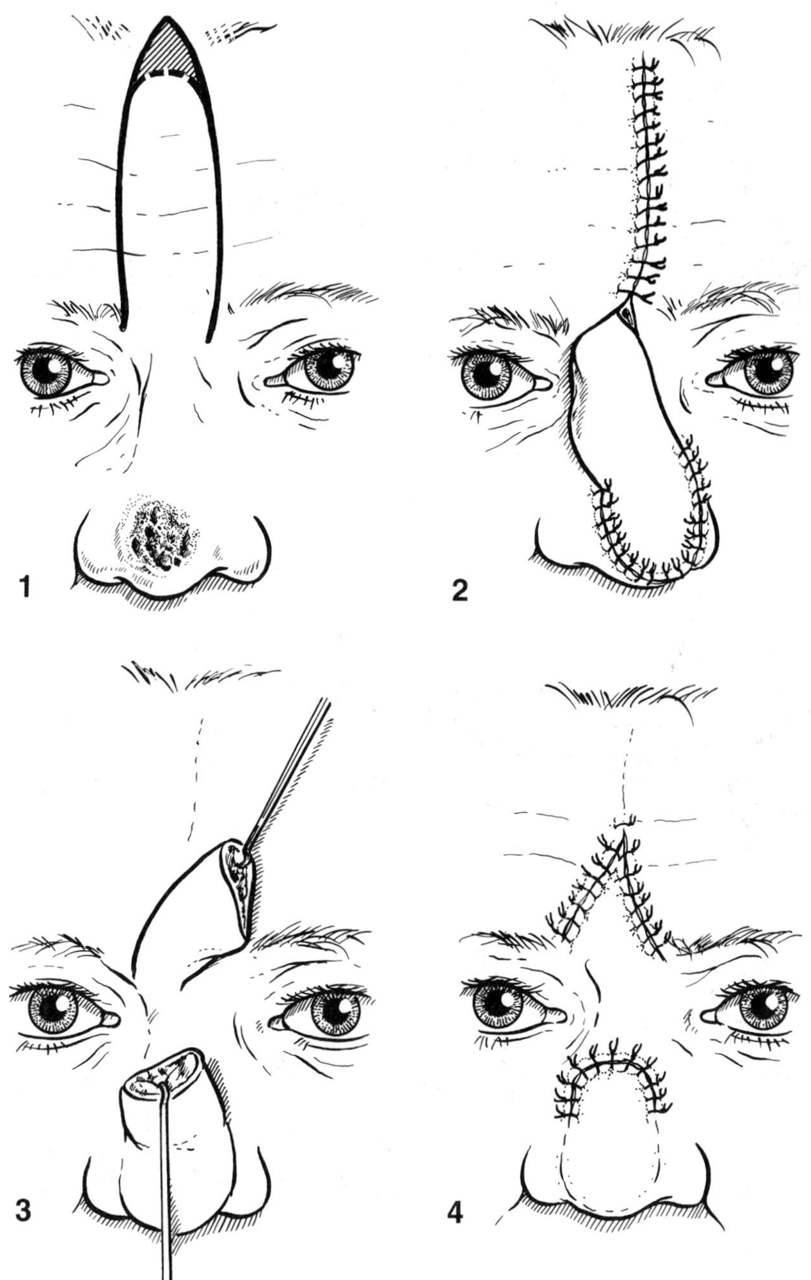

Fig. 10.19 The finger forehead flap, used to reconstruct a midline defect of the nasal tip.

The flap, though midline, can be curved a little to one or other side towards its base (**1**), allowing it to turn more easily, and slightly extending its reach. The effect is to reduce its perfusing system to a single supraorbital : supratrochlear one, but the flap remains a safe one. The entire height of the forehead is usually required to allow the flap to reach the nasal tip. The flap is raised, initially deep to the frontalis muscle system, though often thinned over the segment to be inset to match the depth of the nasal defect, rotated downwards (**2**), and sutured to the margins of the defect, the forehead defect being closed directly. At the second stage, three weeks later, the flap is divided (**3**), part of the bridge segment is discarded, and the remainder is returned to the forehead (**4**), insetting of the transferred segment being completed.

The flap is designed vertically on the forehead if at all possible, because the scar which results is much less obvious than oblique forehead scars. Since the secondary defect on the forehead is closed directly, the permissible breadth of the flap is determined by the degree of laxity of the skin in the midline.

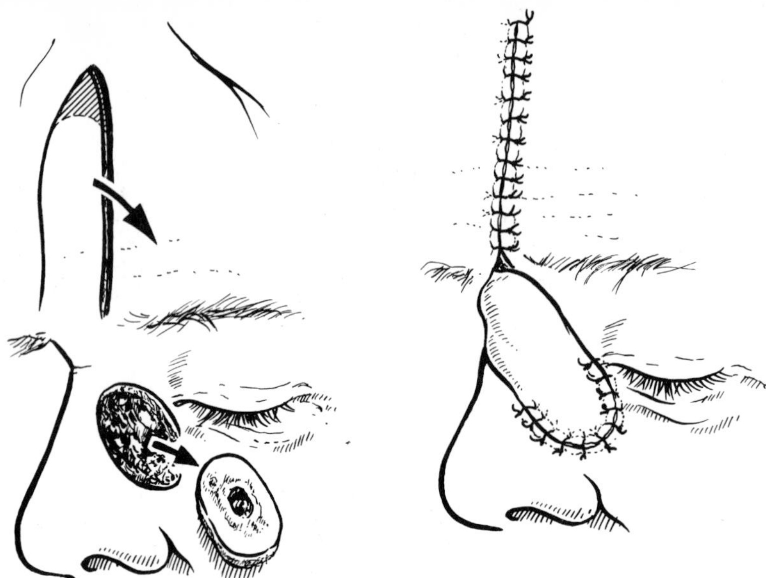

Fig. 10.20 The finger forehead flap used to reconstruct a defect in the medial canthal area which is beyond the reach of the standard glabellar flap.

The site of the defect determines the length of the flap which is required. When the flap is relatively short, the plane of elevation can safely be made more superficial, so that its thickness will match as accurately as possible the depth of the defect.

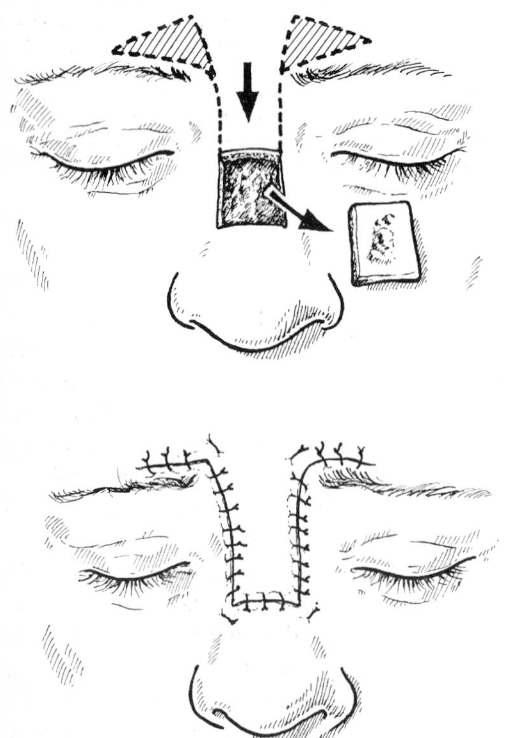

Fig. 10.21 The glabellar advancement flap, used to reconstruct a midline defect of the upper half of the nose.

This reconstruction can only be used when there is an adequate gap between the eyebrows.

The superiorly based nasolabial flap is also a useful method of reconstructing the partial-thickness defect of the upper lip, and here it can be designed inside the beard area when the patient is male. The flap has the considerable virtue of allowing the symmetry of the lip to be maintained.

EAR

In those parts of the pinna where the cartilage and the skin are in direct contact they are adherent to one another, the adherence greater on the lateral surface than the postauricular surface, and increasing towards the external acoustic meatus. On the postauricular surface, adherence decreases towards the postauricular sulcus. The outer surface is the area most prone to develop skin tumours, mainly actinically-induced squamous cell carcinomas, and the strength of the adherence between skin and cartilage there has a strong influence both on resection and reconstruction.

The usefulness of *direct suture* varies in the different parts of the ear. On its lateral surface, the combination of skin fixity and a concavity makes direct suture of a defect of the conchal hollow virtually impossible. On the postauricular

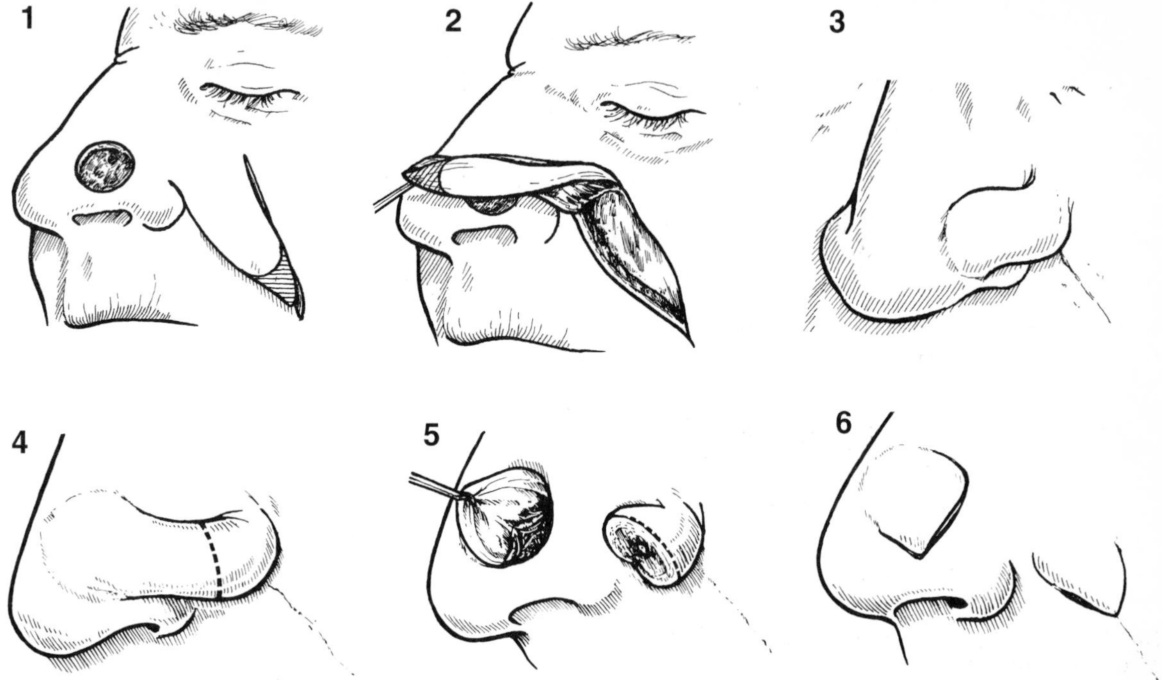

Fig. 10.22 The nasolabial flap, based superiorly, used to reconstruct a defect of the side of the nose.
In the clinical example shown, the procedure was a two-stage one, the defect and the flap being at a distance from one another. **1** Shows the alar defect and the flap, raised and transferred (**2**) to the defect. **3** Shows the appearance three weeks later, with the flap in position filling the defect, ready for division of the pedicle, and the scar of direct closure of the nasolabial defect. **4** Shows the line of division of the pedicle, and **5** the pedicle divided, with insetting being completed (**6**), and the trimmed remnant of the pedicle returned to its original site.

When the defect is close to the base of the flap it may be possible to make the transfer into a single stage one, but the result is often a loss of the nasolabial hollow, and the two-stage method is generally preferable. The thickness of the flap, even allowing for as much thinning as is permissible while retaining flap viability, is also liable to be greater than the depth of the defect, and results in a contour mismatch. Removal of the underlying cartilage, lateral or alar, deepens the defect, equating the depth of the defect to the thickness of the flap. As shown in Figure 10.24, removal of the cartilage may also have the virtue of making depth clearance of the tumour more certain.

surface, the greater skin mobility, coupled with the fact that the ear tolerates being set back closer to the head, increases its role considerably.

For the tumour arising on the margin of the pinna (Fig. 10.23), it is a simple and effective method. After clearance of the lesion, an additional narrow strip of cartilage is excised from the rim to allow the defect to be directly closed without tension. In excising this additional cartilage it is important to make sure that the margin which is left passes smoothly on to the adjoining intact cartilage. Any small prominence left at the junction is liable to form a nodule which, apart from being painful on occasion, can create suspicion of local recurrence. There is some loss of the curve of the margin, but the patients tend to be in the older age group, and find the result acceptable.

Split skin grafts are the standard grafts used in managing tumours of the outer aspect of the pinna, and in using them the 'cartilage tumour barrier' is particularly useful. The adherence of the skin deeply makes it rare to be able to excise a tumour leaving the perichondrium intact, with any confidence of depth clearance, while inclusion of the cartilage (Fig. 10.24) as part of the overall excision makes certain of depth clearance, and leaves an excellent bed for grafting. When there is enough cartilaginous skeleton surrounding the site to maintain the shape of the pinna, the cosmetic result is excellent, and even when the defect is near the margin, and there is some loss of the shape of the ear, the appearance remains acceptable.

Where the tumour is small enough and in a site

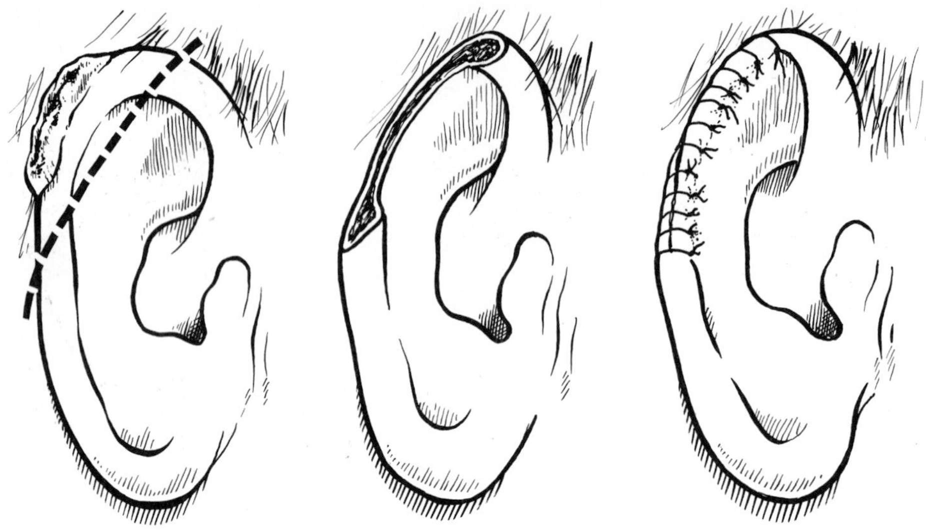

Fig. 10.23 Excision of a tumour of the margin of the pinna with direct closure of the defect. Closure of the defect in this way reduces the curve of the margin of the ear, but not to an unacceptable degree.

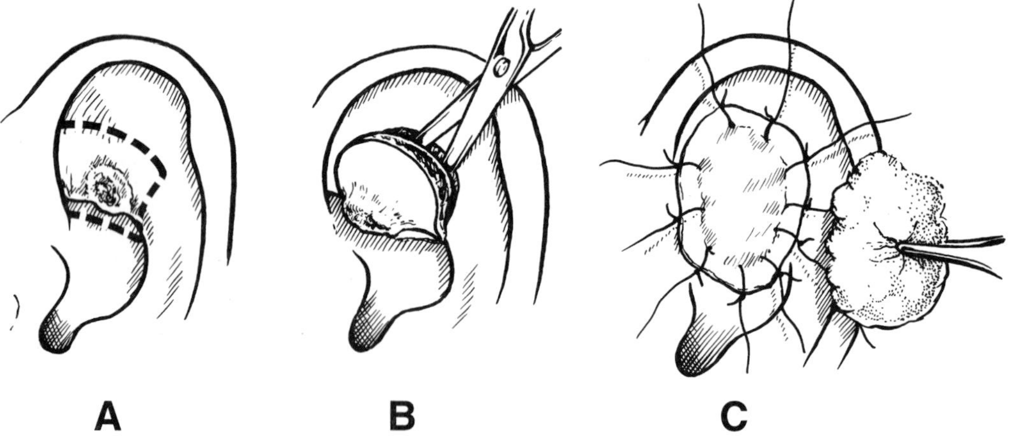

Fig. 10.24 The use of the cartilage tumour barrier in resecting a small squamous carcinoma. The excision of the tumour along with the underlying cartilage ensures depth clearance and also provides a graftable surface.

which allows it to be excised as a full thickness V (Fig. 10.25), the defect can be closed directly in layers. A degree of distortion of the pinna usually results, but in most instances the result is cosmetically adequate.

The lesion whose excision will leave only a remnant of the external ear is probably best managed by total amputation of the pinna. The ear is comparatively easy to replace with a prosthesis and the cosmetic results are good (Fig. 10.1). If possible, the tragus should be preserved, as this makes the fitting of the prosthesis both easier and more cosmetically effective.

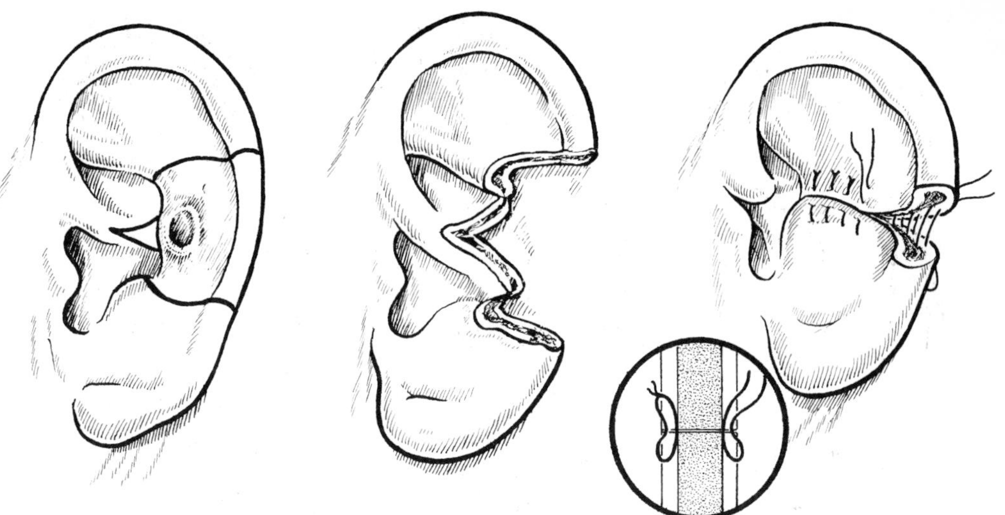

Fig. 10.25 V-excision of the pinna and direct closure.

CHAPTER 11 Hand surgery

HAND INJURIES

In discussing hand injuries consideration will be focused mainly on the methods of providing skin cover. Although other aspects of the problems they present, such as injury to tendons and nerves, or fractures and joint damage, may be equally important in the clinical situation, they are outwith the scope of this book, except to the extent that their presence may influence the type of skin cover selected and the manner of its use.

The provision of skin cover takes priority because the granulation tissue which is produced in the process of 'healing by secondary intention' matures to fibrous tissue, and the presence of a raw surface is a potential focus of infection. Fibrosis and infection are both harmful, and together they are responsible for much of the stiffness seen as a sequel to an injury of the hand. Effective skin cover immediately eliminates infection as a significant factor and the production of granulation tissue largely ceases. Granulation tissue present prior to the provision of skin cover will obviously mature to fibrous tissue, but at least the granulation tissue already present and the scar tissue into which it will mature is not added to.

In a crushing injury, the situation can arise in which the damage is largely confined to the proximal hand, but tissues distal to the site of injury which are otherwise normal, or at least minimally involved, have no circulation because blood flow has been cut off by disruption of the vessels in the zone of crushing. The use of microvascular techniques, discussed in Chapter 4, has changed this situation from one for which nothing could be done to save the devascularised tissues into one where they are potentially salvageable. By the use of vein grafts which bridge the zone of damage it may be possible to restore circulation to the distal tissues. The technique has its main value in the severely crushed hand where the salvage of digits can make a very significant contribution to the ultimate function of the hand. Patients with such an injury pattern should immediately be referred to a centre where microvascular expertise is available.

The method of providing skin cover and the form it takes depends so much on the type of injury that an awareness of the pathological features of the common injury patterns is essential.

Hand injuries are of three main types — **cutting and slicing**, **crushing**, and **degloving and avulsion**. As a rule an injury belongs predominantly to one type, but on occasion it combines the characteristics of crushing, and degloving and avulsion. These three types constitute distinct injury patterns but, from the viewpoint of immediate management, injuries have also been divided into *tidy* and *untidy*, a division which has considerable value, particularly as it relates to the use of the tourniquet.

In the tidy injury, the damage to the skin is clear-cut, and the problems of treatment generally concern more the injury to tendons and nerves. Repair and reconstruction of these structures requires a bloodless field and for this a pneumatic tourniquet is used.

In the untidy injury, the initial assessment involves deciding which tissues are viable, made on the basis of whether or not the structures in question have an active circulation, and the use of an exsanguinating tourniquet is clearly contra-indicated. Assessment of the viability of skin is discussed on p. 144.

CUTTING AND SLICING INJURIES

The extent of a cutting or slicing injury, at least as it involves the skin, is obvious at the outset, and the appropriate method of repair can usually be decided on the basis of the preliminary clinical examination.

If there has been no skin loss, the wound can be closed directly with only sufficient excision of the skin edges to remove any obviously devitalised tissue. Accurate suturing is as vital in the hand as it is in the face if rapid healing with minimal scarring is to be achieved. Skin loss is made good by free skin graft or flap. Split skin grafts are the most frequently used cover, and the small amount of tissue damage means that, if the bed exposed is suitable for grafting, good take can be expected.

When the raw area includes a structure which is unsuitable for grafting, as when the pulp of a finger-tip has been lost and replacement requires more bulk than a skin graft can provide, or a structure such as a tendon requiring subsequent repair or reconstruction is left exposed, flap cover should be provided. The restriction of tissue damage to the plane of the cut makes it often possible to proceed to immediate definitive repair of divided tendons or nerves, or to commence the reconstruction of structures lost as a result of the injury.

The injury resulting in a guillotine amputation of a finger which exposes bone can in theory be grafted, but graft failure, partial or total, is common. If the area is allowed to heal spontaneously, the resulting scar adheres to the bone end and is prone to give trouble subsequently. A better result is often achieved by trimming the phalanx until the soft tissues will close over it without tension.

Although this approach may be justified when a single finger is involved, other factors come into play when the thumb is the digit partially amputated. There are then two contending considerations — the desirability of a full-length opposable thumb, and the need for good sensation and a stable tip. Hand surgery has gone through a phase where preservation of thumb length largely overrode other considerations, but it has become increasingly recognised that many patients cope perfectly adequately with less than a full-length thumb. This has made such an extreme attitude untenable, and the approach of the surgeon should be the commonsense one of assessing how vital a full-length thumb is likely to be, given the patient's work requirements, and also how long he can afford to be off work. Suffice it to say that there should be no excessive trimming of a traumatically amputated thumb to get skin cover, and free skin grafting may be legitimate as a temporary measure pending more definitive management. It is also true as a generalisation that the greater the number of digits injured the greater the need to conserve the length of individual fingers.

Injuries of this type involving the finger-tip often present special problems because of the nail and its bed. Their management is discussed on p. 189.

CRUSHING INJURIES

A crushing injury can vary in severity and extent from the mildest subungual haematoma, through the crush injury of fingers with or without bony damage, up to the power-press injury which leaves a shapeless pulp of devitalised tissue. In such an injury, loss of skin and soft tissue may not be a feature in the literal sense, but the ultimate loss is often much greater even than was immediately apparent because, in addition to the obvious devitalisation of the crushed tissues, disruption of blood vessels adds to the necrosis both of the skin and the deeper tissues. A consequence of this 'hidden' damage is unexpectedly severe oedema postoperatively, and a degree of fibrosis which is responsible for the frequently disappointing final functional result.

In appraising the extent and severity of the injury, the first fact to establish is what structures are definitely not viable. With the caveat already stressed on p. 183 soft tissue structures which are considered to be non-viable should be excised quite ruthlessly. When the obviously non-viable tissue has been excised, the position can be assessed afresh. In this second assessment, decisions have to be made regarding which damaged but viable structures are worthy of retention and skin cover. The detailed decisions involved will take account of such factors as the relative importance of the fingers and the thumb, the age and work requirements of the patient, as well as the extent and severity of the damage.

With the exception of the thumb, where the pressures towards conservation of length carry greater weight, there are two opposing lines of argument. On one side, the more severe the damage to the individual components of a single finger — nerve, tendon, skin, bone — the stronger is the argument for amputation although the finger as a whole may be viable, because the less is the likelihood of a useful digit resulting. On the other side, the greater the damage to other fingers and the rest of the hand, the stronger is the argument for retention of the individual digit, even in the knowledge that it will be stiff. A useless finger can also be considered as a potential source of skin. Filleted, it can be used to cover a defect of adjoining dorsum or palm, avoiding the need for a graft or flap.

Even after scrupulous excision of non-viable structures, tissue is usually left which, although viable, is still showing crush damage. Such tissue provides a less than perfect surface for grafting and take tends to be poorer than in the comparable injury where crushing is not a factor. The crushing probably produces devitalisation of the tissues severe enough to affect adversely the vascularisation of a graft yet insufficient to devitalise them completely.

Compared with a cutting injury of apparently comparable severity, the crushing injury carries a much longer disability period and the end result in terms of stiffness and function generally is much poorer.

DEGLOVING AND AVULSION INJURIES

The distinction between degloving and avulsion injuries lies in the tissue involved.

Degloving is confined to the skin and fascia, the superficial fascia always, the investing layer of deep fascia usually. The important pathological factor is the disruption of the blood vessels in the degloved tissue. To a casual inspection the damage may appear to be minor, but where there is no circulation the tissue will die. Damage to tendon, bone and joint is not part of the typical pattern.

Avulsion involves the deeper tissues, typically as part of a combined degloving/avulsion injury when a digit is avulsed, pulling with it the tendons inserted into it, and plucking them from their muscle bellies, and in a similar manner a length of nerve. It is generally when the degloving force is considerable that it produces avulsion as well.

The management of such a severe mixed degloving/avulsion injury is a matter for the experienced hand surgeon, preferably one with microvascular expertise, since the avulsed digit may be potentially salvageable depending on the severity of the neurovascular disruption it has sustained. Its importance in this respect will also depend on the extent of the damage to other digits.

In both the dorsum and the palm the circumstances of the degloving injury often leaves the degloved flap attached distally, but the differences in the characteristics of palmar and dorsal skin are reflected in their different behaviour subjected to the stress of the degloving injury.

In the palm, the usual degloving plane is between the palmar aponeurosis and the flexor tendons, the skin and the aponeurosis, with their firm attachment to one another, behaving as a single structure. The strength and relative inextensibility of the aponeurosis also protects the circulation of the palmar skin to some extent, and the area devascularised may be less than one might expect from an early assessment.

In the dorsum, the plane leaves the extensor tendons exposed, though generally covered by paratenon, which provides a graftable surface unless it has been allowed to dry out.

The important assessment which has to be made is that of skin viability, the principle of treatment being that skin which is not demonstrably viable must be excised. The difficulty in practice lies in estimating the skin loss accurately immediately after the injury, the mistake generally made being to underestimate. If primary excision has been carried out, and at the first post-operative dressing a fresh area of slough is found to be present, it should be immediately excised and skin cover provided. In this way healing is achieved as quickly as possible. For the surgeon who feels unhappy at immediate excision of skin which appears to be minimally damaged, an alternative is delayed primary treatment, waiting for the necrotic area to declare itself before carrying the necessary excision. This approach is valid as long as the skin excision is carried out as soon as the extent of the slough is apparent. To wait for it to separate spontaneously is not acceptable.

Split skin grafting of the defect is the usual form of cover used at the acute stage, and it is often satisfactory as a permanency. Even when it is considered that subsequent flap cover is likely to be needed, split skin grafting is still generally the cover of choice at the primary stage. Only if the surface exposed is one which will not take a graft, such as bare tendon, bare cortical bone or open joint, should a primary flap be considered.

Degloving of a single finger is a recognised injury pattern, most often involving the ring finger, the ring becoming caught on a fixed object, and degloving the digit as it is forcibly dragged off. The injury may include a phalangeal fracture, and the degloving may be complete or partial depending on whether the skin is stripped off the finger completely or remains attached over the distal phalangeal segment.

Management of the single finger which has been degloved leaving it skeletonised, but with normal tendon and joint function, depends very much on whether or not the surgeon has microvascular expertise. The form which the degloving force takes in this injury is such that, apart from the segment at the site of the skin dehiscence, the blood vessels and nerves in the degloved tissue are liable to be undamaged. If the tissue is still attached distally it may be possible to restore the skin to its original site on the finger and revascularise it by bridging the damaged length of one or both digital arteriovenous systems with vein grafts, at the same time carrying out nerve suture. A successful result can give a virtually normal finger and is certainly worth attempting. If the necessary microvascular expertise is lacking, or the attempt fails, amputation is generally advisable.

When the thumb is degloved, management is quite different. The functional value of the thumb

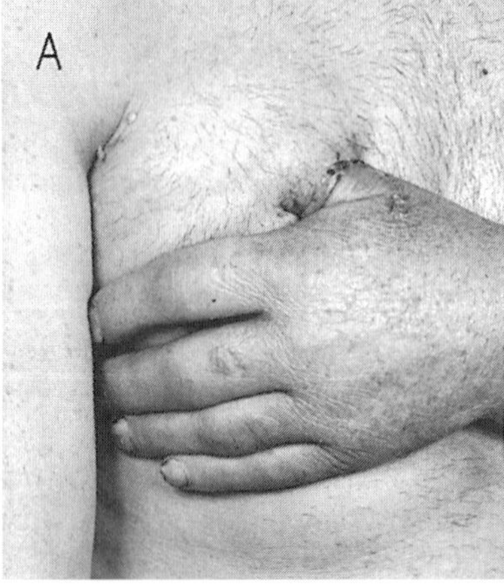

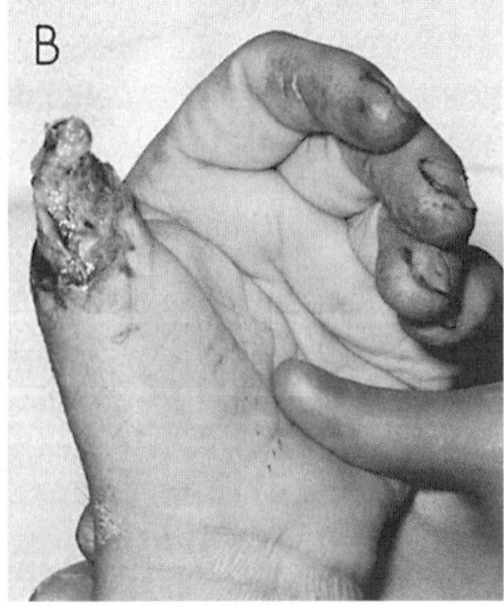

Fig. 11.1 Degloving of the thumb with loss of the distal phalanx, treated initially (**A**) by burying the degloved digit under the chest skin. It is apparent that burial of the digit in this way (**B**) has not provided skin cover. Figure 11.2 shows the method used to provide definitive skin cover.

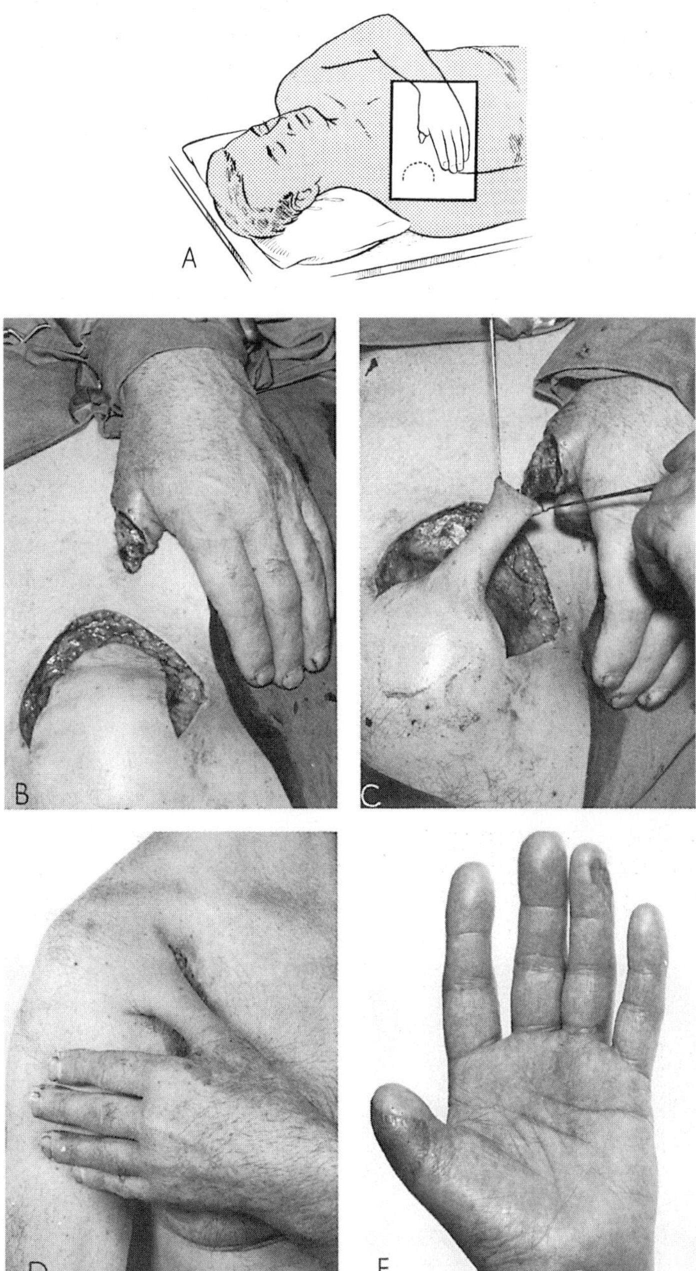

Fig. 11.2 The degloved thumb in Figure 11.1, showing the pectoral tubed flap used to provide skin cover, followed by division of the flap and simultaneous transfer of a neurovascular island flap (see Fig. 11.3) to provide sensation in the thumb tip.

A The position of the flap on the chest.
B, C The flap raised, and tubed ready to have the thumb inserted.
D, E The interval appearance of the tube, and the final result with the neurovascular island flap in position.

in relation to the other digits means that every effort should be made to salvage the skeletonised component, even if it is only of part-length, or is likely to lack independent mobility. The method of temporary salvage which has been described, namely to 'bury' the degloved digit under the skin of the chest or abdomen (Fig. 11.1), may buy time but it does nothing to advance the provision of skin cover. It is preferable to raise a tubed flap and insert the degloved thumb into it. There are several potential sources of such a flap. Examples are the groin flap and deltopectoral flaps, their virtues and adverse qualities discussed on p. 199 *et seq.*, and the pedicled version of the radial forearm flap may also be a candidate. The example shown in Fig. 11.2, using the pectoral skin as a source, is a random pattern flap, but having a length:breadth ration of approximately 1:1, is safe. It has the virtue of providing thin skin, and maintenance of the position post-operatively with a sling is straightforward.

The thumb encased in this way has a poor blood supply, and lacks sensation. The inadequate blood supply results in poor tip healing when the pedicle of the tubed flap is divided, and leads to subsequent cold intolerance. These, combined with an absence of sensation, result in poor usage of the thumb by the patient. Both deficiencies benefit from the incorporation of a neurovascular 'island' flap in the reconstruction (Fig. 11.3). The hemipulp of a functionally less important finger, traditionally the ulnar side of the ring or middle finger, is raised, pedicled on the digital vessels and nerve back to their origin in the palm, and tunnelled through palm and tubed flap to a functionally suitable site near the thumb tip. There it is sutured in position, and the donor pulp defect is free skin grafted. The effect is to bring both sensation and blood supply to the tip of the digit, and the result is a marked improvement both in utilisation and in vascularity. Sensation is projected to the donor finger

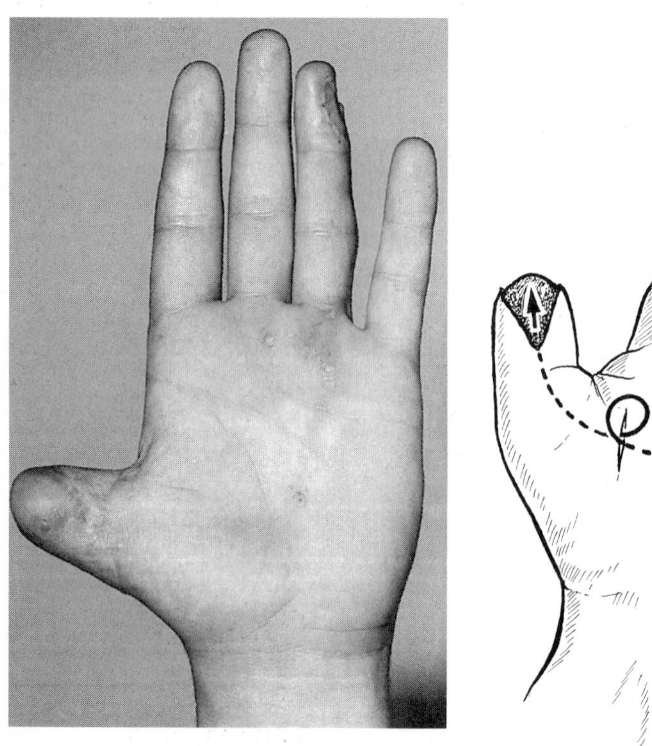

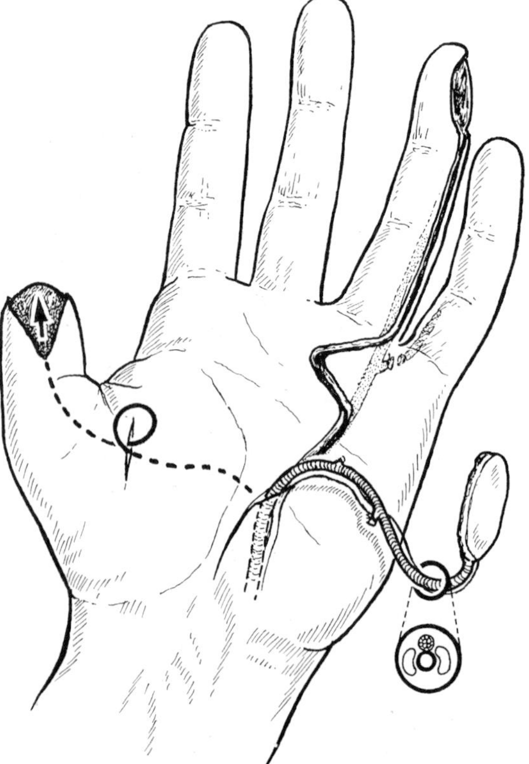

Fig. 11.3 The use of a neurovascular island flap to provide sensation in a thumb resurfaced using a pectoral tubed flap.

to begin with, and persists there indefinitely in most individuals. Despite this, patients adjust remarkably quickly, and do not appear to have difficulty in use.

The use of microsurgical techniques has created alternative methods of managing the thumb which has been degloved with partial amputation, or totally amputated. The great toe or the second toe has been transferred to replace the thumb, and the surgically degloved soft tissue component of the great toe has also been used as being less likely to result in problems with the donor foot. It has to be stressed that these techniques are not for the occasional operator, even one with some microsurgical expertise. Their effective use calls for experience and careful patient selection.

In viewing the indications for thumb reconstruction and the results in terms of usage two conclusions emerge. First, the younger the patient the better the result; secondly, many adults who have lost a thumb from trauma manage remarkably well, and in their healed state would strongly resist any attempt to have a reconstruction inflicted on them.

FINGER-TIP INJURIES

Isolated finger-tip injuries are relatively common, and the influence on treatment of the nail and pulp makes separate consideration of the injury necessary. Integrity of all three elements of the distal segment of the digit, nail, pulp and phalanx, is essential to normality of each component, a fact which becomes apparent when the effects that damage to one component has on the others are analysed. Loss of phalangeal length results in distortion of nail growth beyond the remnant of the phalanx; loss of pulp substance results in similar distortion of nail growth beyond the phalanx, the distal nail curving round towards the pulp, sometimes with almost claw-like growth. The integrity and smoothness of the nail-bed are crucial to a smoothly growing nail. Damage or destruction, partial or complete, of the generative element of the nail, mainly proximal to the nail fold, makes for irregular and patchy growth, progressing with increasing severity of the damage to virtual absence of nail growth. Complete absence, however, is rare, spikes of nail continuing to grow, usually at each side of the original nail site.

Once the effect of damage to the pattern of nail growth has become clinically manifest, the surgeon is largely powerless to rectify the situation, all that he can do being to obliterate those areas of nail growth which are troubling the patient. This makes it desirable to prevent the deformities of growth from developing, although even then success is very partial.

An injury to the finger-tip which occurs sufficiently often to constitute a distinct injury pattern is the partially avulsed finger-tip which is left attached by a pedicle of pulp skin. When the injury has been of the crushing type the nail is usually avulsed from its base with the flap. The ungual process of the phalanx may be intact but denuded, or fractured, the distal fragment as part of the avulsed segment. With a cutting type of injury the nail may be cut transversely, the distal half attached to the avulsed flap.

It is remarkable how small the pedicle need be to ensure survival of the partially avulsed flap, and a decision as to viability should only be made when the flap has been restored to its original position to eliminate the adverse effect of torsion and angulation of the pedicle on the blood supply of the flap. If it is not viable, treatment is as for a guillotine amputation, but with a viable flap the finger-tip should be reconstituted after minimal excision of wound edges and pulp fat. The nail should be retained and replaced in its bed to provide splintage and help to ensure a smooth nail-bed after healing. In this way the likelihood of distortion when the fresh nail grows in is reduced. When the nail has been transected care should be taken to get the edges of the nail, and hence its bed, accurately apposed for the same reason.

When the finger-tip injury has resulted in tissue loss it will involve damage to the pulp with its skin, the phalanx, the nail and its bed, in varying degree. The appropriate reconstruction, whether by shortening of the digit, free skin graft or flap, depends at least partly on the extent of the damage to each constituent. In the extreme case the choice may be clear-cut; it is in the mixed injury that difficulty arises.

Severe crushing which devitalises the nail and phalanx while the pulp is still viable is best treated by amputating the devitalised segment and closing the defect with a flap of the pulp skin. For the slicing injury which removes either pulp skin or distal nail without significantly damaging pulp or phalanx, the obvious measure is a free skin graft, while the more severe injury where there is loss of pulp substance requires a flap to restore the volume lost, and preserve normality of nail growth. The majority of injuries lie between these extremes, however, with loss of pulp and sometimes of bone, and management is less clear-cut.

The finger-tip is one of the very few sites where a full thickness skin graft has been successfully used in primary trauma, but it has no real advantage over a thick split skin graft, the all-important need in grafting being for good take. The common cause of graft failure in this situation is haematoma and in fact haemostasis in a finger-tip injury is not always easy to achieve. There is much to be said for delayed grafting, postponing application for 24 hours to allow for natural haemostasis. It is not even essential to suture the graft in position with a tie-over dressing. Micropore tape can be used most effectively to hold the graft in position. Indeed, tape has a most useful role in minor hand injuries generally, particularly in children where it can sometimes obviate the need for an anaesthetic of any kind. The suitability of a finger-tip defect for grafting can be judged by comparing the area of bare exposed bone with the area of soft tissue; the greater the soft tissue the more suitable for grafting, the greater the area of bone the less suitable for grafting.

Skin grafting apart, various techniques involving the use of flaps have been described for providing cover for finger-tip injuries, ranging from shortening of the digit to allow creation of a flap of flexor surface skin to close the defect, through local flaps advanced to provide skin cover, to pedicled flaps from sites in the vicinity, transferred to the defect. Each has its protagonists, but the fact that none has universal acceptance indicates the complexity of the problem, and the fact that each technique has imperfections. Some of the methods are described on p. 205 *et seq.* The essential primary aims in managing a finger-tip injury are rapid healing, with a pain-free scar and a sensate pulp, and the use of complex reconstructions to achieve desirable as opposed to essential aims increases the possibility of failure to achieve either.

In practice, many finger-tip injuries are allowed to heal spontaneously, and it is remarkable how well most of them do. This applies most of all to children, where the defect in any case is a small one and there is no fear of a tender scar. Indeed, this fact should make the surgeon chary about carrying out elaborate procedures at all in children with finger-tip injuries. It is astonishing too how, with growth, the scar of a finger-tip injury, left untreated in the young child, shrinks in size, and similar shrinkage of a split skin graft takes place.

TECHNIQUES OF REPAIR AND RECONSTRUCTION

The skin of the palm is widely believed to be more rigid than skin in most other body sites, but its rigidity is largely determined by the degree of callosity which is present, and this depends on whether or not the individual is a manual worker. Even when the skin is soft and without any suggestion of callosity, an illusion of rigidity is created by its limited amount of mobility. The limitation is largely due to the pattern of flexure line 'creases' on the palm and the digits. Along these lines the skin is fixed deeply, to the palmar fascia in the palm, and to the fibrous flexor sheaths in the digits, the cushion of fibro-fatty pads which separate them elsewhere being absent. The effect of this deep fixation of the skin along the flexion creases is to limit its mobility in the areas between, particularly where the distance between two creases is short, as between the proximal and distal palmar creases. It also largely restricts the width of the defect which can be closed directly to the small amount of laxity present between adjacent creases.

Along the medial and lateral margins of the palm and the digits the skin loses the characteristics of palmar skin without taking on those of dorsal skin. Lacking hair follicles, but without the 'finger print' pattern of papillary ridges, it provides a 'neutral line' between the palmar and dorsal surfaces, remaining unwrinkled both when the digit is flexed and extended. In the two proximal digital segments the skin is also tethered to the sides of the phalangeal shafts by Cleland's ligaments.

On the dorsal surface the skin is flexible, and moves freely over the extensor tendons. A degree of skin laxity is indicated by the fine pattern of transverse wrinkle lines which is present over almost its entire surface, disappearing when the fingers are flexed. Overlying the site of each proximal interphalangeal joint in the fingers there is a localised area of skin redundancy, with a pattern of coarse transverse wrinkles, oval in outline but becoming circular with flattening of the wrinkling as the redundancy is taken up when the finger flexes. A similar redundancy is present over the interphalangeal joint of the thumb.

SUTURING TECHNIQUES

The skin of the palm is unusual in the way it reacts to suture materials. When many of the standard suture materials are used epithelium tends immediately to grow along the track of the suture, and removal of the suture, even relatively soon after insertion, leaves a cone-shaped keratin plug like a comedo in the path of the suture. This can give rise to discomfort amounting to pain on local pressure, with slight reddening around the site, and the condition is slow to subside. Different materials vary in their proneness to this complication, nylon being among the less prone.

The hand is a site where catgut used as a skin suture has a place. Epithelial down-growth and keratin plug formation do not appear to occur, and when it is used to suture wounds and for tie-over bolus dressings, the fact that it dissolves spontaneously is a valuable attribute in managing grafts and wounds particularly when the patient is a child.

PLACING SCARS

Incisions which cross palmar and digital creases at right angles should be avoided (Fig. 11.4) as contraction of the scar is liable to cause a flexion contracture. The principle also applies to a graft, to the extent that its margin should not run in an unbroken line across a crease, the marginal scar being liable to contract, particularly if there is failure of take at its margin for even a millimetre or two. It is well established that incisions which result in scars running lengthwise along the middle of the palmar aspect of a finger are contra-indicated because of the contracture which almost inevitably results.

In the finger, the lateral line is neutral as regards skin tension, and scars in that line are not subject to contractural problems. Similarly, if grafts and flaps are carried round on to the side of the finger to bring the marginal scar into this neutral line, a minor contracture of the scar becomes of little consequence.

These rules of scar placement, as they relate to the use of the neutral line and crossing the skin creases at right angles, are undoubtedly valid, but the latter particularly represents an extreme situation, and in that respect they are unnecessarily restrictive. Incision lines which cross the line of the flexion creases at more acute angles, or at the neutral line, have been found in practice to be acceptable, and between the flexion creases incisions can be allowed to run in virtually any direction. Examples of incisions which illustrate this approach, and which are frequently used, are shown in Figure 11.5. The scars which follow a properly designed Z-plasty also provide an example of these less restrictive practices.

USE OF THE Z-PLASTY

The Z-plasty can be used to prevent a contracture from developing when a linear incision running proximo-distally over the distal palm and the digit has been necessary to provide adequate surgical exposure, in Dupuytren's contracture for example, as discussed below, or to correct the linear contracted scar resulting from the use of such an incision, closed directly without incorporating a Z-plasty. The technique is most effective when the contracture is linear, well-defined, and narrow. It is unsuitable for the diffuse, broad contracture, for example post-burn, the importation of skin using a flap or graft being required.

Where the contracture crosses more than one skin crease, a multiple Z-plasty is generally required, with a Z to correspond to each crease. As explained in Chapter 2, the lengthening which occurs with each Z is accompanied by transverse

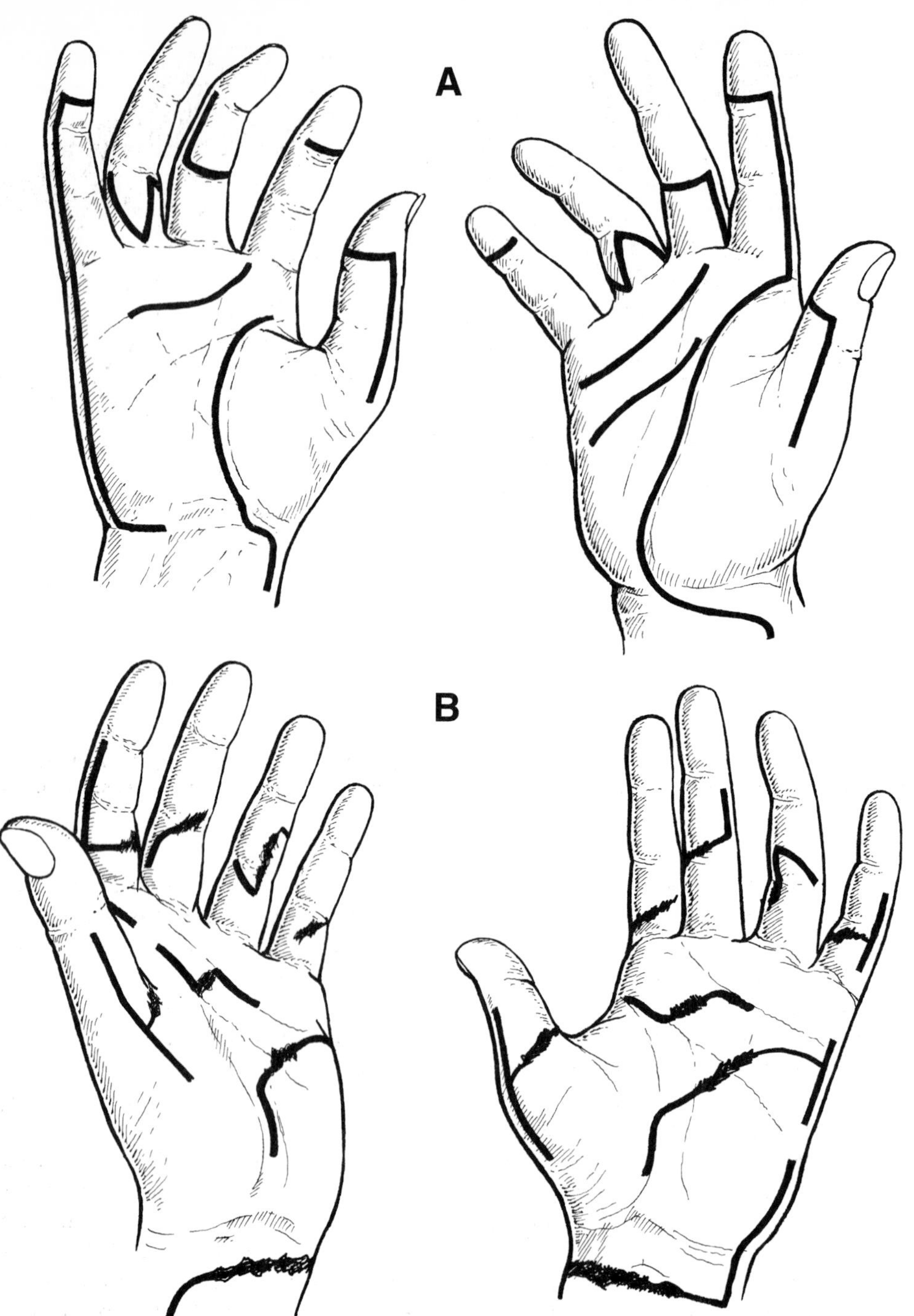

Fig. 11.4 Commonly used skin incisions in the hand (**A**). These may be combined or modified if necessary, *with the proviso that the blood supply of any flap raised must be adequate for its survival.*
Skin incisions, extending existing wounds (**B**), suitable to permit exploration, and repair if necessary, of nerves and tendons.

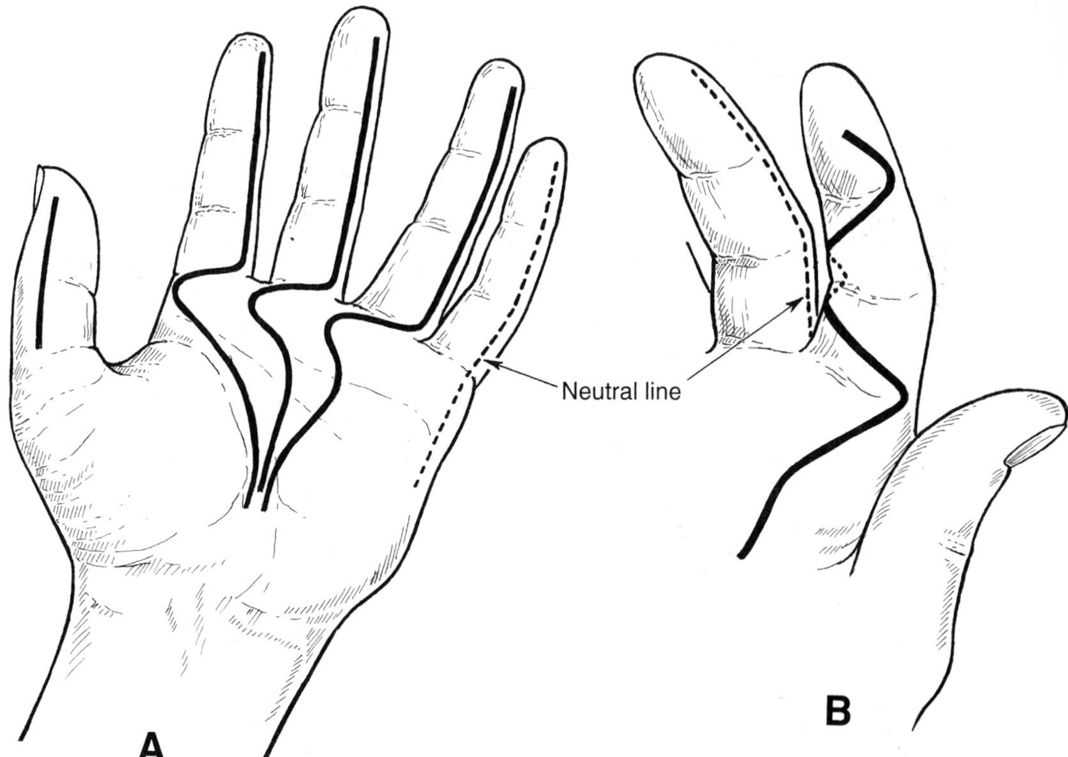

Fig. 11.5 Skin incisions, as described by Littler (**A**), and by Bruner (**B**). Although these incisions do not follow the restrictive dicta illustrated in Figure 11.4, they are entirely acceptable. The lateral line, with an absence of skin wrinkling, is neutral for skin tension.

shortening, and in the hand the amount of transverse slack available is extremely limited. A good working rule is that a Z-plasty of a size which would fit into the adjoining phalangeal segment can be used. This is certainly the largest Z which should be used, and a smaller one may be preferable. Each Z-plasty can be designed individually if desired; more often they are planned as a continuous multiple Z-plasty. The standard 60° Z-plasty is used routinely with the modified flap shape as shown in Figure 2.6 to broaden the tip of each flap. It is possible to make the multiple Zs skew or symmetrical, but unless the presence of previous scarring makes the skew design essential the symmetrical design is to be preferred.

The lines for elective scars in the hand have already been discussed, and the desirability of avoiding unnecessary crossing of a flexion crease. The Z-plasties should therefore be designed wherever possible so that, when completed, each transverse limb lies in a flexion crease.

To achieve this, the Z-plasty has to be planned formally, and drawn out on the skin (Fig. 11.6). The line of each flexion crease is marked as a first step. The key to successful planning of the actual Z-plasty incisions is to ensure that each lateral incision is made to end on the line of the flexion crease. Transposition of the flaps will then automatically leave the transverse limb lying along the crease.

In practice, with the line of the crease marked out on the skin, an equilateral triangle can be drawn on each side of the scar into which the Z-plasty is being inserted so that the apex of each triangle is on the crease already marked. Of the two possible pairs of 60° Z-plasty flaps outlined in this way, the appropriate one can be chosen in the knowledge that, since each incision ends on the crease, completion of the procedure will leave the transverse limb lying along the crease.

A multiple Z-plasty used in the hand leaves a redundancy of skin in passing from one Z to the

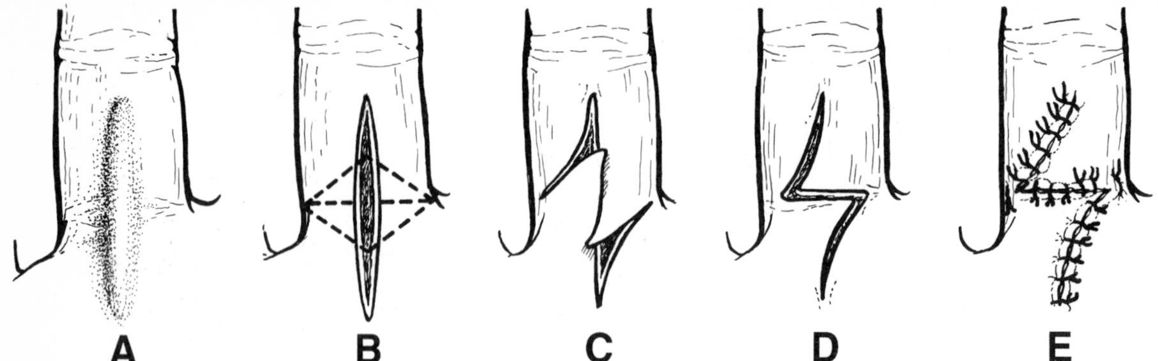

Fig. 11.6 Siting the Z-plasty in the hand to ensure that the transverse limb of the completed Z-plasty lies along a skin crease.

A The scar crossing the line of the metacarpophalangeal skin crease and producing contractural flexion of the joint.
B The triangles constructed on each side of the scar with the intended transverse limb along the metacarpophalangeal skin crease.
C, D The Z-plasty flaps selected, the skin incisions made, the flaps raised and transposed.
E The transposed flaps sutured in position with the transverse limb lying along the skin crease as planned.

Although the triangles on each side of the contracted scar are equilateral, contractural scars in practice are frequently under tension, and release of the tension when the Z-plasty flaps are raised allows the scarred skin to shorten a little. For this reason it may be appropriate for the limbs of a Z-plasty which are part of a contracted scar to be constructed a little longer than the limbs which are not similarly stressed, the limbs becoming equal in length when the contracture is released.

next. There is a temptation to trim this for greater neatness but it should be resisted. Skin is never available to excess in the palmar aspect of the hand and, in any case, if the Zs have been planned as described, the apparent excess will have developed in the middle of a phalangeal segment between the skin creases. There is a natural fullness in this part of a normal finger and the redundancy settles rapidly to a normal and natural-looking bulkiness.

As already indicated, the Z-plasty can also be effective used in Dupuytren's contracture. With conservative fasciectomy now largely standard, its virtues have become increasingly obvious. The contracture often presents as a linear contracture, sometimes confined to the finger or palm, sometimes extending over both. The linear proximodistal incision provides excellent access to the fascia, and the incorporation of a continuous multiple Z-plasty at the same time acts prophylactically to prevent any tendency to subsequent scar contraction (Fig. 11.7). When the finger is markedly contracted, the proximo-distal incision alone should be made in the first instance. Once the fasciectomy has been carried out and the finger is straight, or near straight, it becomes an easy matter to construct the Z-plasty flaps.

A problem which can arise in severe Dupuytren's contracture is the difficulty of excising the contracted fascia without 'buttonholing' the skin on one or other side of the initial longitudinal incision. By waiting until the fasciectomy is complete before designing the Z flaps it is usually possible, if the skin has been buttonholed, to make the 'hole' part of the incision used in designing the Z-plasty flaps without compromising their circulation. The effect may be to leave the transverse limb in a less than ideal line, but in the circumstances this is acceptable.

The method can also be used when the contracture involves more than one ray (Fig. 11.8). The palmar involvement is approached with the standard transverse skin incision, and the contractural element in each digit is exposed using the proximodistal incision already described, its proximal extent brought close to the transverse palmar incision but not becoming continuous with it. The exposure which this combination provides is exemplary and, with the fasciectomy carried out, the Z-plasties in each finger can be completed. Depending on the usual practice of the

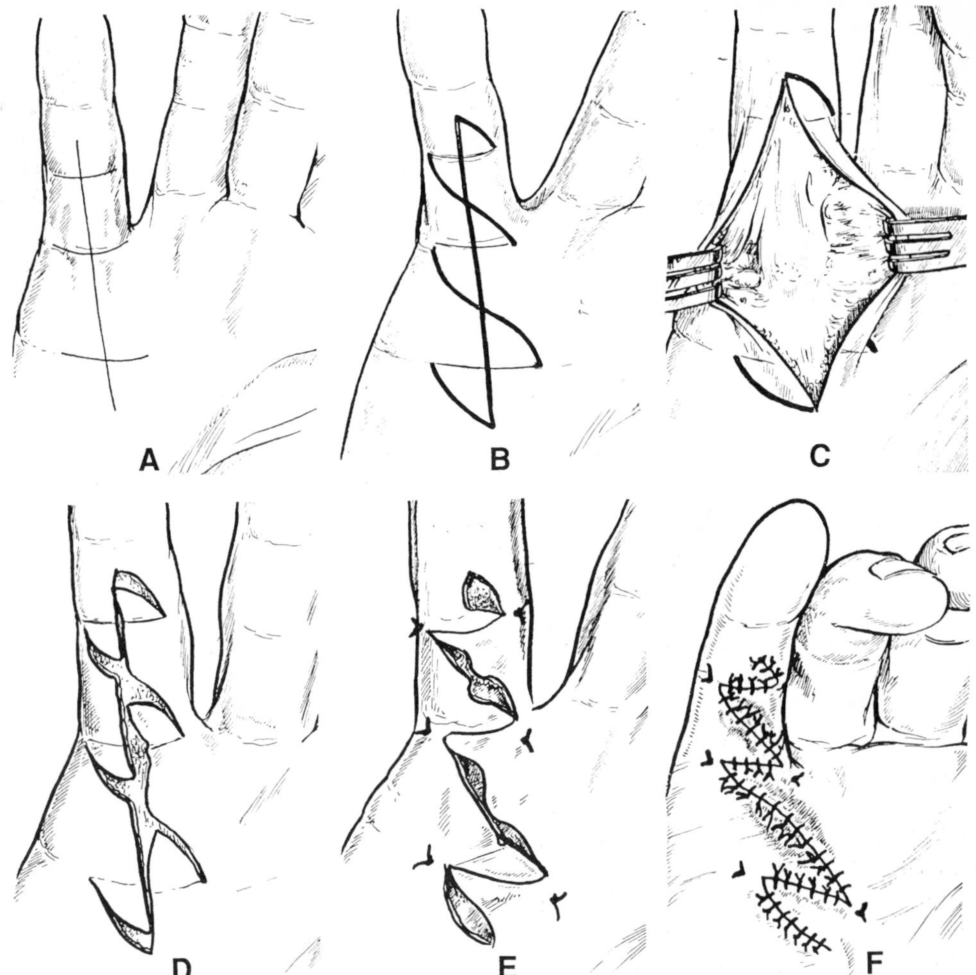

Fig. 11.7 The use of a continuous multiple Z-plasty in carrying out a fasciectomy for Dupuytren's contracture involving a single ray.
A The line of the skin incision, extending over the length of the contracted fascia, with the intended line of the transverse limb of each Z-plasty element in the line of a skin crease.
B The multiple Z-plasty drawn out on the skin to place each transverse limb of the completed Z-plasty in the skin crease, using the method shown in Figure 11.6.
C The exposure provided by the longitudinal skin incision.
D The fasciectomy completed and the Z-plasty flaps cut.
E The Z-plasty flaps in their transposed position, with each transverse limb in a skin crease.
F The completed procedure, with the skin sutured.

surgeon, the transverse palmar incision can either be closed or left unsutured, as in the McCash open palm method. This approach lends itself particularly well to the latter.

The problem of deepening the web (Fig. 11.9) can also sometimes be solved by the use of the Z-plasty. If the web is looked upon as a line of contracture, a Z-plasty can be designed with a dorsal and a palmar flap. Transposition of the flaps has the effect of lengthening the web and in the process deepening it. The method works best where the web is reasonably wide, allowing flaps of a suitable size to be used.

USE OF FREE SKIN GRAFTS

The individual behavioural characteristics of the split skin graft and the full thickness skin graft

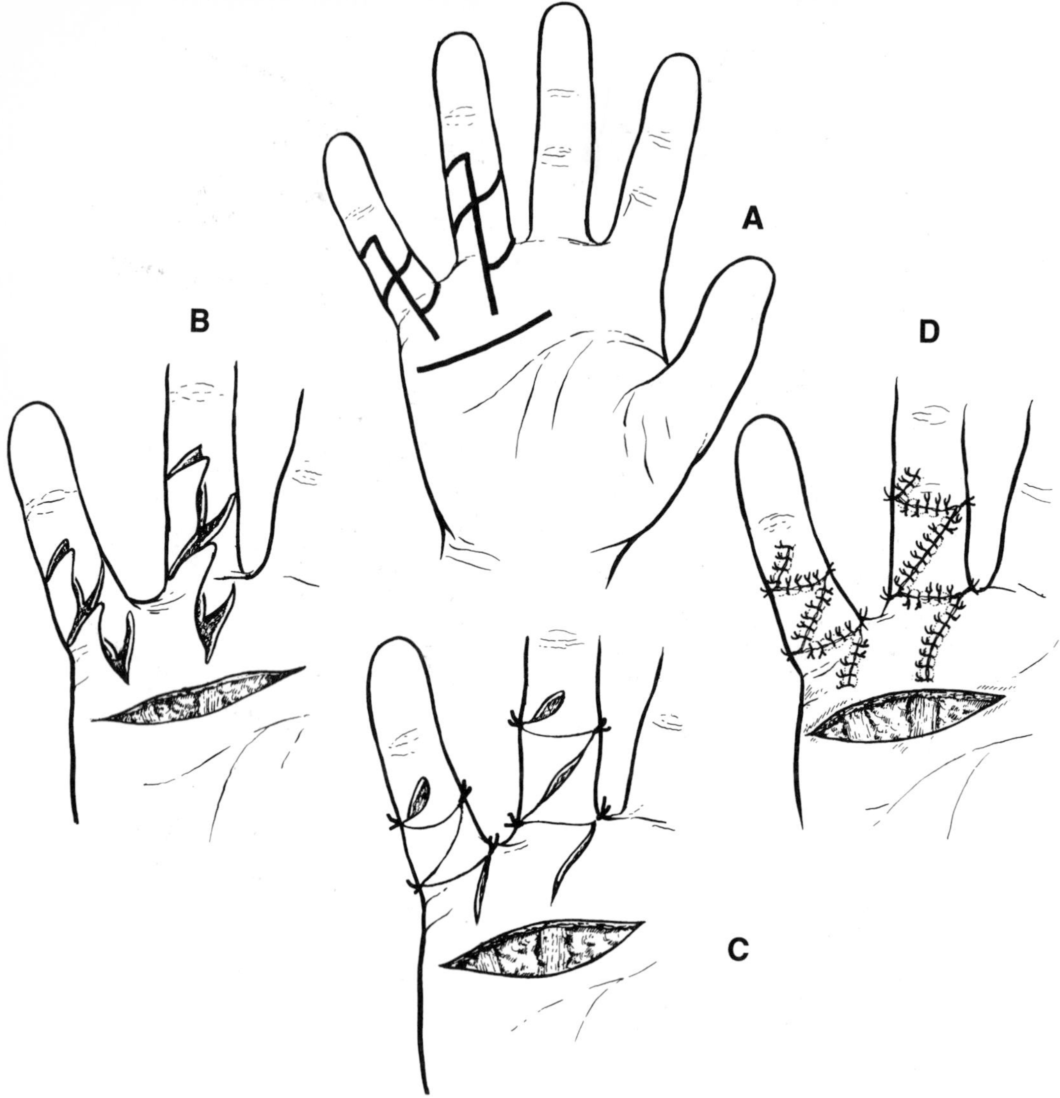

Fig. 11.8 The use of multiple Z-plasties, in combination with the Open Palm technique, in carrying out a fasciectomy in Dupuytren's contracture involving two rays.

A The skin incisions drawn on the skin, with the longitudinal incisions stopping short of the transverse palmar incision.
B The fasciectomy completed, and the Z-plasty incisions.
C The Z-plasty flaps transposed.
D Suturing of the Z-plasties completed, with the transverse palmar incision left to heal spontaneously.

determine their usage in the different sites and the differing circumstances which arise in providing skin cover.

The characteristics which are relevant are that a split skin graft takes more readily in clinical situations where there are adverse factors, but it contracts secondarily if circumstances permit. The full thickness skin graft requires optimum conditions for successful take, but it does not contract secondarily.

When the skin loss is post-traumatic, the all-important requirement is good graft take, and the graft of choice is therefore a split skin graft, even although the surgeon is aware that it will prob-

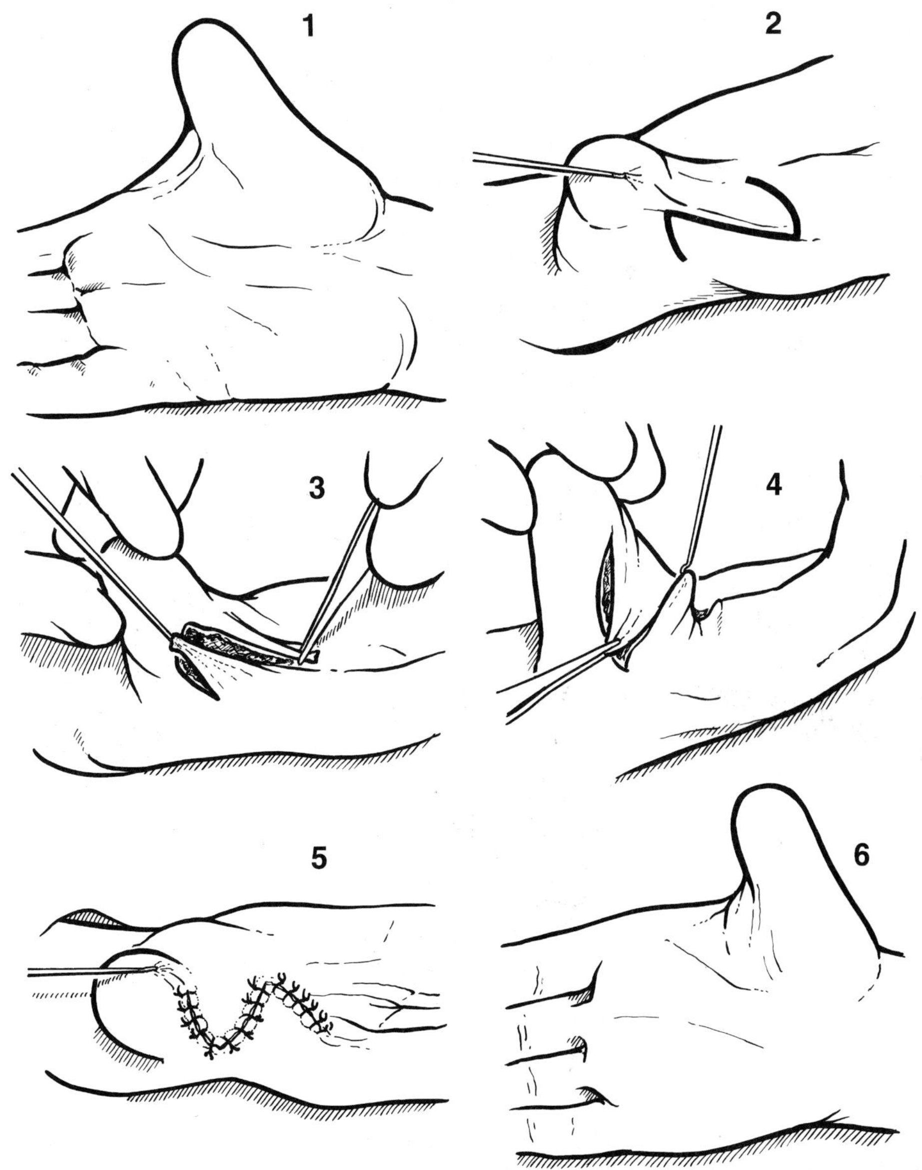

Fig. 11.9 The Z-plasty, used to deepen the web between the thumb and index finger to increase the grasp of a thumb short as a result of trauma.

ably be necessary to replace it subsequently with a full thickness skin graft if contracture becomes a problem. Where the defect has been surgically created, conditions for take can be assumed to be ideal, and the choice of graft type is then determined by how essential it is that the graft should not contract secondarily.

The grafts used for permanent cover in the dorsum and the palm differ because of the differences in their subsequent behaviour in the two sites. The degree of laxity of the skin of the dorsum of the hand and the fingers, coupled with its mobility, allows it to tolerate a degree of graft contraction, though the use of a moderately thick split skin graft, in which the tendency to contract is minor, is still preferable.

A further factor in selection concerns the comparative power of the long extensors and flexors in the hand, and whether or not that power is able to overcome the innate tendency of split skin grafts to contract secondarily. The tendency of split skin grafts to contract secondarily is a temporary phenomenon and, in clinical situations where contraction can be prevented for a prolonged period, the tendency is finally and permanently overcome. The flexor group of muscles appear to be powerful enough to act in this way and prevent significant late contraction. For these reasons the split skin graft can safely be used on the dorsum of the hand and fingers. In the palm the less powerful extensors are unable to prevent late graft contraction and, as a result, full thickness skin grafts are used to resurface palmar defects. In the webs also, where secondary contraction would have adverse effects, a full thickness skin graft is preferable.

Split skin grafts settle remarkably well on the dorsum, both of the hand and the fingers, generally developing a pattern of creases to match the surrounding skin, and weathering to an appearance which makes it virtually indistinguishable from the surrounding skin, particularly if it has proved possible to leave the dorsal pattern of veins intact.

Free skin grafts applied to sites on the tactile surfaces which are used in heavy work have a subsequent tendency to fissure. This disadvantage can be overcome by using one of the glabrous skin donor sites which more nearly match the skin of the palm. The available sites (Fig. 11.10) are limited in area, but where a small graft only is required, excellent quality split skin can be obtained from the ulnar margin of the hand, extending forward from the neutral line, between the distal palmar crease and the wrist crease. The non-weightbearing instep area of the sole of the foot has similar skin, and is capable of providing a greater although still limited amount of skin. Both donor sites heal quickly, and seem to give no problems such as tender scars.

A late problem which may arise following the use of a graft, whether full thickness or split skin, is the development of a line of contraction along the margin of the graft, by a process akin to that

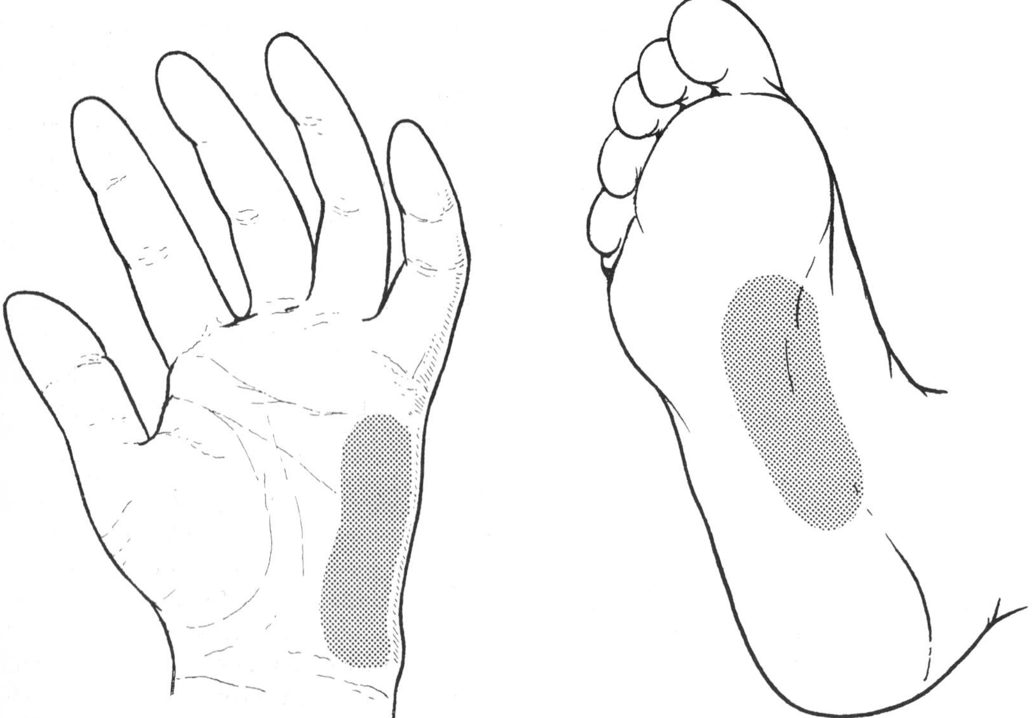

Fig. 11.10 The sites from which small split skin grafts of glabrous skin can be harvested.

which causes scar contraction. The severity of the resulting contracture depends on the site and how rapidly healing at the margin of the graft has taken place. It is not always possible to avoid such contraction but its more severe effects can at least be mitigated by placing the margins of the graft along one of the elective incision lines already described (p. 191). The bringing of the graft margin to such a line may of course mean carrying the graft beyond the obvious defect, if need be excising normal skin to do so. If this is felt to be undesirable, an alternative may be to break the line of any contracture which subsequently develops with a Z-plasty.

The method of applying and suturing the graft is similar to that described for general use. When applying the tie-over bolus and the subsequent pressure dressing, care should be taken to avoid undue pressure on the graft. It is the graft on the dorsum of the fingers and hand which is specifically at risk, and the most vulnerable areas are the prominences caused by the heads of the metacarpals and the proximal phalanges. Failure of the graft in these areas is particularly undesirable, exposure of extensor tendon and joint capsule being a likely result. Marked flexion of the fingers accentuates these prominences, and the hand is best immobilised on the extended side of the position of function.

The application of the dressing will be discussed under the heading of Postoperative Care.

USE OF FLAPS

The flaps used in the hand are either **pedicled** or **free**, and at the outset of any discussion on the pros and cons of their use it has to be recognised that unless the surgeon has the expertise to transfer a free flap, and the necessary facilities, he is restricted to using pedicled flaps.

Pedicled flaps

The pedicled flaps used in reconstructing hand defects are either *local* or *distant*.

The majority of **local flaps** used in practice were designed to cope with specific problems, most often involving either the palmar aspect of digits which were unsuitable for grafting, or the distal phalangeal segment with loss of pulp or part of the nail bed, and they do not have a wider clinical usage. Others make use of the skin of the dorsum of the hand, the deep fixation and physical characteristics of palmar skin making it unsuitable for use as a flap. The only site on the hand which can provide even a modestly sized transposed or rotation type of flap is the area between the wrist and the webs, and as a result the defect which it can cover is a small one.

Distant flaps can be of the *direct* or *tubed axial pattern* type (p. 79), or as a pedicled variant of the *radial forearm flap*, in which the part of its perfusing arteriovenous system distal to the flap is retained as its pedicle. A further flap, the *posterior interosseous* (p. 201), which uses the same principle, pedicled on the posterior interosseous arteriovenous system, has also been described. All of these flaps are capable of being used primarily, and can consequently be used in acute trauma.

In the case of the **direct flap** the very short pedicle reduces the margin for error very greatly, and the transfer has to be planned with considerable care. It also requires immobilisation of the involved part of the hand and arm for a minimum of three weeks, and this is liable to create problems of stiffness not merely of the fingers but also of the elbow and shoulder, particularly in the older age group. In the past, because of the absence of alternatives, it had a significant role in acute major hand trauma. With the alternatives currently available its role has markedly diminished.

The **tubed axial pattern flap** has the advantage of the latitude which its long pedicle permits. Its favourable length:breadth ratio also reduces somewhat the need for careful positional planning and fixation.

The flap most often used is the *groin flap* (Fig. 11.11), and the *hypogastric flap* is an alternative. With either flap the position is a comfortable one for the patient, but both sites can be undesirably fat, the hypogastrium more so than the flank, and this might influence the surgeon in his choice. The hypogastric flap also transfers skin which is often hairy while the groin flap uses skin which is usually free of hair even in the most hirsute. The secondary defect of the groin flap is less con-

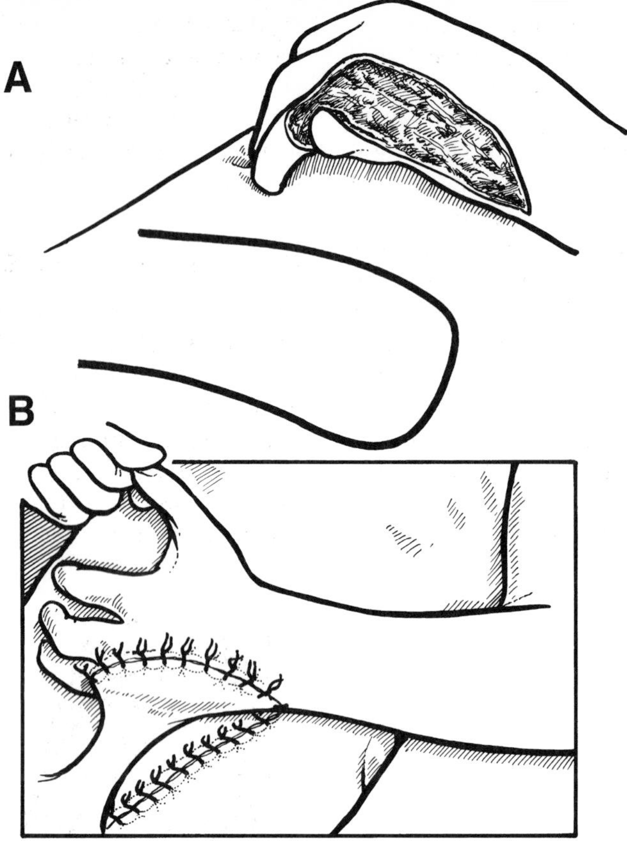

Fig. 11.11 The groin flap, used to resurface a defect of the ulnar side of the hand.
A The defect of the hand and the groin flap outlined.
B The groin flap raised and transferred, with the secondary defect closed directly.

spicuous, and it can usually be closed by direct suture. Both flaps involve a degree of dependency of the hand and, as a result, carry a potential for postoperative oedema. The severity of the problem largely depends on the degree to which the type of the injury and its extent preclude the early institution of a full regimen of active exercises. Oedema has proved to be less of a problem when the flap is used in secondary reconstruction, and active exercises can be instituted from the outset.

The *deltopectoral flap* (Fig. 11.12) is also capable of providing a considerable area of thin flexible skin. It maintains the hand in an elevated position, and on that basis might be expected to counter the development of oedema. In practice, the ease with which the hand can be brought to the chest and maintained there depends on the physical characteristics of the patient, easy when the

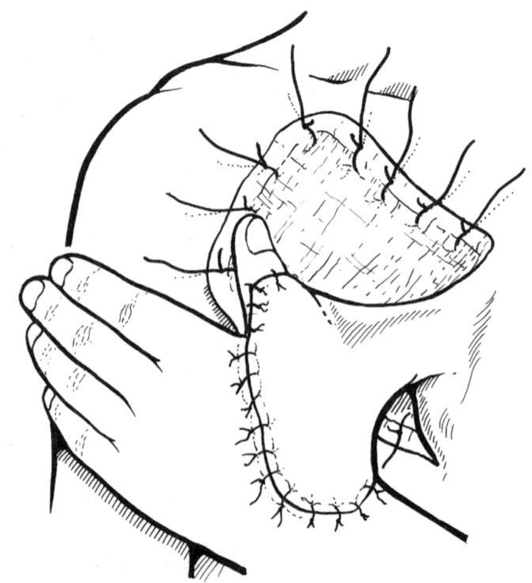

Fig. 11.12 The use of the deltopectoral flap, showing the way in which the site of the flap helps to maintain the hand in an elevated position.

patient is thin, difficult in the case of the short, broad-chested individual. This is an aspect easily tested, and would be part of the selection process. The role of the deltopectoral flap has historically been in head and neck surgery, but for the hand surgeon restricted to the use of pedicled flaps it is worthy of consideration.

The skin transferred in the *pedicled version of the radial forearm flap* has similar characteristics to those of its parent free flap. To have a vascular pedicle long enough to permit transfer to a hand defect, the flap has to be sited in the proximal forearm, with a skin incision made from the distal border of the flap in the direction of the wrist to allow mobilisation of the vessels forming the pedicle. Depending on the site of the defect the distal extent of the vascular pedicle may be in virtual continuity with it; if it is not, the forearm incision is extended to bring it into continuity with the defect. A key element in the safety of the flap lies in ensuring that the pedicle is of adequate length, and is not subjected to external pressure.

Posterior interosseous flap

The posterior interosseous flap (Fig. 11.13) is sited a little above the middle of the forearm on its extensor aspect, and is based on the posterior interosseous artery and its venae comitantes. The vessels emerge proximally from under supinator into the intermuscular septum lying between extensor carpi ulnaris and extensor minimi digiti and pass distally in the septum, reaching the dorsal

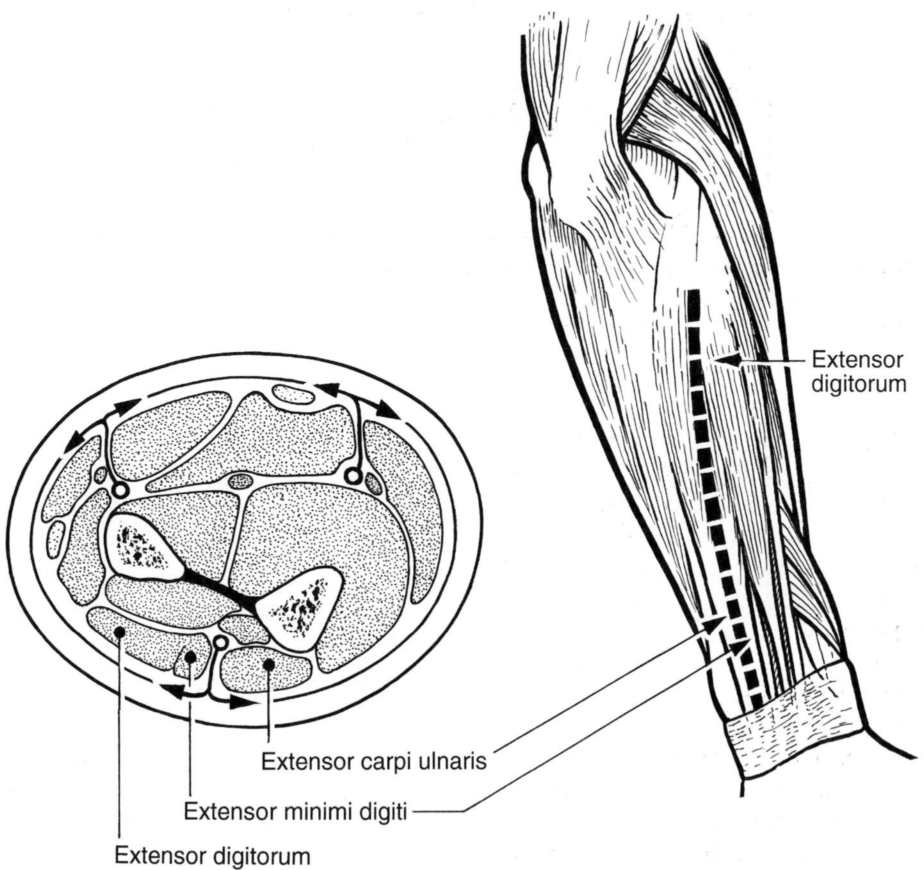

Fig. 11.13 The posterior interosseous flap.
The line of emergence of the perforating vessels which perfuse the flap, and the line of dissection in mobilising its vascular pedicle, lies between extensor carpi ulnaris and extensor minimi digiti. The distinction between the two is greater distally, and it is there that the dissection to separate them is begun.

carpal vascular arch, and anastomosing with the anterior interosseous vessels at the level of the wrist. Branches are given to the adjacent muscles and the ulna, and also to the investing layer of deep fascia, through it perfusing the overlying skin. In the process of elevating the flap the vessels proximal to it are divided, and blood flow becomes retrograde with reliance on the dorsal carpal arch and the anastomosis with the anterior interosseous vessels, the site of which provides the pivot point of the flap.

In planning the transfer of the flap, the surface marking of the septum, a line joining the lateral epicondyle of the humerus and the head of the ulna with the arm fully pronated, is drawn on the skin, and the flap is outlined as an ellipse positioned with its axis proximo-distal and its centre approximately 9 cm from the lateral epicondyle. The flap is designed with its long axis proximo-distal. Its width is limited by the desirability of closing the defect directly, 5 cm being an approximate maximum though, with the defect consisting of muscle belly, split skin grafting should present no problems.

The margin of the flap and the line of the septum distal to it are incised, and the musculotendinous structures are dissected free from each side of the septum with its vessel content. Dissection is carried out from distal to proximal because the structures involved are superficial in the distal forearm and easier to identify, in contrast to the situation proximally where the vessels lie deeply, hidden between the two muscle bellies. With an artery whose external diameter is approximately 1.7 mm, and branches which are correspondingly smaller, the dissection involved is a delicate one, and cannot be hurried.

The relative shortness of the vascular pedicle restricts its use mainly to defects of the dorsum of the hand. On the palmar aspect it cannot reach much beyond the wrist. For defects of these sites it provides thin skin of excellent quality. It has the further virtue of not requiring the sacrifice of a major perfusing source for the hand, a factor which may be relevant in a mutilating injury.

Free flaps

In free flap selection, desirable attributes are that the skin which it provides should be adequate in area, thin and flexible. There is obvious advantage in having the donor site in the same arm, thus confining dressings to a single limb, and making for easy mobilisation both of the patient and his hand.

The flaps which fall into this category are the *radial forearm* (p. 111) and the *lateral upper arm* (p. 114). Of the two, transfer of the radial forearm flap is technically easier, and is generally more popular. As discussed on p. 114, the ulnar forearm flap is a potential alternative, used both as a free flap, and pedicled distally.

Before either of the forearm flaps is used, the effect of the injury on the various perfusion sources of the hand must be assessed with care, since the process of transfer involves division of one of the two major axial arteries in the proximal forearm.

PREPARATION OF THE DEFECT

In preparing the defect, its margin should always be excised to healthy tissue, and this applies with equal force to a granulating area. Only with adequate marginal excision, removing any spread epithelium, can the flap be soundly sutured to good surgical material. As has been pointed out in relation both to scars and free skin grafts in the hand, and for the same reasons, ideally the margin between a flap and the hand is best placed along one of the elective lines for scars. This may involve bringing the flap beyond the obvious defect and, if the resection required is small, is worth doing.

When a flap is being transferred as a preliminary to a reconstructive procedure, e.g. of tendon, it may be advisable to have the transfer complete and the area healed before treatment of the deep structure is begun, particularly if sepsis is seen as a potential hazard.

DEFECTS PROXIMAL TO THE WEBS

If a defect of the dorsum is small, a rotation or transposed flap is occasionally a possible method of repair (Fig. 11.14). Planning has to be careful, since the amount of 'slack' available is deceptively small, and free skin grafting of the secondary defect is almost always needed. In practice, cases suitable for such a local flap seldom occur.

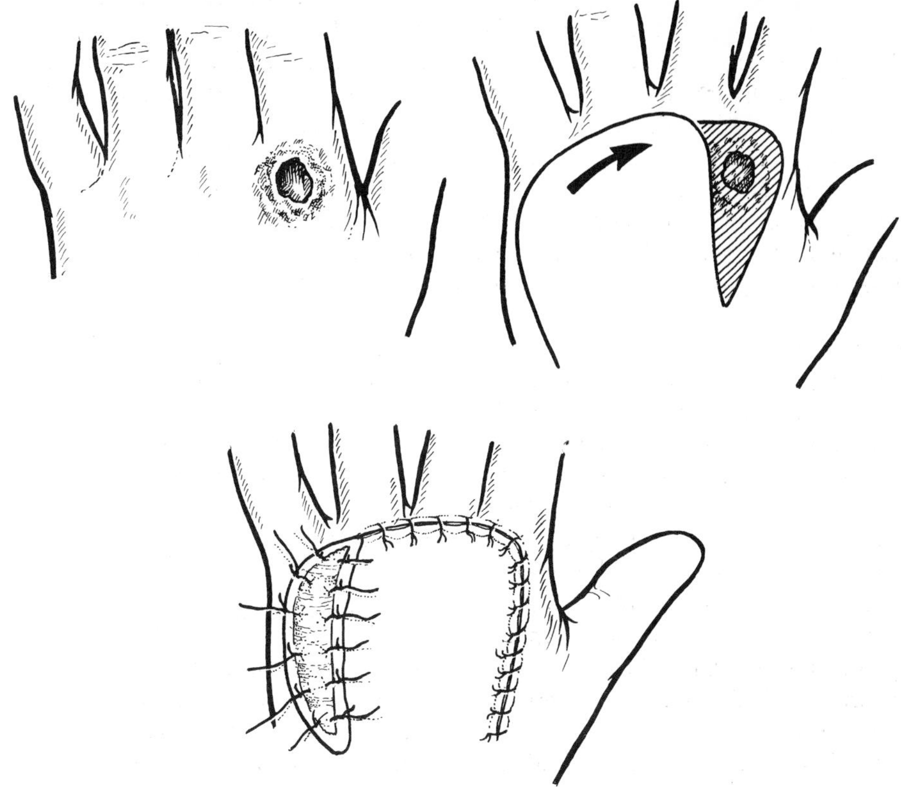

Fig. 11.14 A transposed flap, used to provide skin cover for a localised deeply penetrating ulcer of the dorsum of the hand.

Its use in the older age group is generally unwise. Ageing, atrophic skin makes poor surgical material, and is apt to necrose.

When a distant flap is required, the decision regarding the appropriate source depends very much on the size of the defect. For the defect of intermediate size near the radial or ulnar side a direct flap from the opposite forearm is a possibility (Fig. 11.15). A very real factor in limiting the value of such a cross-arm flap concerns the fact that the patient will be unable to look after his toilet requirements. The upper arm is also a potential source, used in correction of the adduction contracture of the first web by filling the gap created when the contracture has been opened up (Fig. 11.16). The hand with the web opened fits particularly well around the upper arm, and the position is a comfortable one for the patient.

When the defect is more extensive, the facilities available and the expertise of the surgeon are likely to determine whether a free transfer such as a radial forearm flap or one of the pedicled transfers already described is chosen.

DEFECTS DISTAL TO THE WEBS

The defect may be of one finger only or of several fingers and according to circumstances a local flap from the same or an adjoining finger, or a distant flap from the arm or trunk, may be used for cover. The first choice should generally be a local flap, but its use implies a localised defect. It is when the defect is more extensive or involves more than one finger that the larger area of tissue a distant flap provides is unavoidable.

Distant flaps

Because of their size, most distant flaps are unsuited for the average defect involving a single

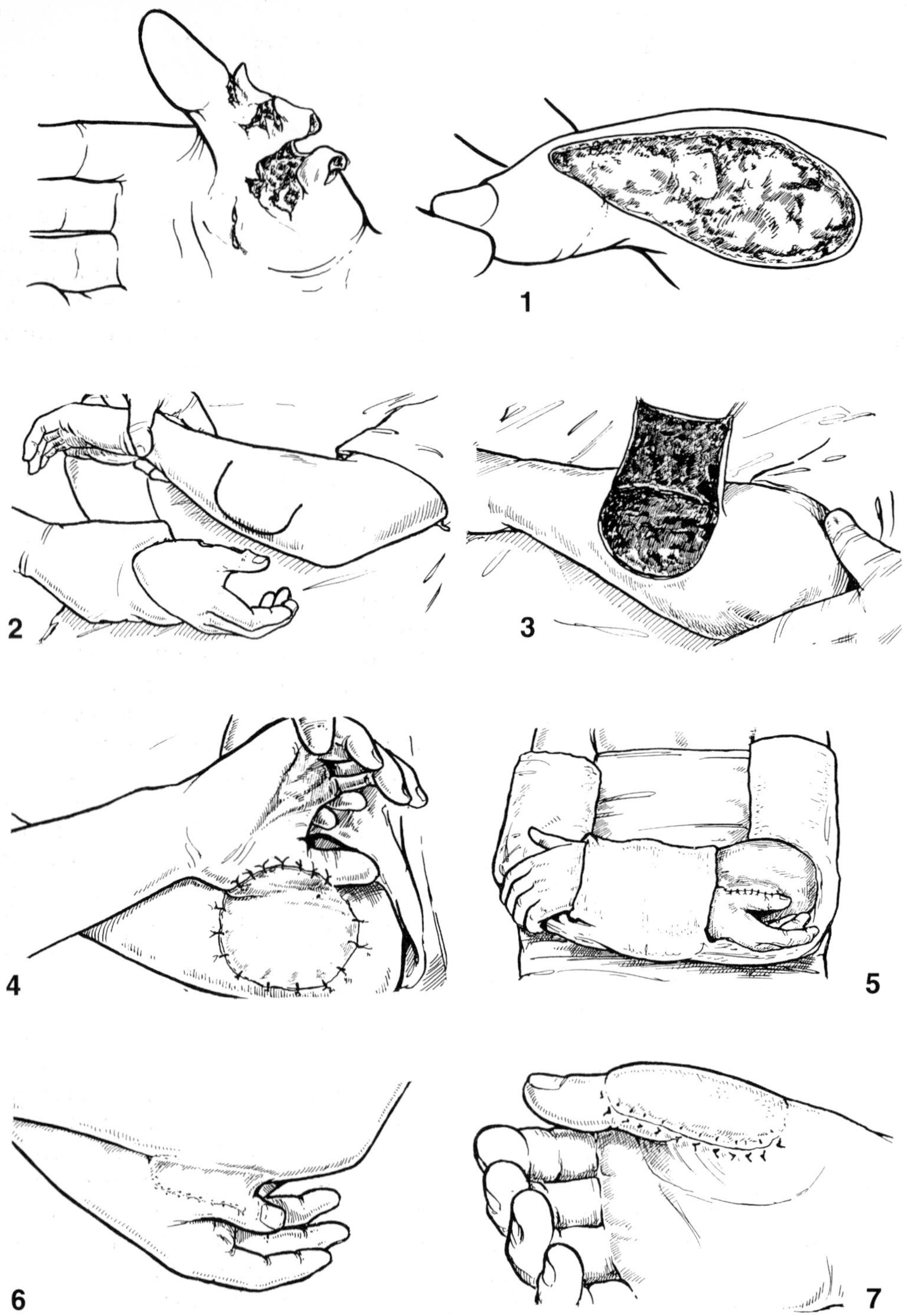

Fig. 11.15 The use of a cross-arm flap in repairing an injury of the thenar eminence. The injury, involving the metacarpophalangeal joint, prepared (**1**) to receive the flap after excision of all damaged tissue, and in position to receive the flap, outlined on the forearm (**2**), and raised (**3**). The split skin graft applied to the secondary defect is extended to line the bridge segment of the flap (**4**), with plaster of Paris fixation of the arms (**5**). **6** shows the flap at three weeks, immediately prior to division, and 7 the flap divided with insetting completed.

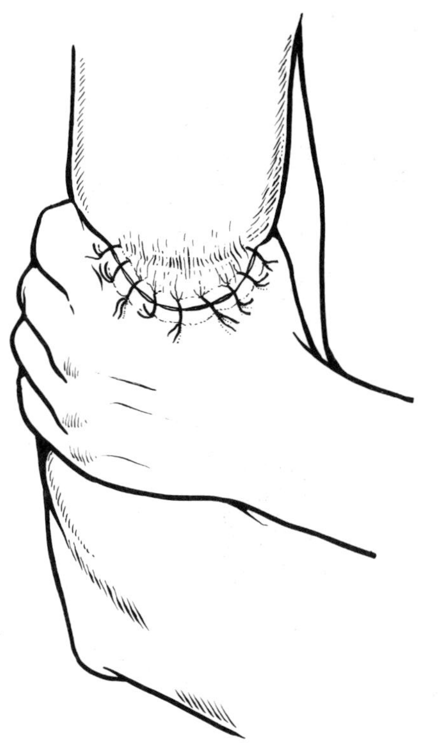

Fig. 11.16 Cross-arm flap raised on the upper arm, used in correction of a 1st web contracture, showing how the hand fits round the upper arm, helping to maintain the correction of the contracture while the flap is attaching to the defect.

digit. It is in managing defects which involve several digits that they can be of value. When it is possible to convert the small individual defects into a single larger defect by suturing the adjacent margins of each defect together, creating a temporary syndactyly, it can become a candidate for a single distant flap (Fig. 11.17).

The subsequent management of such a reconstruction provides certain problems once the flap has been successfully transferred, relating to the management of the syndactyly. If a pedicled flap has been used, it is probably best to divide the pedicle before dividing the syndactyly, to allow mobilisation of the fingers. It is when the fingers come to be separated that difficulties arise because of the thickness of the flap, as demonstrated in Figure 11.18. The simplest solution is to remove the flap in its entirety, and split skin graft the raw surface on each digit. In contrast to the surface exposed at the time of the injury, which would not have accepted a graft, the coverage provided by the flap creates a surface which, when the flap is removed, can be grafted without difficulty.

Local flaps

Local flaps have their greatest value in managing defects on the flexor aspect of the fingers which are unsuitable for grafting, often because they extend deeply to expose the flexor tendons, and in managing certain guillotine amputations of the distal phalangeal segment.

Cross-finger flaps

These flaps are raised on the dorsal aspect of a finger, most often to provide cover for a defect of the palmar aspect, occasionally the tip, of a nearby digit. The defect of the flexor aspect considered suitable for the technique usually involves the middle and/or proximal phalangeal segments. Shorter defects increase the length:breadth ratio of the flap to an undesirable extent, while the technical difficulties of the transfer increase if the area to be covered is much longer than this.

The flap is side-based in most instances (Fig. 11.19), though a distal pedicle is generally required in the rare instances when the flap is used in order to preserve the length of a finger, as in Figure 11.20. In designing such a distally based flap, it is important to avoid encroaching on the nail bed of the donor finger. The index finger is the one which is most likely to sustain an injury suitable for this particular flap.

When the defect is of the thumb, the fact that its distal phalangeal segment lies alongside the proximal segment of the index finger means that the site of the defect suitable for the reconstruction can extend well on to the distal segment of the digit. The patient may also find the position more comfortable with the middle rather than the index finger used as the donor digit (Fig. 11.21), and a preoperative trial should be carried out to test this before proceeding to design the transfer.

The flap must be raised to leave the extensor expansion of the donor finger covered with paratenon, and in the case of the side-based

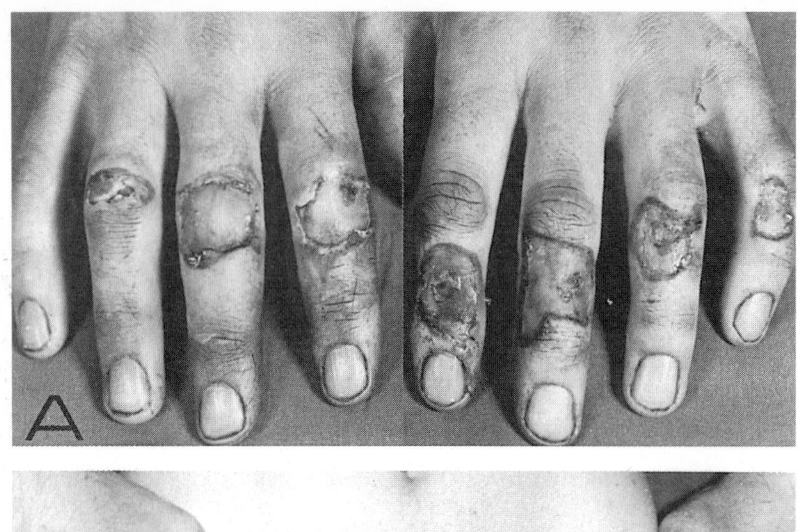

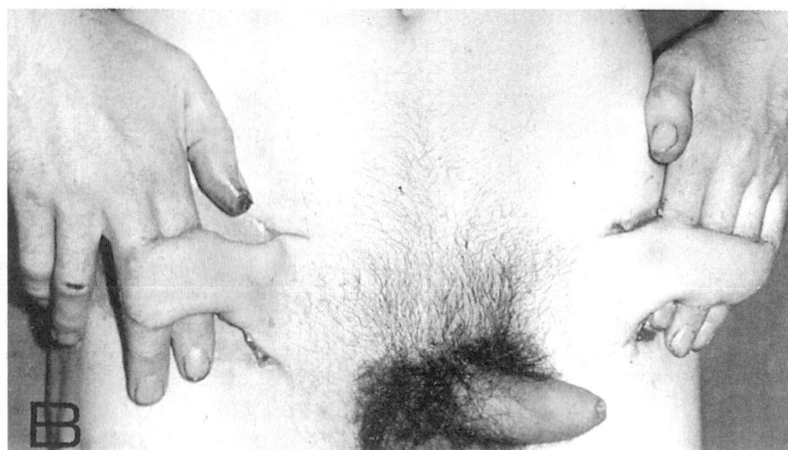

Fig. 11.17 The conversion of an injury involving several fingers into a single defect to facilitate the provision of flap cover.
The injuries of both hands (**A**), consisting of full thickness skin loss burns of the dorsal aspects of several fingers, with damage to the underlying extensor expansion, were converted (**B**) in each into a single defect and covered with a groin flap.
The subsequent management of this patient is shown in Figure 11.18.

design to avoid baring the digital nerve and artery. The secondary defect on the donor finger is covered with a thick split skin graft, extended to line the bridge segment of the flap, using a bolus tie-over dressing.

The reach of a side-based cross-finger flap can be increased if a point is made of dividing Cleland's skin ligaments (Fig. 11.19 C,D). These ligaments, as they appear in this surgical procedure, combine to form a fibrous septum just dorsal to the neurovascular bundle, and they bind the skin of the neutral line to the side of each phalanx. Their division frees the skin of the neutral line and adds considerably to the mobility and reach of the flap itself. The pedicle of the flap is divided at 3 weeks. If it is felt that the attachment of the flap is too tenuous for comfort, insetting can be postponed for a further week.

V–Y flaps

Following a guillotine amputation it may be possible to cover the finger-tip defect by advancing distally a V-shaped flap of the pulp skin, approximating the skin on either side to close the residual pulp defect (Fig. 11.22). The effect is to convert the initial V of the flap into a Y-shaped suture line.

The V is designed on the pulp skin so that its apex reaches almost to the distal interphalangeal crease, and the width of its base distally should equal that of the nail. The incision along the

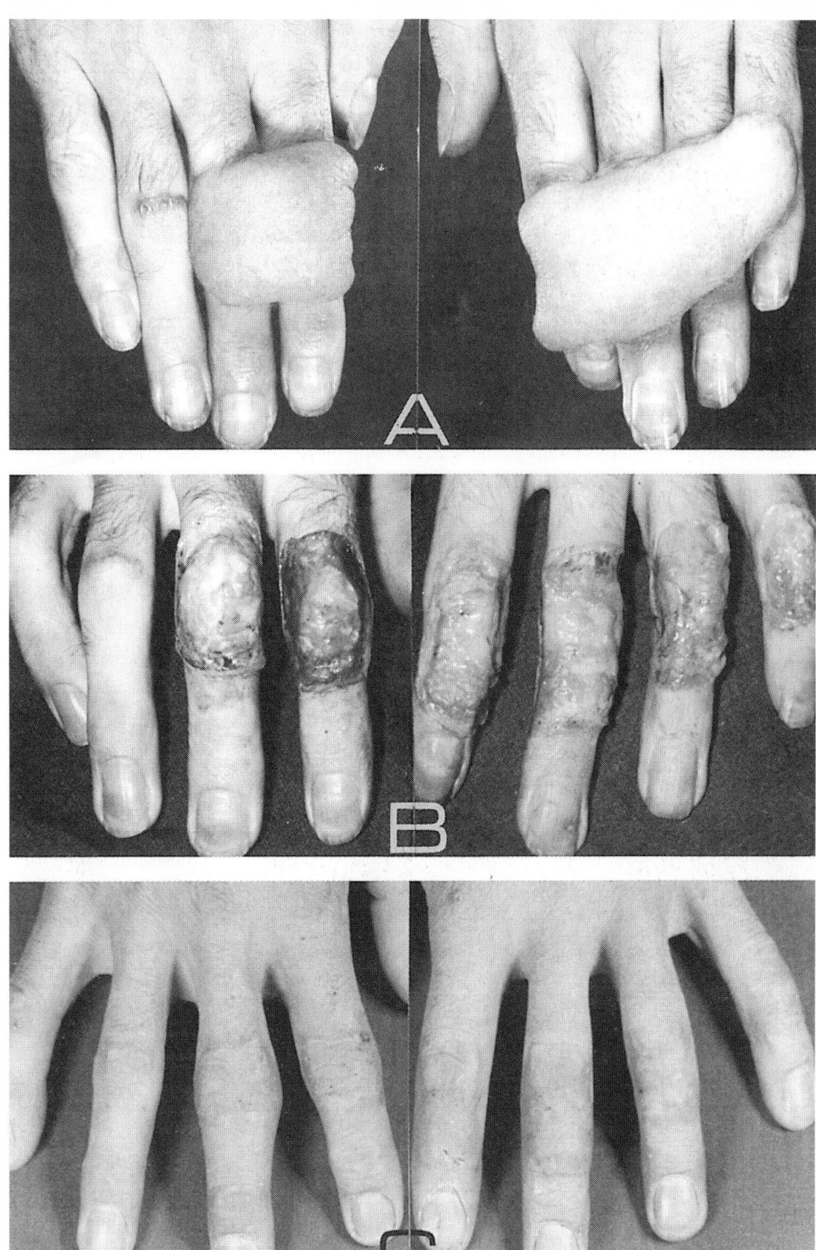

Fig. 11.18 The subsequent management of the injured digits shown in Figure 11.17, using the 'crane' principle.

A The groin flaps divided at three weeks following application, to allow full mobilisation of the hand, elbow and shoulder as early as possible, leaving the temporary syndactyly.
B The surfaces left following excision of the flap from each hand, ready for split skin grafting.
C The end result following split skin grafting.

The concept of using a flap to provide temporary cover for a defect in order to convert a surface, initially unsuitable for grafting because of tissue damage, into one suitable for grafting by making use of the reparative capacity of the vascular content of the flap, as in the patient illustrated, is referred to as the 'crane' principle.

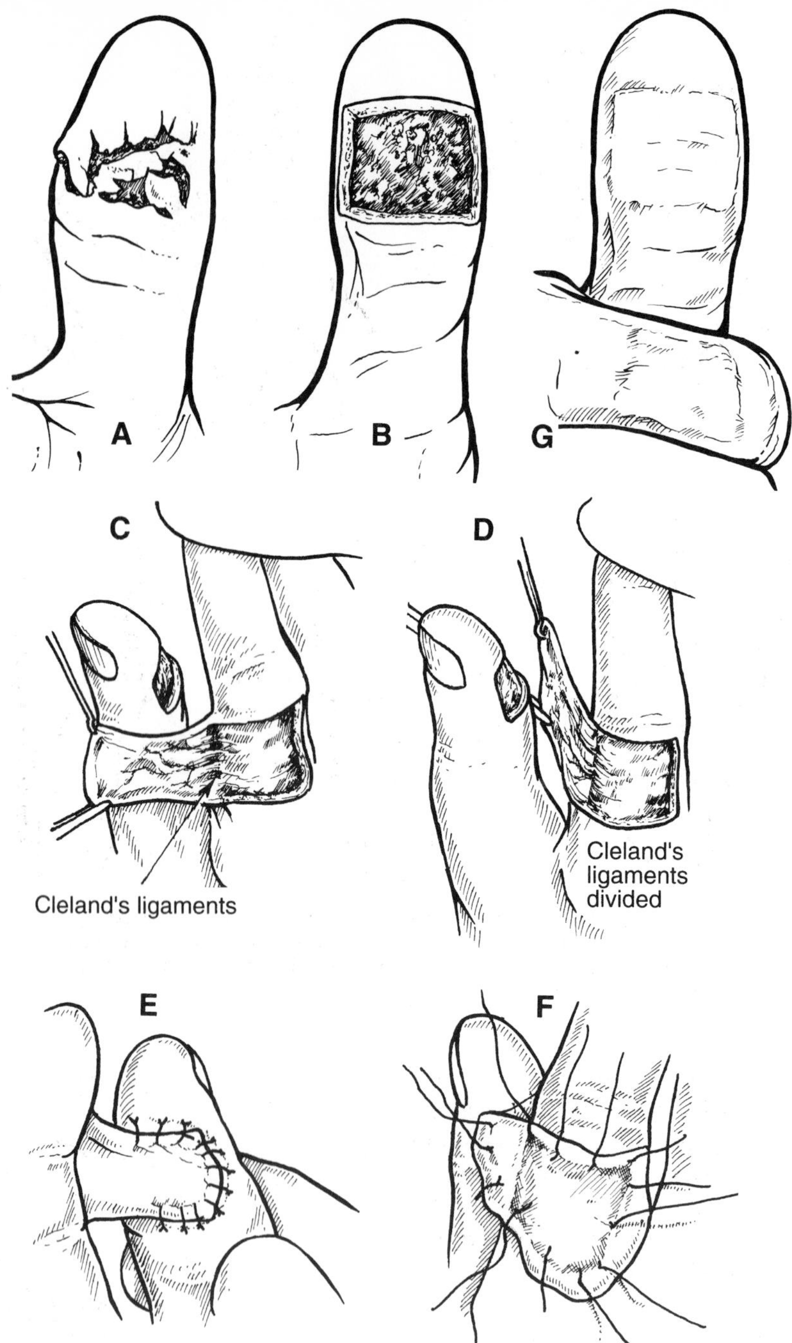

Fig. 11.19 Cross-finger flap used to resurface the pulp of the thumb.
The injury of the pulp (**A**), and the defect prepared to receive the flap (**B**). The flap, laterally based, raised and turned back, before dividing Cleland's ligaments (**C**), and after dividing the ligaments (**D**) to provide the flap with additional reach. The flap is sutured to the defect (**E**), and the split skin graft applied to the secondary defect (**F**), ready for the tie-over bolus to be applied, with the final result (**G**), following division and insetting of the flap.

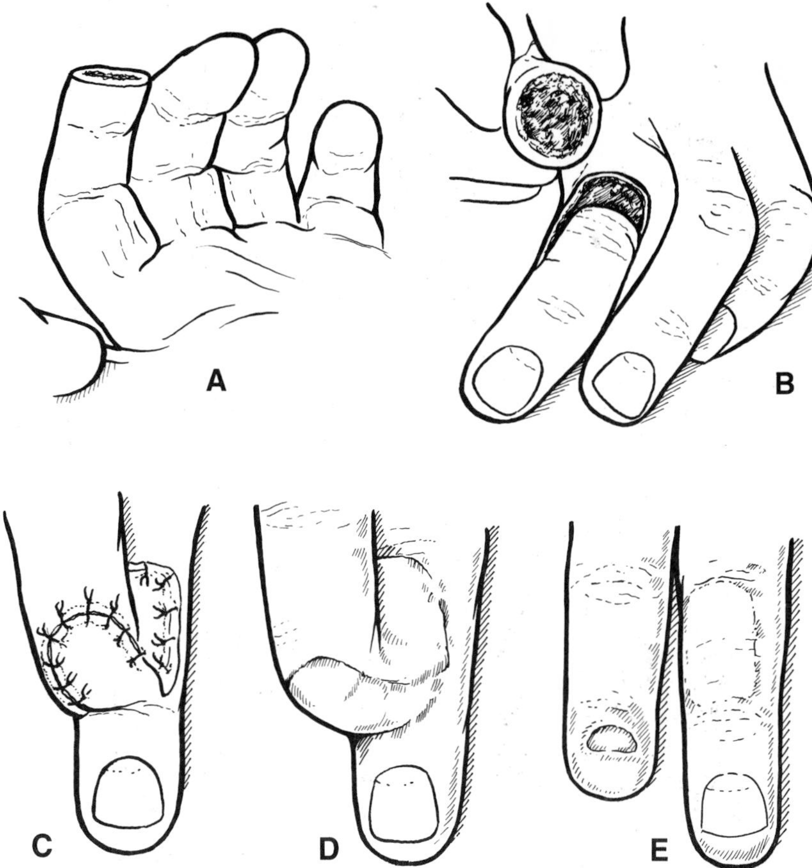

Fig. 11.20 A distally based cross-finger flap used to cover a guillotine injury of the index finger-tip.
The injury (**A**), and the distally based flap (**B**) raised on the dorsum of the middle finger. The flap sutured in position (**C**), with a split skin graft applied to the secondary defect, and the appearance (**D**) 14 days after the transfer of the flap. The final result (**E**) after division and insetting of the flap.

limbs of the V goes through skin alone. Thereafter, sharp-pointed scissors are thrust carefully into the pulp fat and gently opened, mobilise the flap without destroying its nerve and vascular attachment to the proximal finger. Freeing of the flap deeply is carried out by dividing its fibrous attachment to the distal phalanx and the distal fibrous flexor sheath close to these structures. Mobilised, the flap is advanced distally and sutured to the margins of the pulp defect with fine sutures. Suturing around each side of the flap proceeds until the lines meet at the apex of the V and continues proximally, converting the suture line into a Y.

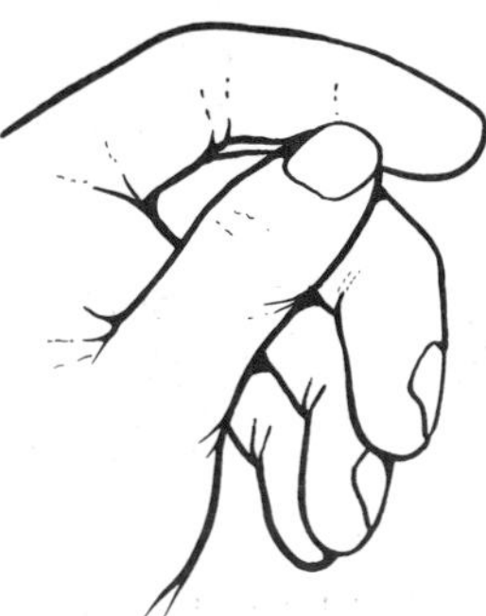

Fig. 11.21 The middle finger can be a potential donor for a cross-finger flap to the thumb, depending on the site of the defect and its extent, as demonstrated by the ease of the position when the two are placed together.

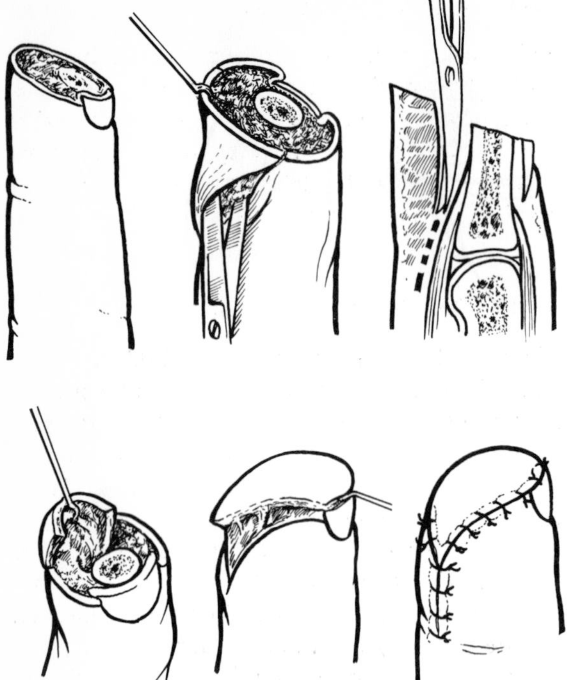

Fig. 11.22 The V–Y pulp advancement flap, as applied to a guillotine amputation of the finger-tip, showing the various steps in the technique.

The flap is really neurovascular and the mobilisation necessary to achieve the required degree of advancement is best carried out under magnification. The method works best when the obliquity of the injury leaves more of the pulp than the nail.

An alternative version (Fig. 11.23) of the technique makes use of two side-based flaps similarly advanced using the V–Y principle. With both versions it may be necessary to trim sharp edges of the exposed distal phalanx to facilitate the transfer.

Both techniques are best carried out under magnification, to ensure that the neurovascular bundles are demonstrated to be intact, and before either can be used there must be no element of devitalising crushing. Enough soft tissue of the phalangeal segment should also remain to allow a flap, or flaps, of adequate size to be constructed, capable of allowing closure free of tension. The single flap works best when the injury is an oblique slicing one which leaves more pulp than nail. The double flap is more effective when the obliquity leaves less pulp than nail, but each of the two flaps is smaller than the single flap, and this increases the possibility of necrosis as a result of too much undermining.

SENSORY FACTORS IN THE USE OF FLAPS

A factor in assessing the usefulness of the various flaps which have been described, and one which has not received the emphasis it deserves, concerns the sensation which they eventually develop.

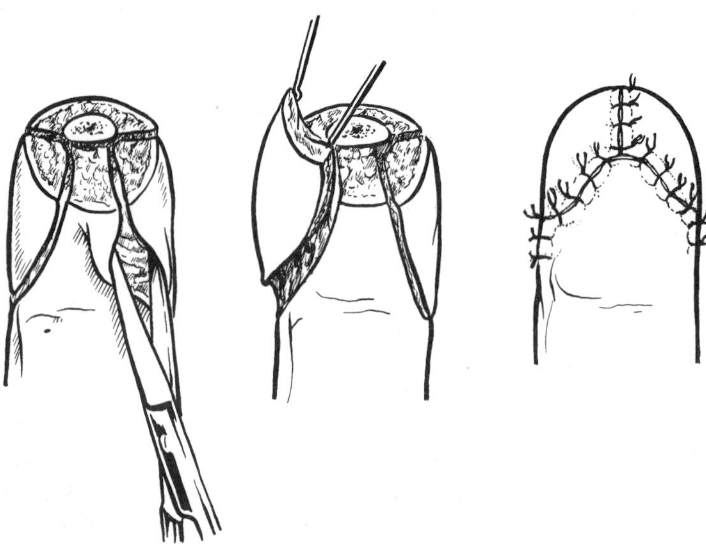

Fig. 11.23 Bilateral V-Y (Kutler) advancement flaps, used to provide skin cover for a guillotine amputation of the finger-tip.

Each of the two flaps is smaller than the single flap shown in Figure 11.22, and the added potential for loss of one or both of the flaps makes the desirability of carrying out the undermining and mobilisation under magnification even greater. The method works best when the obliquity of the amputation leaves more of the nail than the pulp.

Different areas of the hand vary in the sensory demands which the patient places on them. The important areas are the pulp segments, and in this the different fingers vary in comparative importance. Thumb and index finger in their normally apposing surfaces, the 'pinch sites', are of prime significance. Thereafter comparative importance diminishes from the radial to the ulnar side of the hand, subject to the proviso that the ulnar side of the little finger is comparatively important. The radial side of the other fingers is more important than the ulnar, this side being the one most likely to be used in prehensile movements.

While the relative importance of these sites is valid in the normal hand, they require to be appraised afresh in the mutilated hand, and the assessment should be reflected in the selection of the donor and recipient sites for any island flap which may be contemplated.

The originators of free flaps seldom fail to stress the presence of a nerve supply in the flap they are describing, which has the potential for use in providing sensation in its transferred site, but the quality of sensation achieved, as far as value in hand function is concerned, is generally poor. In the areas of greatest demand, where it really matters, it would be of little value.

The return of sensation in those flaps which have to rely for reinnervation on the ingrowth of axons from its surroundings, deep and marginal, is extremely variable. It depends, among other things, on the quota of nerve fibres in the bed of the flap and the severity of the scarring present at the interface between flap and bed. At best it is unlikely to be more than protective. Its functional adequacy depends of course on the site, and the demands put on it. In the most demanding areas, the pinch sites, its quality even at best is not remotely adequate. It is for this reason, among others, that neurovascular island flaps (p. 188) have proved such a valuable adjunct to the conventional flaps transferred to the pulp areas of the thumb and index finger. In areas where tactile discrimination is less important, and protective sensation is sufficient, the amount which returns may be adequate, though return cannot be guaranteed. It is wise to warn the patient to be careful, and avoid burning the flap while it lacks sensation.

POSTOPERATIVE CARE

Following a surgical procedure in the hand, a period of immobilisation is generally desirable, and this is provided by the dressing, on occasion reinforced by plaster of Paris. At the same time measures should be taken to prevent oedema developing in the hand.

POSITIONING OF THE HAND

When the hand has to be immobilised, it should be in a position which will allow a full range of movement to be restored as rapidly and completely as possible. The position frequently recommended is the so-called **position of function** — the position which the hand takes up in holding a glass. When the immobility is for a short period, e.g. following the application of a skin graft, this is adequate, but when immobilisation is to be for a longer period, e.g. after tendon grafting, it is preferable to immobilise the hand with the metacarpophalangeal joints flexed and the interphalangeal joints extended — the **position of immobilisation**.

Positioning of the hand is often discussed solely in terms of the finger joints, but the position of the wrist can be just as important, because of the strong influence which it has on the positions the fingers take up spontaneously. It exerts its influence through the effect which extremes of flexion and extension have on the relative tensions of the long extensors and flexors in the forearm. With the wrist extended, the natural tendency of the metacarpophalangeal joints is to move into flexion; with the wrist flexed, the tendency is for the metacarpophalangeal joints to move into extension.

When the hand develops oedema, the wrist tends to drop into flexion as the most comfortable position, and fingers take up the undesirable position of metacarpophalangeal joints in extension and interphalangeal joints in flexion (Fig. 11.24). This position is one which must be countered as quickly as possible, since it fixes with disturbing speed and, once fully established, can be corrected only with difficulty, and often only partially. The surgeon thinking in terms of prevention should make extension of the wrist his

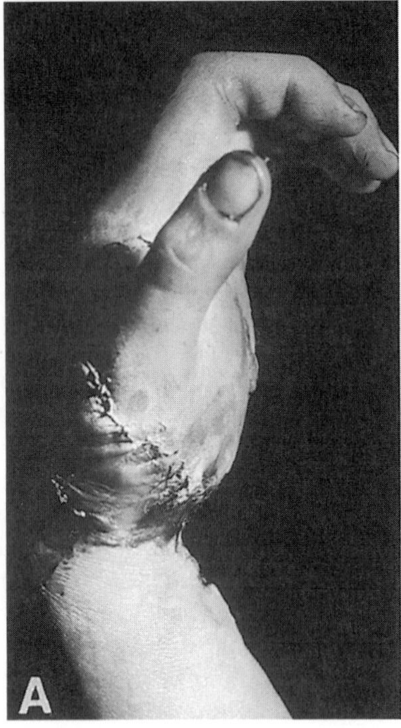

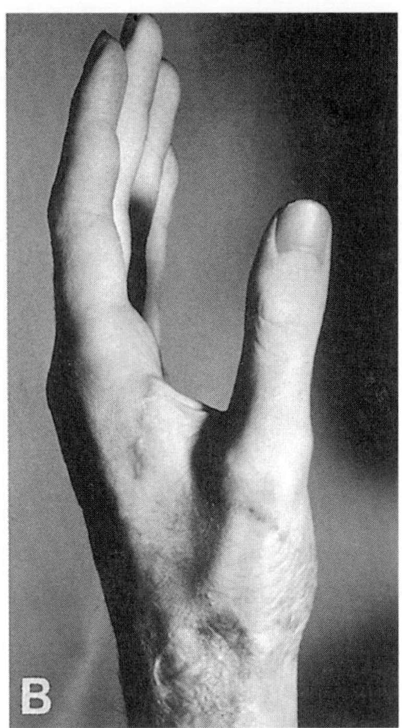

Fig. 11.24 The position of immobilisation.

A The hand at the time of referral, 10 days after a crush-degloving injury, showing the adverse effects of failure to position the hand properly, allowing the wrist to become flexed, and the metacarpophalangeal joints to extend to an undesirable extent, with associated flexion of the interphalangeal joints, particularly the proximal joints. Skin loss was confined to the area obviously present at the level of the wrist joint.

B The appearance after debridement of the area of skin loss and split skin grafting, with full function.

An initial general anaesthetic was necessary to correct the wrist flexion, and this, followed by a regimen of vigorous active finger exercises, prevented the original position of the fingers from stiffening into permanency.

first step, and the same is true of correction if the situation has been allowed to arise.

DRESSING OF THE HAND

If a graft has been used, it is usually wise, regardless of the site, to immobilise the entire hand in the position of function. The areas of maximum hazard lie over the metacarpophalangeal joints, and to a lesser extent over the proximal interphalangeal joints, the former in particular forming a marked prominence when the finger is in flexion. Withdrawal from extreme flexion reduces the prominence, and it is for this reason that the position of function is preferable to the position of immobilisation when the area is being grafted.

Following the tie-over dressing, careful padding of the whole hand, in the webs and between the fingers, must be carried out before applying the circumferential crepe bandages. The aim in padding is to convert the hand into a cylinder so that pressure is evenly distributed. Failure to pad the palm and dorsum adequately causes undue pressure on the radial and ulnar sides of the hand, and sores can result. The finger-tips are left visible to indicate the vascular state of the hand.

When no graft has been used, absolute immobilisation may be less necessary, and the regimen can be suitably relaxed.

The positioning required to get a flap to lie properly may be unsuitable from the point of view of joint function, and this may have to be accepted as a hazard. Awareness of the fact that the position is not the ideal one will at least remind the surgeon to maintain it for the shortest possible time, and redouble his encouragement to subsequent mobilisation of the joints. The problem is less likely to arise when the forearm has provided the flap, whether free or pedicled.

PREVENTION OF OEDEMA

Oedema fluid provides the raw material of stiff fingers, and elevation of the hand is used with the aim of reducing its occurrence or preventing it completely. An exception to this is the hand where a free flap has been used in the reconstruction, when positioning on a pillow at approximately the level of the heart is more appropriate.

Various methods are used to achieve the elevation. A well-padded plaster of Paris cast encircling the arm as far proximally as the upper humerus, so that weight is taken on the upper arm and not on the wrist and hand, may be used, but its weight tends to make it unpopular with the patient. The plaster may be confined to below the elbow and the elbow supported on a pillow, suspension merely keeping it vertical. Suspension with Tubegauz works equally well, and can be extended up the arm to the axilla so that any traction is spread as widely as possible. Whatever the method used, the plaster must not be allowed to hang free and constrict the wrist.

In more minor procedures elevation on a pillow or in a sling without plaster of Paris is adequate. The sling should be such that the hand is as high as is consistent with comfort.

When a distant flap has been used, elevation is naturally not possible, and its role as a prophylactic against oedema should then be replaced by a vigorous regimen of active exercises, every joint not of necessity immobilised being regularly put through a full range. If such a regimen is applied dependency is less likely to create problems.

CHAPTER

12 Maxillofacial injuries

The maxillofacial bony complexes are the **mandible**, **maxilla**, **zygoma** and **nose**, the last three constituting the **middle third of face**. These complexes (Fig. 12.1) roughly correspond to their anatomical counterparts, and each complex has its distinctive fracture patterns. While a fracture pattern may occur on its own, several patterns may exist together either in a single complex, or in more than one at the same time. In the most striking example, a fractured maxilla may occur alone or along with fractures of one or both zygomas and/or nose. In either case it is generally referred to as a **middle third fracture**.

When the mandible or the maxilla is fractured, it is not uncommon for teeth to be loosened, quite apart from those in the line of the fracture. These result from **alveolar fractures**, due to localised fractures of the alveolar plates in relation to the loosened teeth.

Fractures of the facial skeleton can be grouped into those of the zygoma and nose, which do not involve the dental occlusion, and those of the mandible and maxilla, where the normal occlusion of the teeth is disturbed by the fracture (Fig. 12.2). The objective in treating fractures which involve

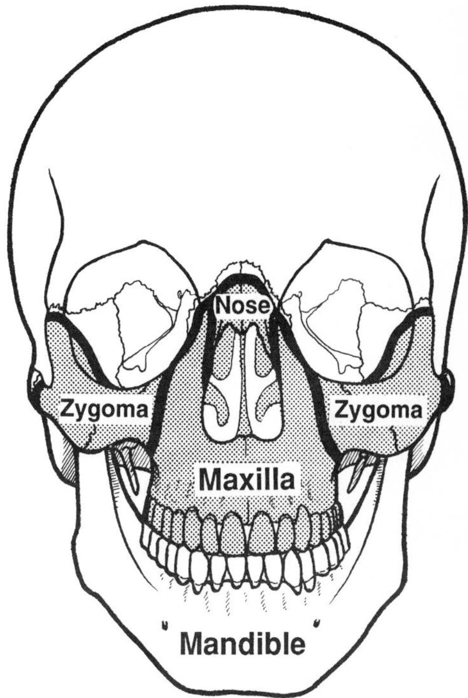

Fig. 12.1 The maxillofacial bony complexes – maxilla, nose, zygomas, mandible. The stippled segment indicates the middle third of the face.

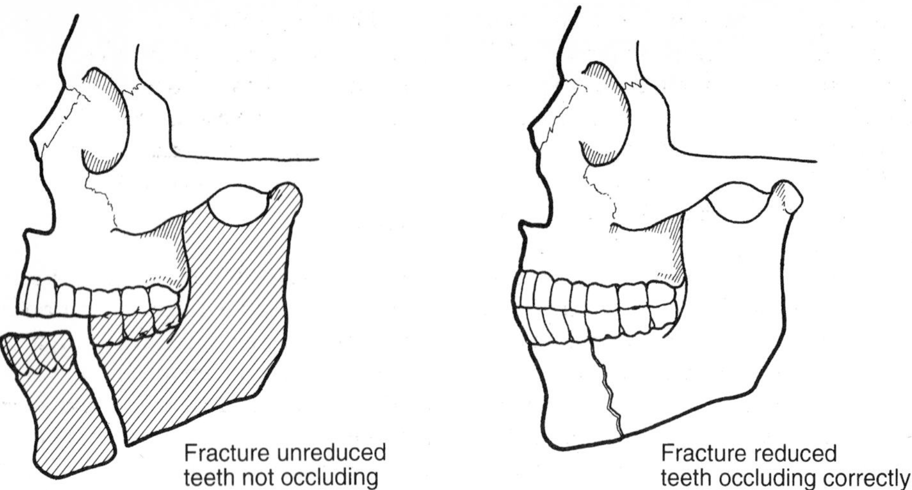

Fig. 12.2 In a fractured mandible the fracture can be presumed to be displaced if the teeth are not occluding properly. Restoration of correct occlusion indicates that the fracture is reduced.

the teeth is the restoration and maintenance of correct dental occlusion, and the surgeon treating such a fracture in the absence of dental help will go far to prevent permanent and largely irreparable deformity if he makes wiring of the teeth of the upper and lower jaws together in correct occlusion the first step in local treatment.

EARLY CARE

A maxillofacial fracture can occur as an isolated injury or as part of a multiple injury. The maxillofacial element of a multiple injury, particularly when it includes a middle third fracture, may be its most dramatic component, and on that score might appear to demand priority of treatment but, *except when it interferes with the airway*, it is not life threatening. It is seldom a real emergency, and in most instances it requires no special primary care other than adequate and repeated gentle cleansing of the mouth to make the patient as comfortable as possible. Any bleeding usually stops once a clear airway has been provided. Pain is not a problem with middle third fractures and, even with mandibular fractures, discomfort due to mobility of the fracture is less than might be expected.

The steps required to provide a clear airway depend on the severity of the problem. Patients with maxillofacial fractures often breathe more easily sitting up, but if this is not possible it has been found that the safest position of the patient is prone with the head to one side. Suction should always be available. Allowing the patient to lie flat on his back can lead to respiratory distress, with the tongue falling back and blocking the airway, and blood and secretions passing back into the pharynx. If provision and maintenance of a clear airway is proving difficult, a close watch on the patient is essential, and the possible need for a tracheostomy has to be constantly in the mind of the surgeon. If a tracheostomy is regarded as 'probably necessary', it is much better done early than late. Respiratory embarrassment tends to build up quickly, and an emergency tracheostomy is always something to avoid.

ASSOCIATED INJURIES

A maxillofacial injury can occur in isolation, or as part of a multiple injury. Occurring as an isolated injury, its various elements are treated together in an integrated manner. When it occurs as part of a multiple injury, management involves the organisation and timing of the treatment of its various elements, with the maxillofacial component taking its place in the queue. When the priorities for treatment in such a situation are being assessed, the maxillofacial fracture can generally wait for a longer period of time before being treated definitively without significant detriment to the final result, compared with the other injuries which are commonly sustained in such circumstances. Indeed, allowing the facial swelling to subside generally simplifies operative treatment.

To such a generalisation the combination of a maxillofacial fracture and chest injury may prove an exception. Each element in such a combination may be contributing to respiratory embarrassment, although not individually to an extent to require tracheostomy, but their combined effect may be to tip the scales in that direction. The presence of an intracranial injury resulting in unconsciousness may also influence management towards tracheostomy, an aspect discussed below in greater detail.

Unless the fracture has been fixed internally, the mandible and the maxilla are usually wired together as the final step in fixation, and this may have implications for the anaesthetist when the injury is a multiple one. If it seems probable that more than one anaesthetic will be required the anaesthetist may argue for the use of a tracheostomy since, with the jaws wired together, the alternative for any subsequent anaesthetic will be a blind nasal intubation. This is a procedure fraught with difficulties and possible danger in the circumstances. It can also provide an argument for fixing the fracture internally since such fixation may avoid the need to wire the jaws together.

The injuries whose management have most often to be integrated with a maxillofacial fracture are **soft tissue facial injuries**, **cranial injuries** and **orbital injuries**.

Soft tissue facial injuries

The management of the soft tissue part of a maxillofacial injury is seldom significantly influenced by the simultaneous presence of the fracture, except to the extent that use may be made of any lacerations present to provide access to the bony skeleton for the purpose of plating bony fragments. The blood supply of the soft tissues of the face and of the bones of the middle third is so good that infection is seldom a problem, even when the fracture is compound. From the point of view of its blood supply, the mandible is more vulnerable, but even here infection arising from the soft tissue element of the injury is most unusual. It is more likely to result from pre-existing periodontal disease and poor general oral hygiene.

Cranial injuries

The mechanisms which result in maxillofacial fractures have much in common with those which produce head injuries, and the association of the two is not unusual.

When the patient is unconscious, treatment of the fracture is generally postponed until he is considered fit for anaesthesia. When techniques which hold the fracture reduced by fixing the teeth and wiring the jaws together are being used, treatment may have to wait even longer since these methods require the active cooperation of the patient.

If the patient is deeply unconscious, and on this score alone would be considered for assisted airway management by intubation or tracheostomy, the added breathing difficulties which a fracture of maxilla or mandible may cause add further weight to the argument for tracheostomy. Even where the level of unconsciousness would not itself merit tracheostomy, there should be no hesitation in carrying one out if the fracture is adding significantly to the difficulties of management.

The cranial injury can result in tearing of the dura in the vicinity of the cribriform plate as part of the fracture of the skull base. The effect is to bring the subarachnoid space into direct continuity with the nasal cavity, allowing escape of cerebrospinal fluid. This manifests itself clinically as rhinorrhoea, with water-clear fluid dripping from the nose, its volume sometimes increased by straining or bending the head forward.

Left untreated, the majority of cerebrospinal fluid leaks stop spontaneously when the fracture is reduced and fixed, and there is no further trouble. Some leaks appear to stop, but meningitis develops after a variable and sometimes quite long period of freedom from all symptoms. Some leaks continue from the outset, with the eventual development of meningitis, despite fixation of the maxillary fracture.

The majority of leaks are managed by reduction and fixation of the fracture under antibiotic cover, the patient being watched carefully thereafter. With this regimen most leaks stop spontaneously, and give no further trouble. Where the leakage is large in volume or persists, the help of a neurosurgeon should be enlisted. In a small percentage of patients the source of the leak has to be exposed by frontal craniotomy, and the dural leak sealed off. This is achieved most frequently by use of a fascia lata graft.

Although this is the standard method of management, the use of craniofacial techniques in the primary management of maxillofacial injuries has altered the approach in some centres. The direct craniofacial exposure of the skull base to reduce and fix the fracture is extended to the frontal area and cribriform plate, allowing the dural repair to be carried out as part of the overall fracture treatment.

Orbital injuries

Injuries to the eyeball and/or the optic nerve are remarkable for their rarity, but when such injuries do occur they are usually irreparable, with either disruption of the contents of the eyeball or crushing of the optic nerve. When such damage is suspected, the opinion of an ophthalmologist should be sought without delay, not so much from a therapeutic point of view, for there is seldom much to be done to save sight if this has already been lost, but to insure against the development of sympathetic ophthalmitis.

When the fracture involves the bony orbit, bleeding into the orbital fat is almost invariable, showing clinically as an area of subconjunctival haemorrhage without a visible posterior margin. Such a haemorrhage is generally viewed merely as an integral part of the injury, and is allowed to subside spontaneously, without requiring special treatment.

When the floor of the orbit is fractured as part of the injury, orbital fat may be forced through the defect downwards into the antrum. Such herniation reduces the volume of fat left within the orbit, and results in enophthalmos. Fracture of the orbital floor may also occur as an isolated injury, the so-called 'blow-out' fracture. Comparable herniation of fat may take place through the medial orbital wall when it is comminuted as part of a fracture involving the naso-ethmoidal complex, but its occurrence is much more rare.

REDUCTION AND FIXATION METHODS

Fractures of the facial skeleton are currently managed in two distinct ways: traditionally, by **using the teeth as a means of indirectly fixing the jaws**, and more recently, by **direct exposure of the fracture and internal fixation**.

Managed in the 'traditional' way, the fracture is reduced by manipulating the fragments into a position of correct dental occlusion *vis à vis* their counterpart on the opposing alveolus, and maintained in that position until the fracture is stable. The fracture site is not approached directly, treatment being based on the assumption that if the dental occlusion is correct the fracture will have been reduced accurately. When the mandible is fractured, reduction is on to the maxilla. When the maxilla is fractured, reduction is on to the mandible. The maxilla is sufficiently stable to provide a secure anchorage for the fractured mandible in the reduced position. Stabilisation of the fractured to the unfractured bone in this way is referred to as **intermaxillary fixation**, the term a relic of the time when there was an upper and lower maxilla rather than a maxilla and mandible. In the case of a middle third fracture, an additional source of stability is often considered necessary. For this **skull fixation** is used, with a separate mode of fixation, independent of that used for intermaxillary fixation.

These methods work satisfactorily in the less severe injuries, but they are less satisfactory when both mandible and maxilla are fractured, and also when the middle third fracture involves the upper part of the maxilla and orbits. They are capable of restoring occlusion adequately, but are less effective in reducing and fixing the circumorbital element of the injury, particularly when the glabellar bone and the immediately adjoining medial orbital wall are the sites involved.

The development of craniofacial techniques, during which these sites are routinely exposed, surgically manipulated and fixed in position, initially with wires but increasingly using plate-

and-screws, has provided the impetus to the use of the method in maxillofacial injuries.

Initially used in the more severe injuries, it has become more and more the standard approach to the management of maxillofacial injuries generally. Used primarily, it frequently eliminates the need for intermaxillary fixation because of the stability which the plates provide.

INTERDENTAL METHODS

When the teeth are used as the means of fixing the fracture in the reduced position, the methods used are **eyelet wires**, and **arch bars**. In the edentulous patient, an alternative method is used, but one which embodies the same principle, namely **Gunning splintage**.

Eyelet wiring

The fixing device used in this method (Fig. 12.3) is a 0.4 mm diameter length of stainless steel wire which has been doubled on itself and twisted, leaving a small eyelet at the end.

The double wire is passed inwards between the necks of two adjacent teeth until the twisted segment is lying between the necks with the eyelet on the outer side. The wire is then separated into its two strands, one being turned forward and one back, and each is passed outwards through the next interspace so that a loop is formed round the necks of the two adjoining teeth. The loops are completed by bending the wires towards one another, passing one through the eyelet, and finally twisting them tightly together before cutting off the excess, and turning in the end so that it will not catch on tongue or cheek.

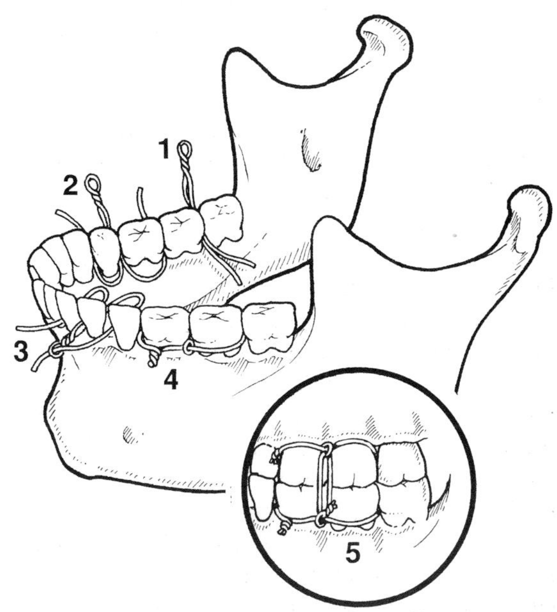

Fig. 12.3 The steps in eyelet wiring.

Several sets of these wires are applied at intervals round the alveolar arch, and also at corresponding points on the opposite jaw. When the fracture has been manually reduced and the mandible closed on to the maxilla, it is held in that position by looping further wires through the eyelets which are opposite one another, and twisting them tightly together.

Arch bars

This technique (Fig. 12.4) is an alternative to eyelet wiring and uses a malleable metal bar made of flattened soft German silver wire. The bar is moulded around the alveolar arch on its outer aspect, at the level of the necks of the teeth, to which it is then wired. With an arch bar similarly applied to the maxilla, the two can be fixed together with wires. Alternatively the arch bar on the fractured bone can be fixed to eyelet wires on the unfractured alveolus.

A logical development of the simple arch bar is to have cleats at intervals along its length, so that the upper and lower bars can be more easily wired together and eponymous splints have been produced along these lines (Fig. 12.4 B,C).

Gunning splintage

This method is used in the edentulous patient. It will be appreciated that if such a patient's dentures could be fitted, and the fracture reduced on to the denture with the upper and lower dentures occluding correctly, the fracture would be accurately reduced. When the patient has well-fitting undamaged dentures, this can be done, but even when the denture has been broken, is lost, or fits so badly as to be useless, the principle can still be used. Dental impressions are taken and 'dentures

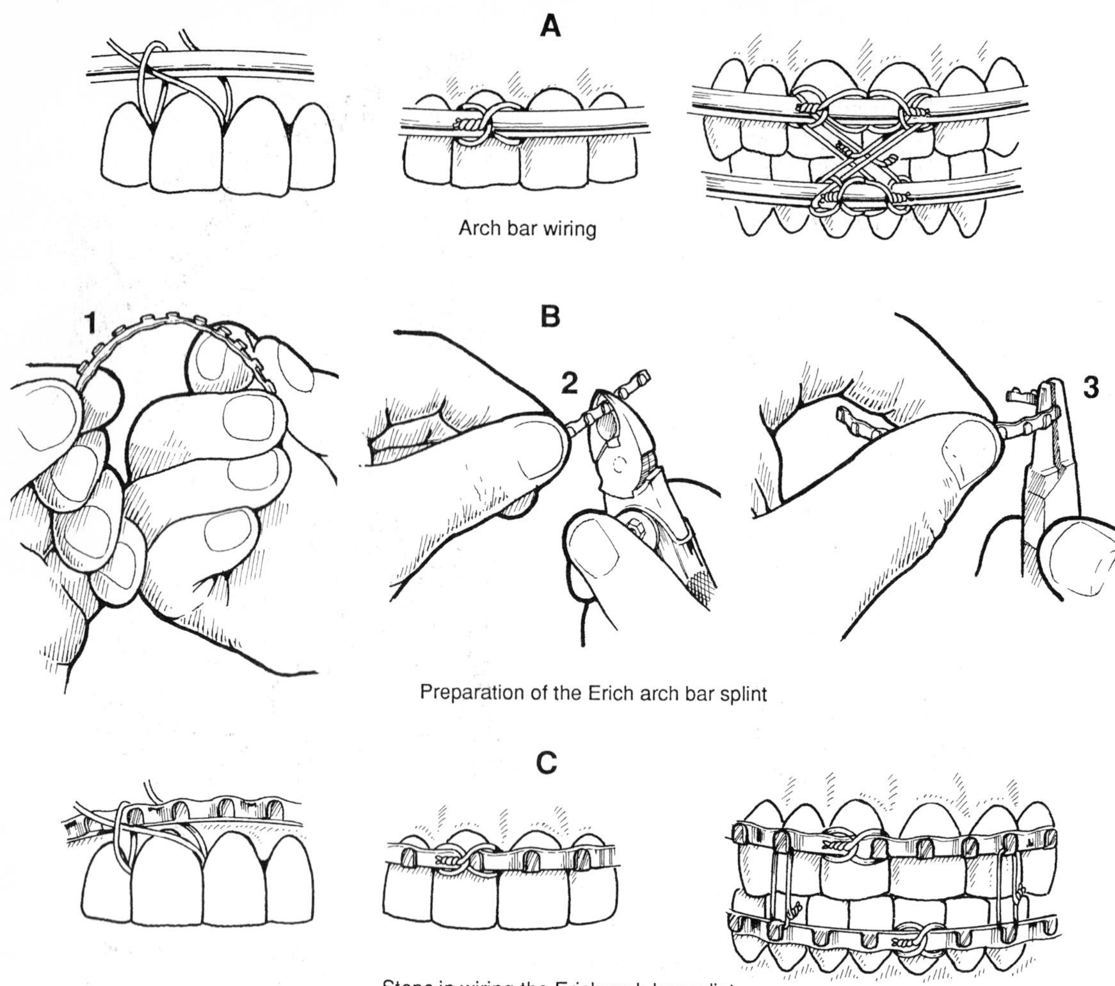

Fig. 12.4 The steps in arch bar fixation.

A The method of fixing the simple arch bar to the upper and lower alveoli.
B The preparation of the Erich arch bar, one of the modified versions of the simple arch bar, with cleats along its length. The bar is bent to match the curve of the alveolus (**1**), and an appropriate length of bar is cut (**2**), with final moulding of the shape (**3**).
C The bar is wired to the alveolus and, making use of the cleats, to the bar wired to the opposite alveolus.

without teeth', so-called **Gunning splints**, are made, wired circumferentially on to the upper and lower jaws (Fig. 12.5), and to each other, to produce the necessary fixation. When the fracture is minimally displaced, and particularly in the elderly patient, it is often enough merely to fit the splints and support the mandible against the maxilla with a firm bandage, without the need for circumferential wires. The absence of teeth makes it less essential to get absolutely accurate reduction, for a denture can subsequently be fitted to compensate for any slight irregularity of alveolar alignment.

Skull fixation

The point has already been made that while a maxillary fracture is reduced on to the mandible in proper occlusion, the final anchoring fixation is to the skull. This is provided by **supraorbital pins** (Fig. 12.6), the technique involving the insertion of a self-tapping pin into the hard cortical

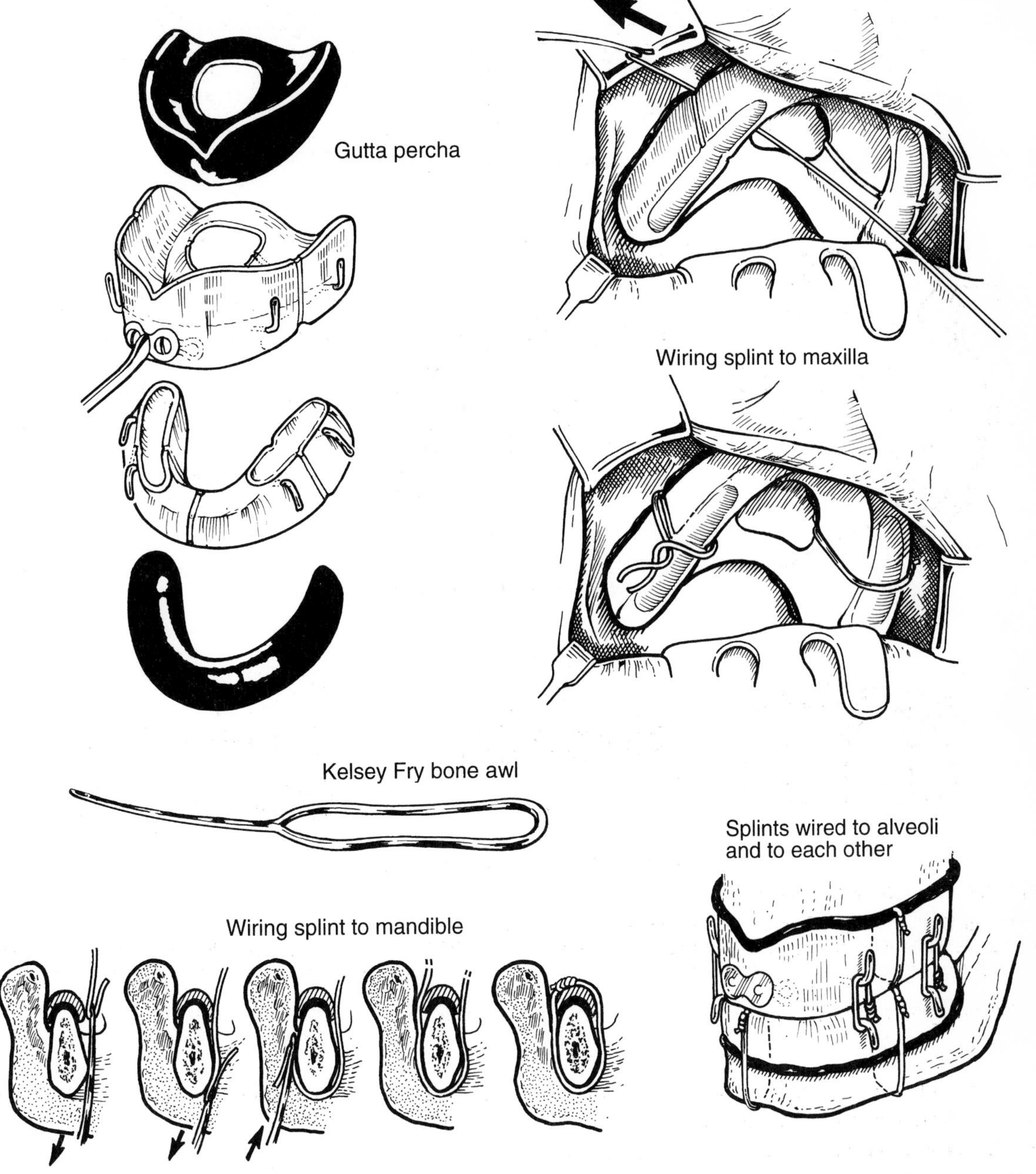

Fig. 12.5 Gunning splints, used in fractures of the edentulous mandible.
The splints, dentures without teeth, are prepared with various modifications which facilitate subsequent fixation to the alveoli, upper and lower – cleats to allow wiring of the splints together, a central hole in the upper splint to allow wiring to the maxilla, and grooves to hold the wires on the splints. A layer of gutta percha is used to line the splints. The splints are wired to the maxilla and mandible, using the Kelsey Fry bone awl and then wired to one another.

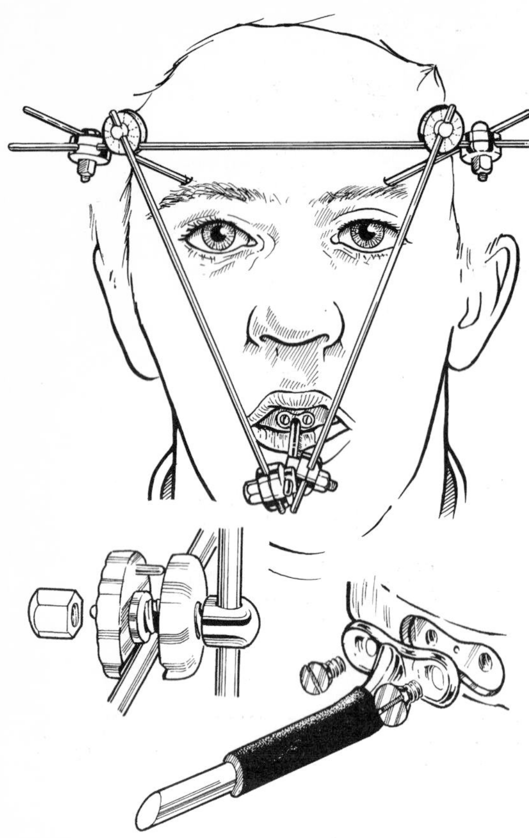

Fig. 12.6 Fixation of the splint to the skull.
Using a system of rods and universal joints, the Gunning splints are fixed to self-tapping pins inserted into the cortical bone of the supraorbital margin.

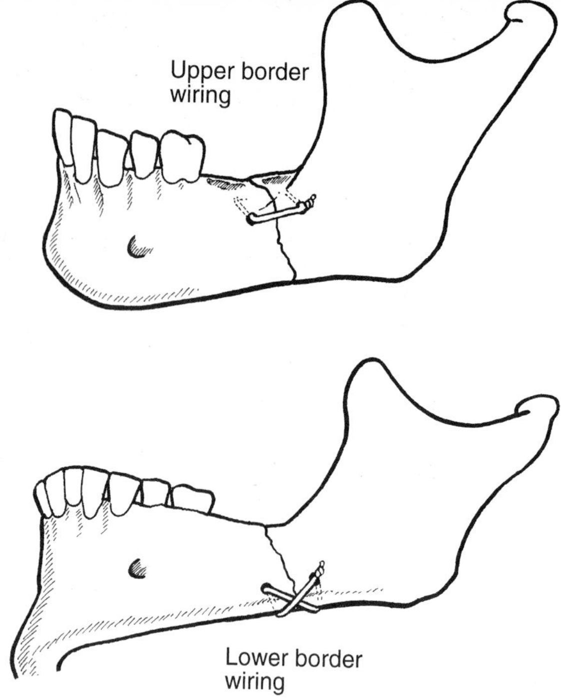

Fig. 12.7 Upper and lower border wiring, used in fixing fractures of the mandible. This method is generally used in conjunction with other fixation methods.

bone of the orbital margin above each orbit. To this solid base the maxillary splint is attached with a system of rods connected to one another by universal joints. When the fracture has been reduced and the dental splints wired together, the final fixation is achieved by tightening the universal joints to make the whole system rigid.

INTERNAL FIXATION

Direct fixation of fractures of the facial skeleton, particularly of the mandible, using wires (Fig. 12.7) to fix fractured segments in a reduced position, was originally used in addition to the standard methods of dental fixation when the fracture was unstable. Its use to fix osteotomised bony segments in craniofacial surgery then led to its use instead of, or in addition to, interdental fixation. Recognition that the use of **plate-and-screw** gives a much more effective fixation has resulted in its replacing wiring in many situations, the fixation which it provides being sufficiently positive to be used as the sole method, without the need for intermaxillary fixation.

Maxillofacial fractures can involve sites, such as the mandibular body, which are loadbearing, or sites, such as the orbital margin, which are not loadbearing. Where the site is not loadbearing, plate-and-screw fixation, using mini- or micro-plates (Fig. 12.8) is effective. These plates can also be used in loadbearing sites, but **compression plating**, an alternative form of plate-and-screw fixation which provides more positive fixation, is also used in these sites.

Compression plating (Fig. 12.9) is effective in the hands of those expert in its use, but the method is a demanding one. It is extremely precise and, when not carried out with a proper awareness of the principles which underlie it, is unforgiving. It makes use of plate-and-screws and lag-screws, whichever is appropriate in the cir-

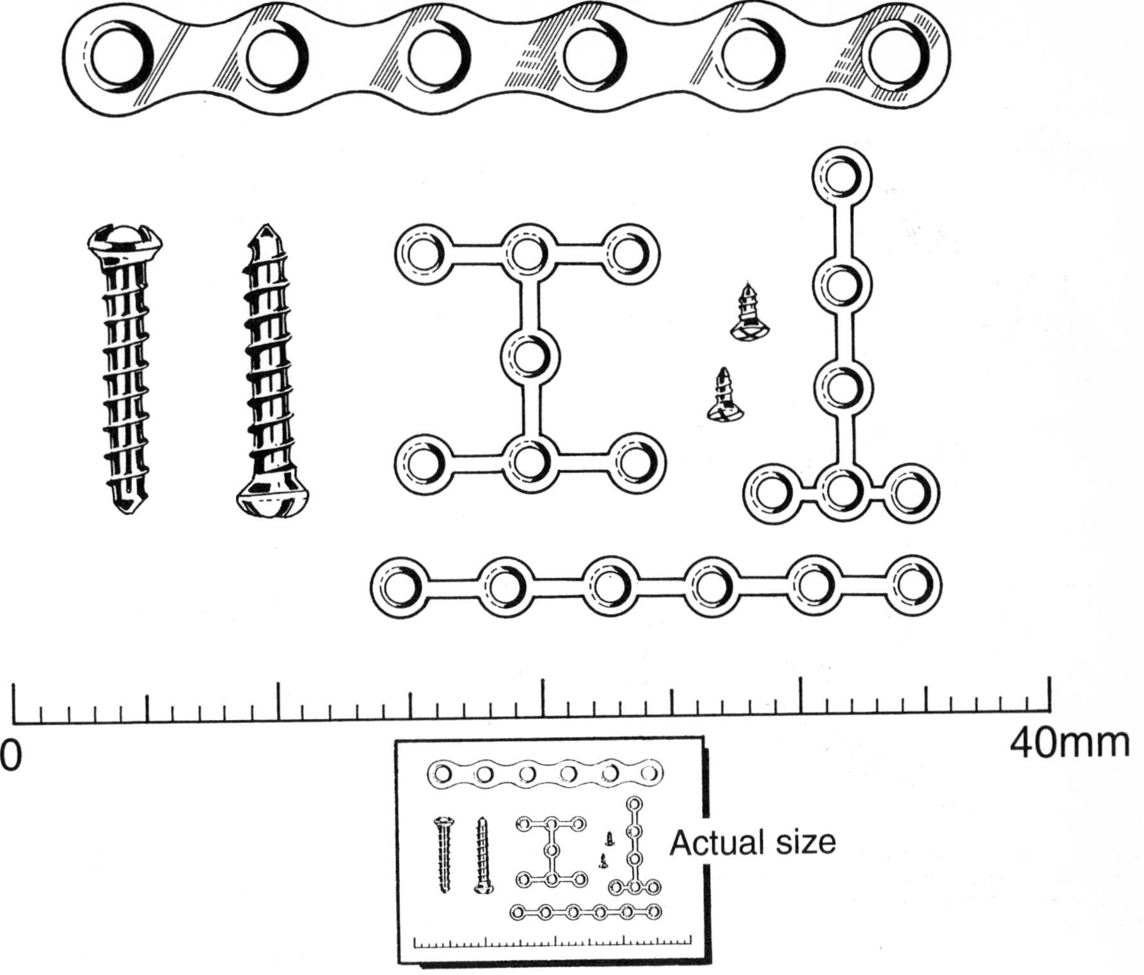

Fig. 12.8 Mini- and micro-plates, used for internal fixation of maxillofacial fractures.

cumstances, to fix and compress the fracture site, adapting the methods developed by carpenters in preparing the holes for inserting screw nails in cabinet making. Extremely precise instrumentation has been developed, which allows holes to be bored in the bone with a precise diameter in an exact direction to permit the screw either to pass through without engaging the cortex, or in the appropriate part of the bone for the screw flange to engage and fix the bone. In maxillofacial fractures the usual hole has a 2 mm diameter for an engaging screw of 2.7 mm.

Using these methods, the fracture is first reduced into proper dental occlusion and held in that position using arch bars with intermaxillary fixation. It is essential, when the plate is being applied, that it should accurately match the contour of the bone, so that when the screws are being tightened the bone is not pulled out of its reduced position. To achieve this, a preliminary template is constructed using a strip of malleable metal, and using this as a basis the plate is shaped to match the contours of the bone on each side of the reduced fracture. The fracture is then fixed in that position with the compression plate. When the fracture has been adequately stabilised in this way the intermaxillary fixation is removed, but it is usual to leave the arch bars in position in case they are required at any time while bony union is taking place.

When internal fixation is used in middle third fractures, the fracture sites are approached from

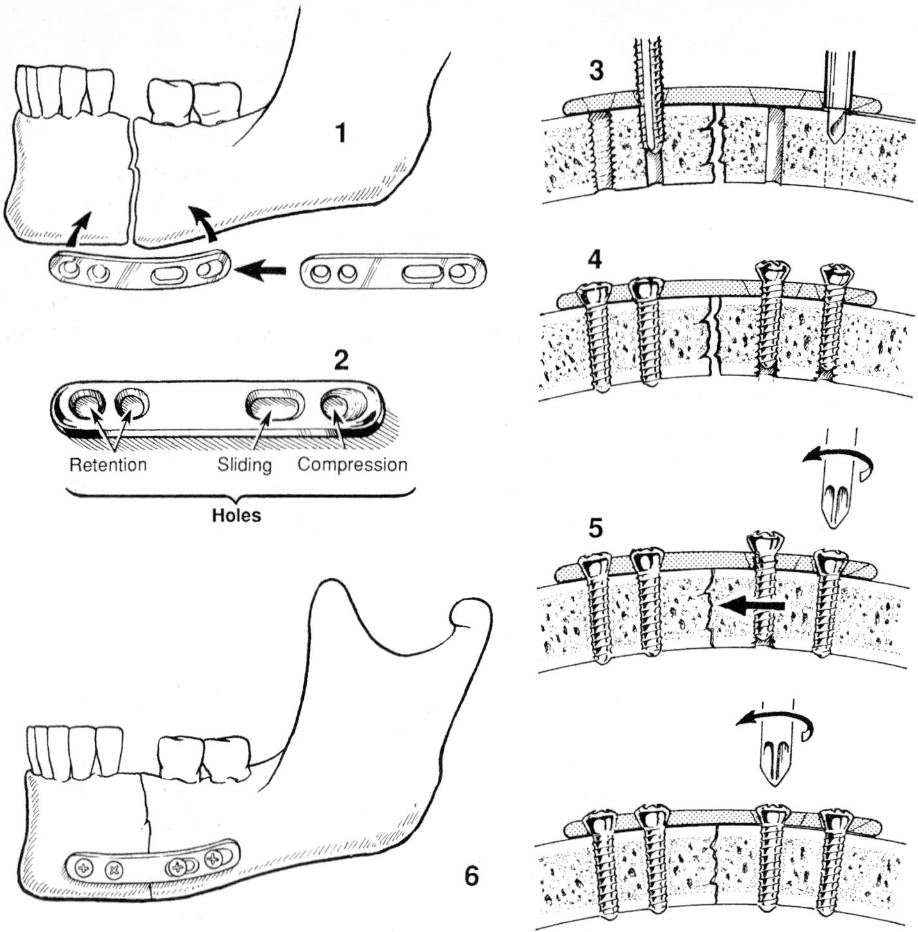

Fig. 12.9 Compression plating of a mandibular fracture.

1 Contouring the plate to the mandible.
2 The compression plate showing the retention, sliding, and compression holes.
3 The holes being prepared for insertion of the screws, the initial hole drilled, followed by the provision of a thread using a hand screw tap.
4 The retention screws inserted and tightened, the sliding and compression screws inserted but not tightened.
5 The compression screw tightened, compressing the fracture ends.
6 The sliding screw tightened, completing fixation.

above and below. From above, a bicoronal scalp incision is used, stripping the soft tissues off the frontal bone down to the orbital margin and into the orbit if necessary, the glabellar area, and the zygomatic arch. The lower maxilla and infra-orbital area are approached from below, using an upper buccal sulcus incision with the soft tissue stripped off the bone. Direct exposure in this way allows the fracture/s to be reduced, so that fracture reduction and plate-and-screw fixation can be carried out directly.

CLINICAL USAGE

For the average fracture of the zygoma or of the mandible, and for most isolated fractures of the toothbearing segment of the maxilla, internal fixation is unnecessary. The standard methods using the teeth for fixation are adequate. Its place is in the management of the patient with major facial trauma, particularly when this is part of a multiple injury. The facial fractures, definitively stabilised in this way, allow management to be concentrated on the patient's other injuries, and they may also allow a tracheostomy to be avoided.

ZYGOMA

Fracture patterns (Fig. 12.10)

In the **simple fracture**, the bone remains in a single piece, the line of fracture in the cheek running from the infraorbital foramen downwards and laterally over the anterior wall of the antrum. Displacement is usually medial, with a medial or lateral tilt, and impacted. The infraorbital nerve is compressed in its bony canal and the branches of the superior dental nerve which cross the fracture line are torn. When the fracture is **comminuted**, the pattern is generally similar, but in addition the floor of the orbit is comminuted and depressed. A depressed, comminuted fracture of the orbital floor, and herniation of orbital fat into the antrum can also occur as an isolated injury, the **blow-out** fracture, classically from direct force by a blunt object, e.g. a fist, on the eyeball. Fracture of the **zygomatic arch** produces a localised depression of the arch. In its medially displaced position, it tends to impinge on the coronoid process of the mandible.

Clinical picture (Fig. 12.11)

Swelling and bruising of the overlying soft tissues is very variable. Sometimes it is almost totally absent; sometimes it is severe enough to

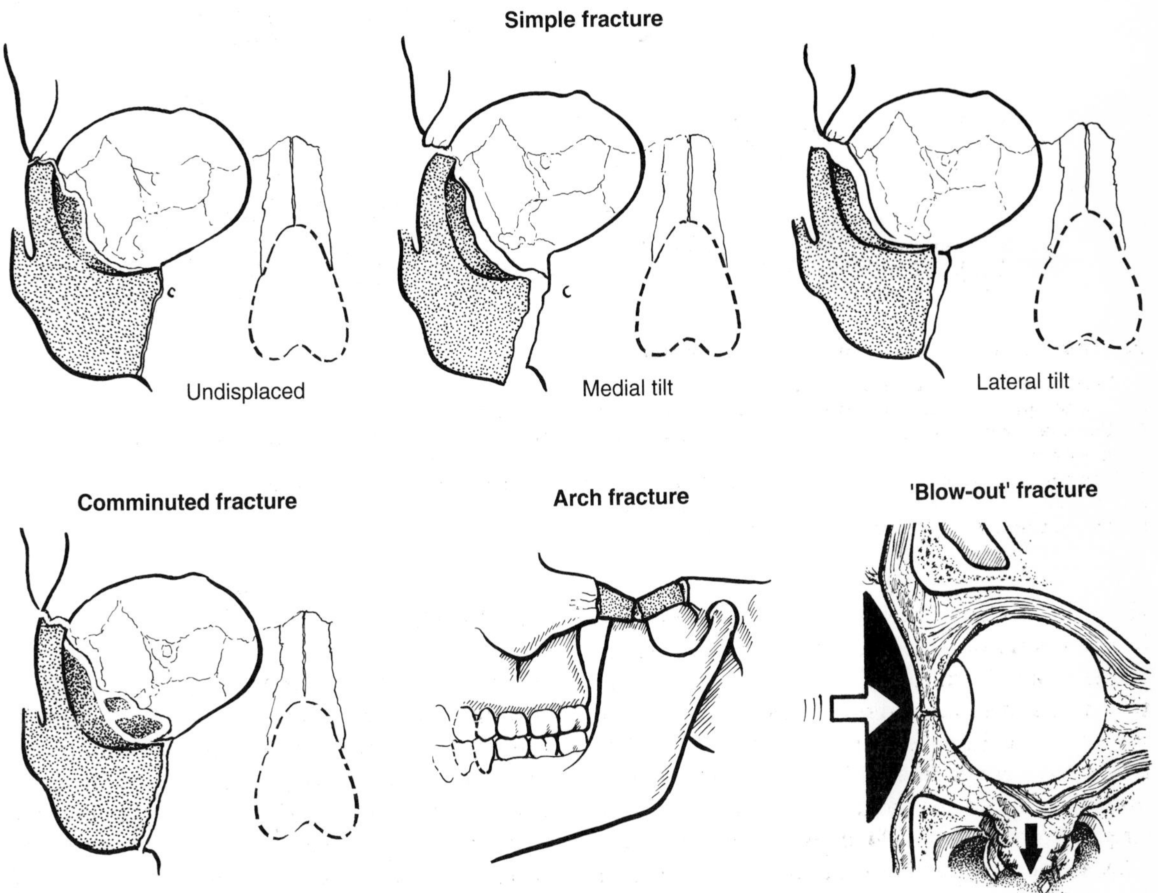

Fig. 12.10 The patterns of fracture of the zygoma.

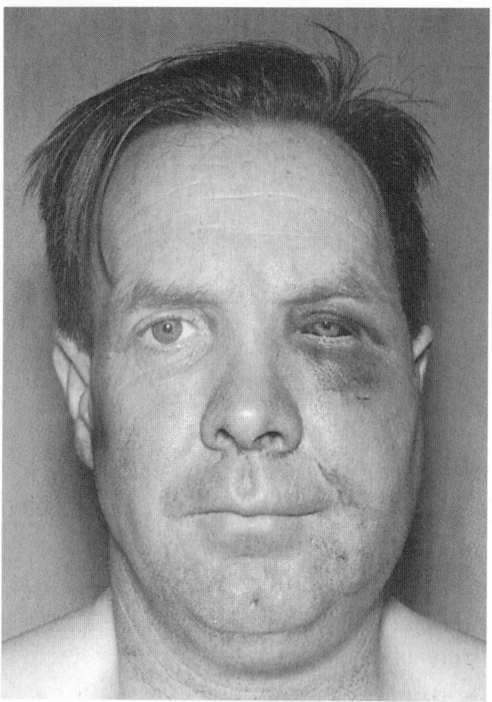

Fig. 12.11 The typical clinical appearance resulting from a fracture of the zygoma.

virtually close the eye and mask any underlying bony deformity. Subconjunctival haemorrhage is regularly present, typically lacking a visible posterior margin, the result of spread forward of bleeding into the orbital fat.

Alteration of bony contour is usually in the direction of flattening of the cheek prominence. A step in the margin of the bony orbit at the infraorbital foramen can be felt as a rule unless there is severe overlying soft tissue swelling.

Sensory loss of the structures supplied by the nerves injured is readily detected, division of branches of the superior dental nerves by the fracture making the teeth of the affected segment anaesthetic to percussion. The extent of the area affected by the damage to the infraorbital nerve is variable, but the two areas regularly involved are the upper lip and the alar region of the nose. The sensory loss can vary from mild paraesthesia to complete anaesthesia. The mechanism appears to be similar to the compression syndromes seen in the upper limb, sensation often beginning to return when the patient wakens from the anaesthetic. Recovery is then invariably speedy and complete. In a minority of patients recovery is slow and incomplete, the injury having then presumably damaged the nerve in the infraorbital canal more severely, to the extent even of dividing it completely.

Enophthalmos is indicative of reduction in the volume of the orbital fat, the result of herniation into the antrum through the fractured floor. This, occurring on its own, is the classic picture of the blow-out fracture, but it can also be part of the standard fracture of the zygoma, where the floor has been fractured, allowing the orbital fat to herniate.

Diplopia may occur as a transient phenomenon in the simple fracture. When it persists postoperatively it is usually found that there has been comminution and depression of the orbital floor, either as part of the overall fracture pattern or as a blow-out fracture. It is caused by entrapment of the inferior rectus muscle, preventing upward rotation of the eyeball with resulting diplopia on looking up.

Trismus is variable and tends to be more severe if there is much depression of the zygomatic arch. In the localised arch fracture, the clinically obvious local depression apart, trismus with marked restriction of lateral movements of the mandible may be the patient's sole complaint.

The clinical picture when the zygoma is fractured can be very variable, and probably the most useful single diagnostic point is the presence of infraorbital anaesthesia. Every patient with a 'black eye' should be tested for diminution of infraorbital sensation, and a positive finding is presumptive evidence of a fractured zygoma.

X-ray diagnosis

The view used routinely is the 30° occipitomental projection, but minor degrees of displacement can be demonstrated more readily by increasing the obliquity of the view to 60°. The points to look for are irregularities or definite fracture lines near the infraorbital foramen, the zygomatic arch, and the lateral wall of the antrum. The line of the orbital floor should also be compared with the normal side, and blood in the antrum may make it appear opaque. A CT scan will demonstrate depression of the orbital floor and confirm herniation of orbital fat.

Management

The presence on X-ray of a fracture of the zygoma does not invariably mean that surgical treatment is necessary. The need or not for surgery is decided rather on the basis of the clinical findings. Infraorbital anaesthesia, trismus, diplopia, enophthalmos, obvious flattening of the cheek prominence — any or all of these are an indication for surgery. When the merest suggestion of flattening of the check is the only positive clinical finding, the decision whether or not the fracture needs to be reduced can be very difficult, but fractures of the zygoma rapidly fix in their impacted position, and the decision should not be delayed.

Another difficult decision concerns the patient with an undisplaced fracture or even an apparently normal X-ray, but with infraorbital anaesthesia. These are probably best 'elevated', even though no actual movement of the zygoma is felt, because once treated recovery of sensation is uniformly rapid and complete. Many would doubtless recover sensation spontaneously, but there is the remote possibility of the non-recovering nerve developing an intractable neuralgia.

Where the fracture is simple and the zygoma in a single piece, capable of being reduced by leverage on the anterior part of the zygomatic arch, **temporal reduction** is the method generally adopted. The arch fracture also falls into this category. In most instances the fracture is stable in its reduced position. The presence of comminution reduces the effectiveness of the temporal approach, and to reduce and stabilise the fracture **direct exposure and internal fixation** may be needed. Internal fixation may also be required if the fracture remains unstable after temporal reduction.

Temporal reduction (Fig. 12.12) is based on the anatomical fact that while the temporal fascia is attached along the upper border of the zygomatic arch the temporalis muscle runs under it. This makes it possible for a lever inserted between fascia and muscle to slide down deep to the arch and exert outward leverage. An oblique skin incision is made over temporalis, taking care to avoid the superficial temporal vessels, and deepened to the temporal fascia. Positively identified, the fascia is incised and McIndoe's scissors are inserted under the fascia to act as a pathfinder, and slid down under the arch. Various levers have been devised to elevate the bone, but the orthopaedic Bristow's periosteal elevator is both effective and available in most operating rooms. Once positioned under the arch, it should be brought forward as far as the arch allows to get anterior to the fracture line, and also allow leverage to be exerted anteriorly if necessary as well as laterally. The leverage required depends on the degree of impaction, but a considerable amount is often required. The fracture is virtually always stable in its disimpacted and reduced position. In closing the incision it is only necessary to suture the skin. The great majority of zygomatic fractures in practice are of the simple type and are suitable for temporal reduction.

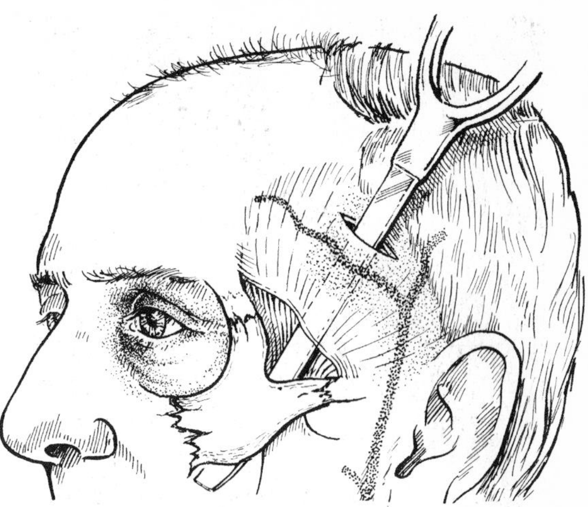

Fig. 12.12 Temporal reduction of a simple fracture of the zygoma.

Internal fixation (Fig. 12.13) is required when the fracture is unstable after reduction, and when the fracture is comminuted, as a result of which temporal elevation can reduce only part of the bone. It is also used when the fractured zygoma is part of a middle third fracture where the overall management is going to be by internal fixation. In the isolated fracture the sites are exposed with small incisions in a skin fold or wrinkle directly overlying the fracture sites, one

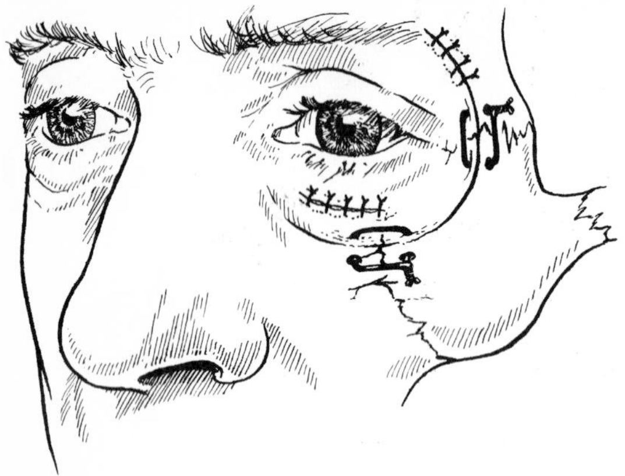

Fig. 12.13 Fixation of an isolated fracture of the zygoma using interosseous wiring at the infraorbital and zygomaticofrontal fracture lines.

in the lower eyelid, and one over the zygomatico-frontal fracture line. With the bone exposed subperiosteally the fracture is reduced and held in position either by wiring or plate-and-screws.

Internal fixation will not of course reduce and hold the comminuted orbital floor or return the herniated fat to the orbit and release any tethering of the inferior rectus muscle. **Exploration of the floor** (Fig. 12.14) is necessary to restore its integrity. The material used to line the floor and seal the opening into the antrum has varied through bone and cartilage to synthetic materials such as silastic sheeting.

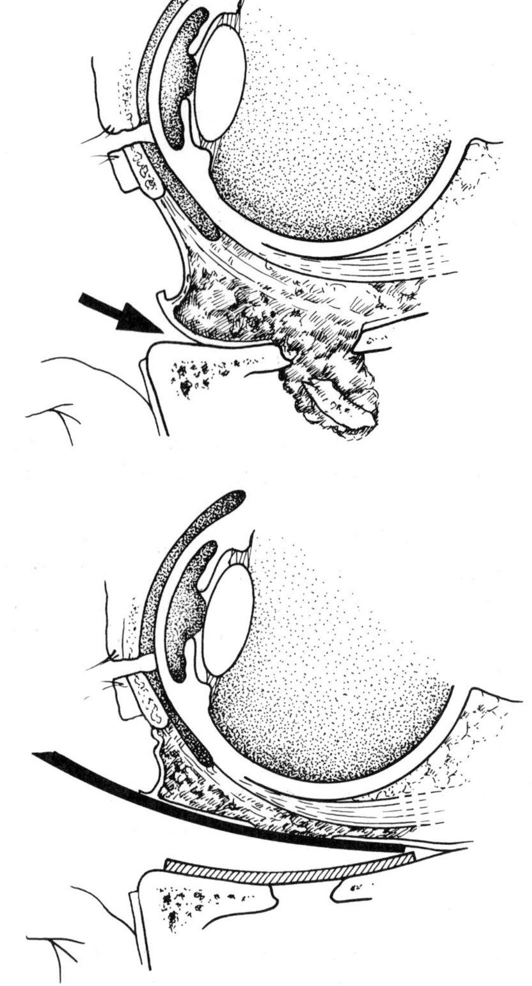

Fig. 12.14 Exploration of the orbital floor, reduction of the herniated orbital fat, and sealing of the defect with a silastic sheet.

NOSE

Fracture patterns (Fig. 12.15)

Lateral violence involving the nose, as it increases in severity, produces fracturing of the nasal bone on the side of the injury, displacing it towards the septum, followed by deviation and then fracture of the septum, and finally fractures the nasal bone on the side away from the injury, so that the entire nasal complex is deviated. The degree of comminution is very variable.

Head-on violence causes backwards displacement and splaying of the nasal bones, creating a saddle deformity and broadening of the bony complex. The backwards displacement also damages the septum, resulting in either buckling or fracture. Dislocation of the lower attachment of the septal cartilage with buckling of its columellar margin can also occur, usually giving rise to deviation of the nose towards its tip.

As part of the septal injury there may be a submucosal haematoma, creating bulging of the septal mucosa, either unilateral or bilateral. Its presence should always be looked for even when the nose is not appreciably deviated or depressed.

Clinical picture

Some nasal swelling is inevitable in patients in

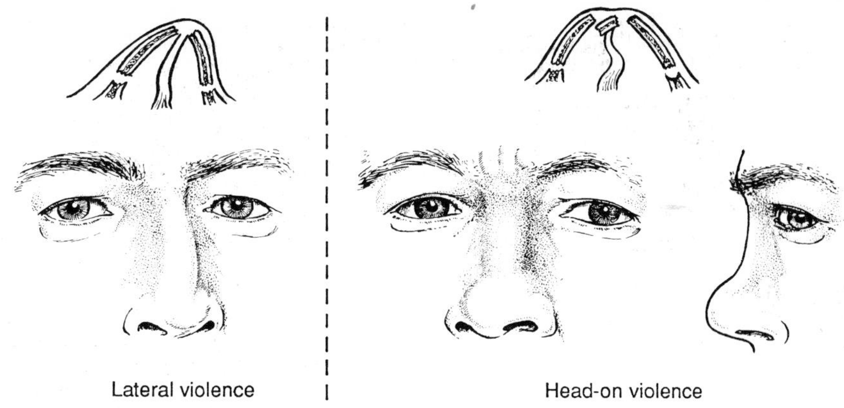

Fig. 12.15 Patterns of nasal fracture.

whom the diagnosis of nasal fracture is being considered, but it is a change of bridge contour or a new asymmetry which is diagnostic, and the best judge of this is often the patient himself. A nasal fracture, apart from its septal element, is treated on the grounds of appearance. In the absence of associated deformity, an X-ray which shows a fracture line is of no significance.

X-ray diagnosis

The fracture is treated on the basis of the clinical examination and X-rays are not essential.

Management

Nasal fractures tend to fix in their displaced position within days and they should be treated with the minimum of delay. The surgical approach used depends on whether the fracture has resulted in **deviation** or **collapse** of the nasal bones.

Deviation can sometimes be corrected by simple thumb pressure (Fig. 12.16), particularly if the fracture is very recent, but it is apt to reduce only the nasal bone which has been pushed out, leaving untouched the side depressed by the fracture. Manipulation using Walsham's nasal forceps is then required (Fig. 12.17). With the forceps appropriate for the side of the nose being manipulated the slim blade is inserted into the nostril and the broader blade outside, the latter covered with rubber tubing to protect the skin from undue local pressure. With the blades closed over the nasal bone, it is disimpacted with a rocking movement of the forceps, first laterally and then medially.

With both bones mobilised, finger manipulation is able to mould them into a symmetrical

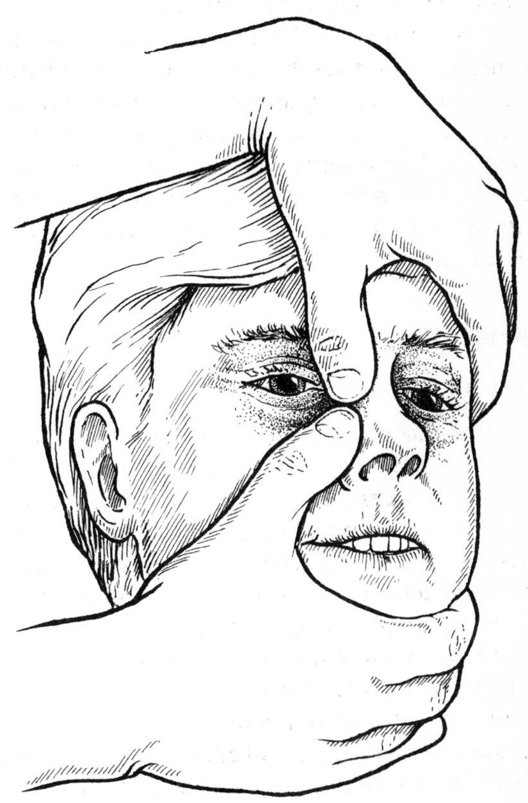

Fig. 12.16 Reduction of a laterally displaced nasal fracture by simple thumb pressure.

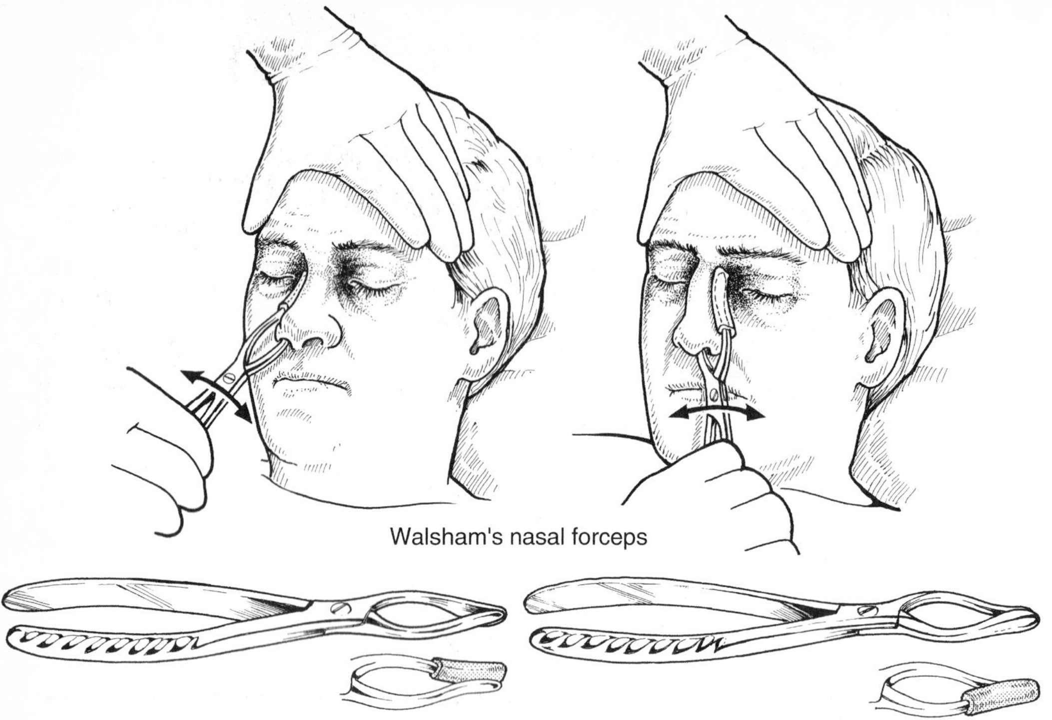

Fig. 12.17 Manipulation of a nasal fracture using Walsham's nasal forceps.
Rubber tubing is used to cover the broader of the two blades of the forceps to protect the skin from undue pressure during the manipulation.

position. The septum should be inspected and if necessary manipulated as described below. In practice, reduction of the nasal bones often reduces the septal displacement simultaneously.

Collapse is the result of head-on violence and, from the viewpoint of treatment, it is essential to recognise that it is a combined injury of nose and septum. The nose cannot collapse without simultaneous buckling or fracture of the septum, and straightening or reconstitution of the septum has the effect of also correcting the bony collapse. Walsham's septal forceps are used for this purpose. The instrument is so constructed that the blades of the closed forceps remain apart, leaving a gap which corresponds to the thickness of the septum. With a blade inserted into each nostril along the nasal floor the forceps are swung up towards the nasal bridge (Fig. 12.18). As they reach the bridge they lift the bridge line forward from its collapsed position. Correction may only be partial at the first attempt, in which case the manoeuvre is repeated. Any associated broadening of the nasal bones can then be corrected by finger pressure, if necessary after mobilisation with Walsham's nasal forceps.

It is in this type of nasal fracture that a septal haematoma is most likely to occur. It should be evacuated by incising the mucosa, if necessary on both sides.

Petroleum jelly gauze packing of the nostrils is advisable. The pack provides support for the septum in its reduced position, and helps to prevent recurrence of haematoma. It also provides counter pressure for the plaster of Paris splint, immobilising the nasal bones and preventing them from collapsing inwards. It can be removed in 48 hours. The plaster of Paris splint (Fig. 12.19), moulded to the nose, should be left in place for a week, and worn at night for a further week or so.

When it occurs as part of a severe middle third fracture, the comminution of the nasal bones may be so gross that the fragments cannot be maintained in a narrow and forward position with splint and packing alone. A through-and-through suture tied lightly over a strip of padded metal or rubber tubing to prevent cutting in with

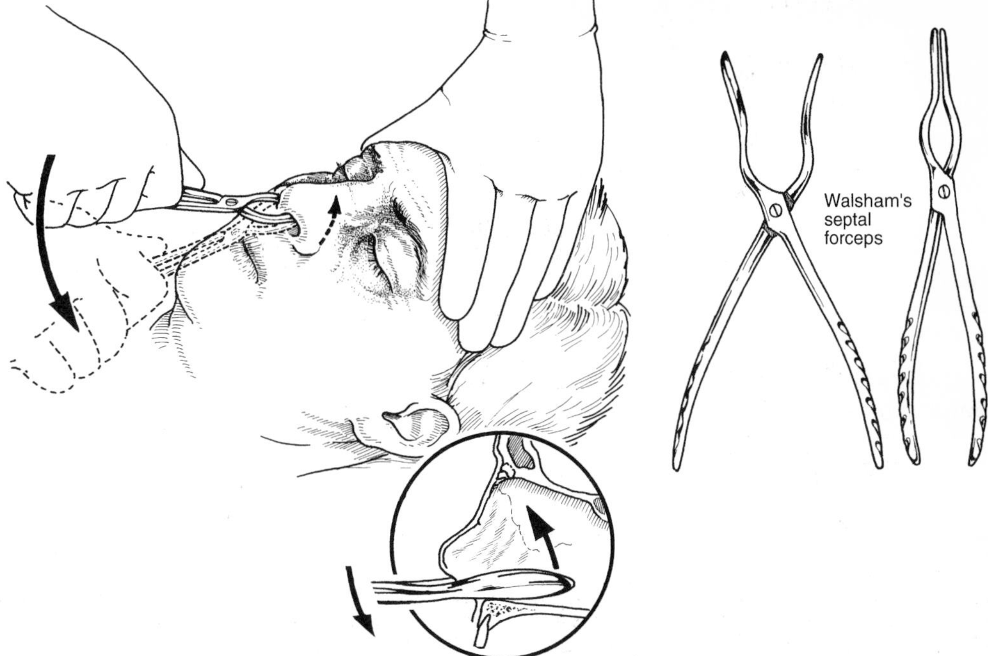

Fig. 12.18 Walsham's septal forceps used to straighten the nasal septum. Straightening of the septum in this way has the simultaneous effect of reducing the collapse of the nasal bones.

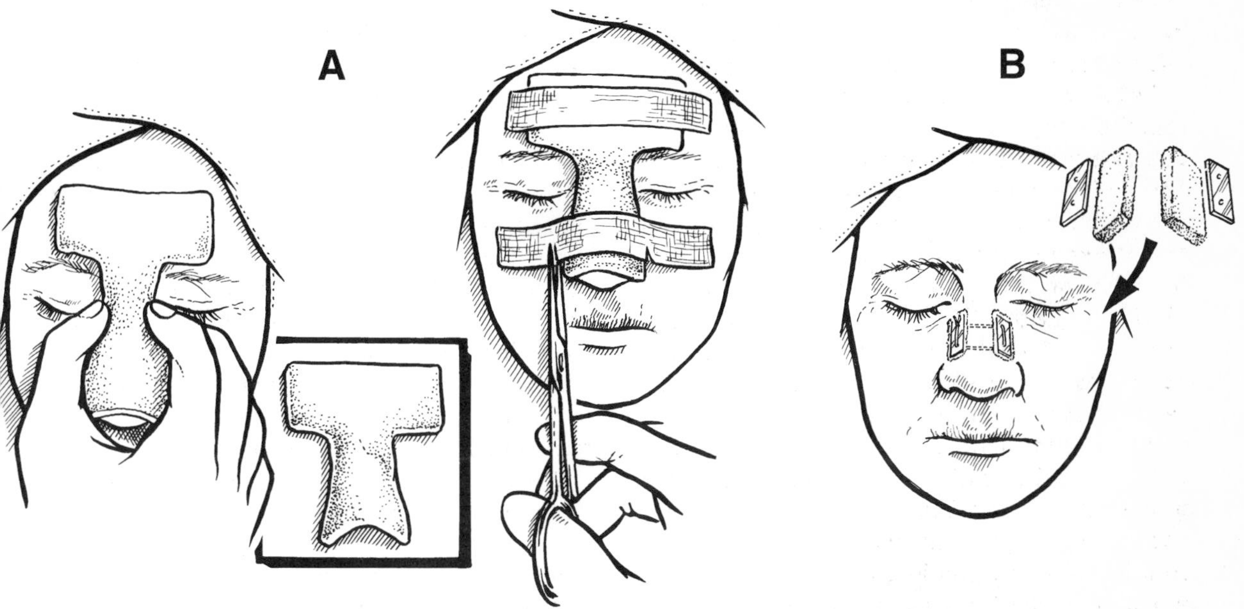

Fig. 12.19 Plaster of Paris splintage used to protect a nasal fracture following reduction (**A**), and the use of a through-and-through suture to stabilise the fracture in the case of gross comminution (**B**), when plaster of Paris is ineffective.

postoperative oedema (Fig. 12.19B) is very useful is such circumstances.

When a fracture is seen too late for primary reduction, or the result following reduction is unsatisfactory, the nose should be left until all reaction has settled, when a formal rhinoplasty can be considered.

MANDIBLE

Fracture patterns

The usual fracture sites are **condylar neck, angle, body near mental foramen** and **symphysis** (Fig. 12.20A). Fractures at these sites may occur singly or in several combinations, typically **both condyles, both angles, body and opposite angle, body and opposite condyle** and **both sides of body** (Fig. 12.20B).

The displacements which result may be caused by the direction of the violence, but they are also dependent on muscle pull. The muscles which elevate the mandible — masseter, medial pterygoid, temporalis — are all inserted behind the first molar; the muscles which directly depress the mandible — geniohyoid, mylohyoid, digastric — are all attached in front of the first molar (Fig. 12.21). The tendency is thus for the posterior fragment to displace upwards and for the anterior fragment to displace downwards, although the direction of the fracture line, particularly near the angle, has considerable influence on the amount of displacement, either permitting or preventing it (Fig. 12.21).

The condylar fracture is a special case. The condylar head is pulled forward by the lateral pterygoid muscle and when both condyles are fractured the displacement of both heads causes the patient to gag on his molars producing an open bite (Fig. 12.22).

Clinical picture

The site of fracture is usually indicated by swelling and local pain on movement or manipulation of the mandible. A sublingual haematoma is common. In the tooth-bearing segment, displacement may be clinically apparent with an obvious break in the line of the teeth, or the patient may volunteer the information that 'the teeth don't

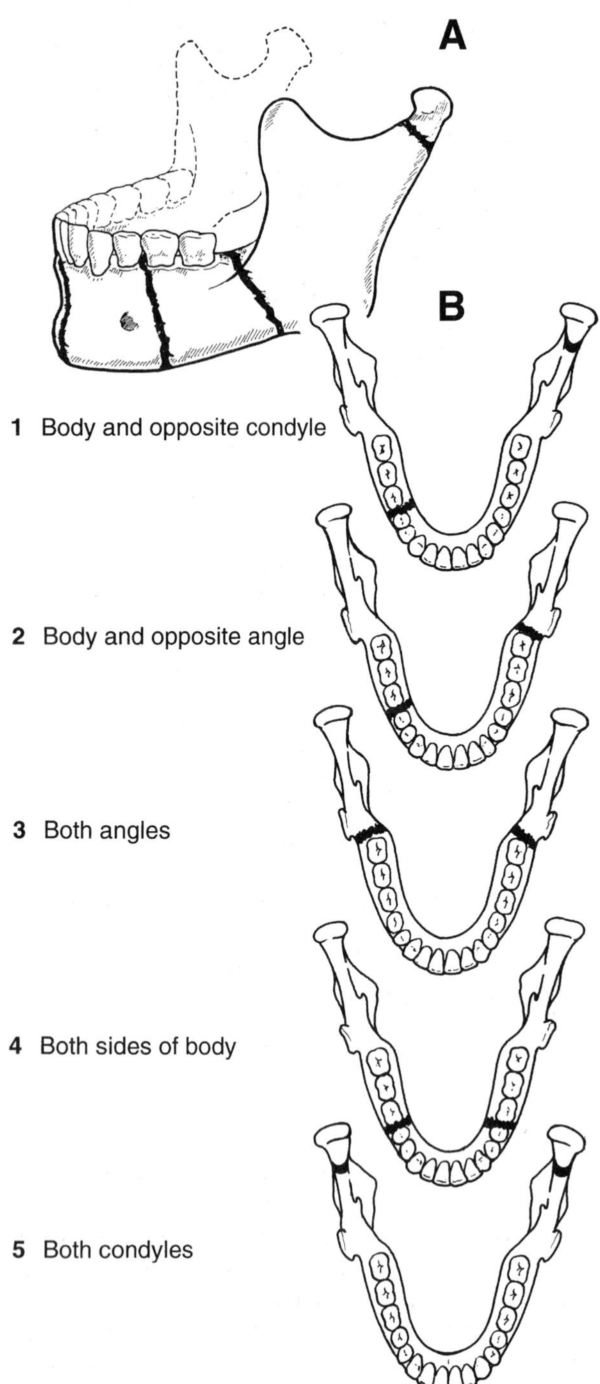

Fig. 12.20 The common sites of fracture of the mandible at a single site (**A**), and (**B**) the common patterns of bilateral fractures in order of their frequency.

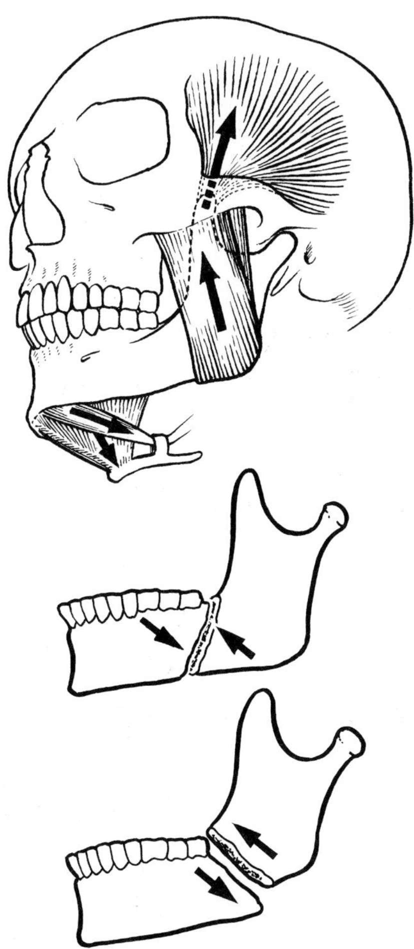

Fig. 12.21 The influence of the direction of the pull of the muscles attached to the mandible on the displacement patterns of mandibular fractures.

Masseter, temporalis, medial pterygoid exert an upward pull on the mandible; geniohyoid, mylohyoid, digastric exert a downward pull on the mandible. With the actions of these muscles as a background, the direction of the fracture line in a fracture of the angle plays a significant part in determining the degree of displacement of the fragments which occurs.

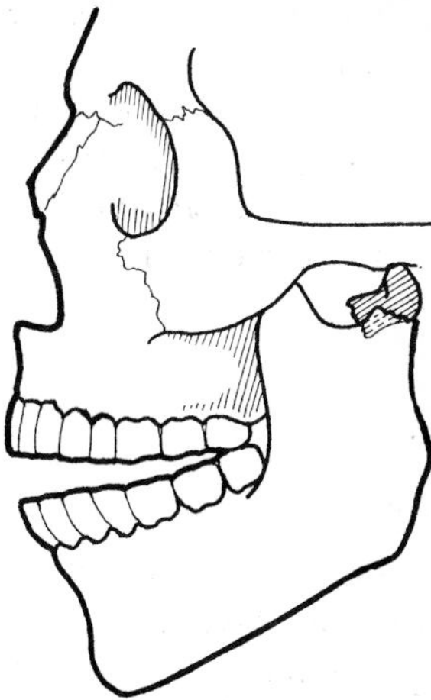

Fig. 12.22 An 'open bite' produced by a bilateral condylar fracture.

close properly'. If the fracture is between the mental foramen and the lingula, with displacement of any degree, anaesthesia of the lower lip may be present, due to damage to the inferior alveolar nerve in the mandibular canal.

A condylar fracture is less clinically obvious, and the only sign may be pre-auricular pain with or without swelling. Evidence of its presence is restriction of movement and deviation of the mandible to the damaged side on opening. Most patients with a fracture elsewhere in the mandible who complain of pain in the vicinity of the temporomandibular joint are found to have a fracture of the condylar neck. The presence of an open bite is typical of the bilateral condylar fracture.

When a fracture of the body of the bone is suspected, a most useful method of clinical examination is bimanual intra- and extraoral palpation, feeling along the lingual and buccal plates of the bone intraorally, and the lower border extraorally (Fig. 12.23). Local swelling and tenderness are suggestive of fracture, and an actual step in the bone is diagnostic.

X-ray diagnosis

Of the possible views used to demonstrate particular parts of the mandible the two most generally useful are the **posteroanterior projection** and the **lateral oblique projection**, in combination with an **orthopantomogram**. If further views are considered necessary it is best to specify to the radiographer the particular parts of the bone which it is desired to demonstrate.

Management

When the fracture is of the **toothbearing segment**, treatment depends very much on the preferred method of the surgeon involved. When displacement is minimal, eyelet wiring with inter-

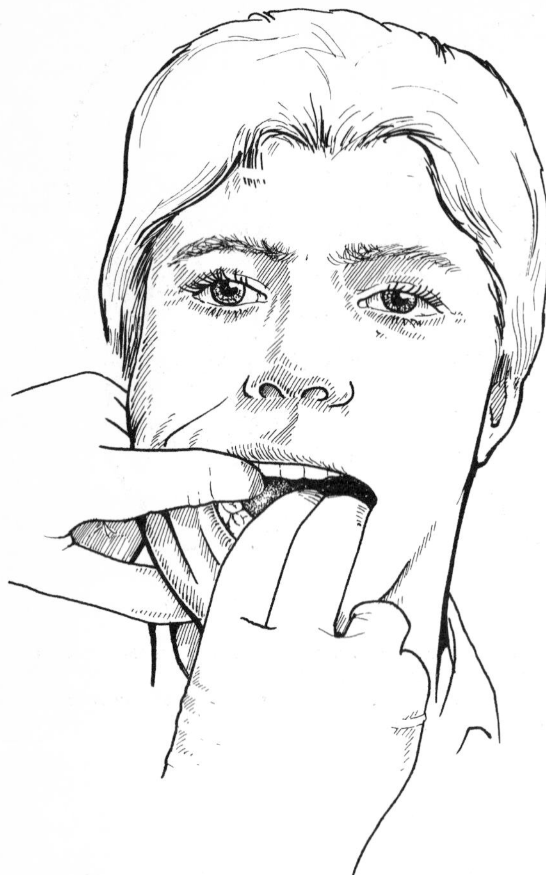

Fig. 12.23 Intra- and extra-oral palpation used in the examination of the mandible for fracture.

maxillary fixation is adequate. In the fracture with greater displacement, arch bars provide more effective fixation, usually with the addition of intermaxillary fixation. When there is instability of the fracture, internal fixation of the fracture has become standard.

With **condylar fractures**, it is not essential to reduce the fragment, regardless of whether the condyle is in the joint or dislocated. The 'joint' can be treated as a pseudarthrosis, and re-education of the muscles relied on to establish good function. When the fracture is of the body and condyle, the body fracture dictates treatment.

Some patients have minimal upset with a single condylar fracture, and are able to chew soft foods fairly quickly, with or without a period of rest depending on the degree of initial discomfort. If pain is severe, intermaxillary fixation with eyelet wires may be necessary for 2–3 weeks. Bilateral condylar fractures require correction of the open bite, either manually or by elastic traction on the fixing splints, followed by active exercises of the mandible in 2–3 weeks.

Fractures are usually tested for union in 4 weeks. If there is clinical union, fixation can be removed but, if the fracture is still springy, fixation should be continued until union is clinically apparent. Fractures of the symphysis, and those which have become infected, tend to be slow to unite. X-ray evidence of union may not be present for many weeks. Sensation of the lower lip usually recovers slowly.

Fractures involving the toothbearing segment are frequently compound into the mouth, despite which infection is surprisingly rare. When internal fixation has been used, its occurrence may necessitate removal of the plate.

MIDDLE THIRD

Fracture patterns

The fracture patterns met in clinical practice result from the interplay of the site and direction of the violence, and the lines of weakness in the bony complex. The patterns (Fig. 12.24) are categorised as **Le Fort fractures 1, 2 and 3**, named after the man who described them.

In the **Le Fort 1 fracture**, the palatal segment of the complex shears off the remainder of the maxilla through a horizontal line corresponding in level to the floor of the nose and the lower part of each antrum. The palate as a whole is displaced backwards and impacted. When the violence has been predominantly unilateral, the fracture may involve only half of the maxilla, with an added fracture line running back along the midline of the palate. The fractured segment tends then to be displaced upwards with impaction into the antrum.

In the **Le Fort 2 fracture**, the fracture line runs upwards and medially on each side, across the anterior wall of the antrum towards the infraorbital foramen, and across the nasal bones to meet in the midline in the glabellar region. The fractured segment is usually displaced backwards, and the inclined plane of the fracture line has the effect of forcing it also downwards, pushing the

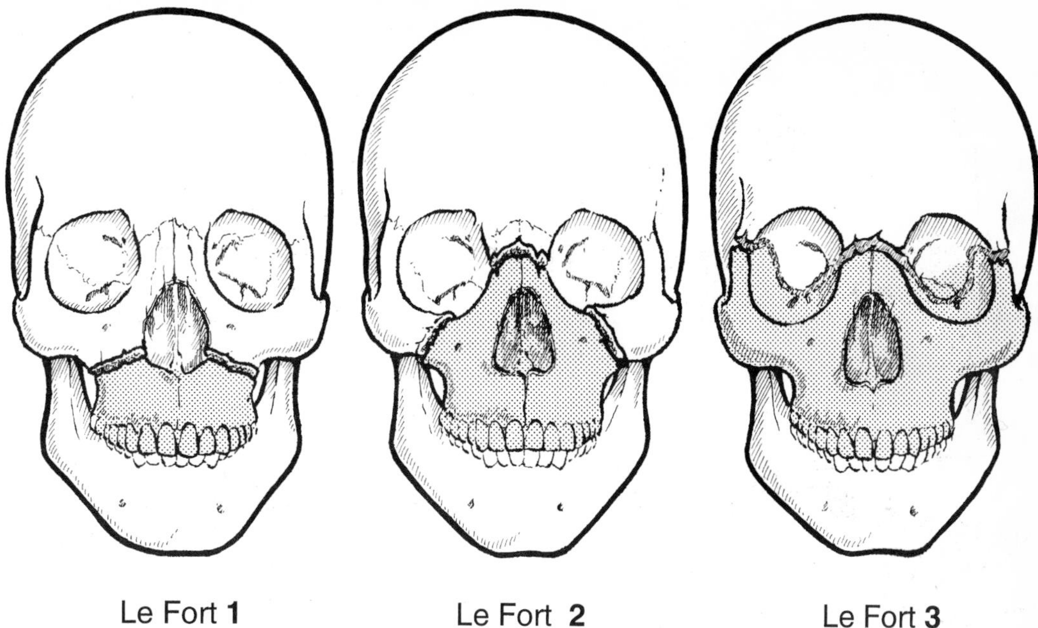

Fig. 12.24 The patterns of middle third fractures, categorised as Le Fort 1, 2 and 3 after the man who demonstrated the lines of structural weaknesses in the complex of bones which together constitute the middle third of the face.

In addition to these patterns of fracture, the individual components, maxilla, zygomas and nose, can also fracture in relation to one another and although these fractures are generally bilateral, they can also involve one side only.

mandible down and creating an open bite, with the patient gagging on his molars. The degree of impaction varies greatly, from the severely displaced and impacted fracture to the so-called 'floating' fracture where impaction is minimal.

In the **Le Fort 3 fracture**, the line of fracture extends approximately along the zygomatico-frontal suture line on each side and across each orbital floor to meet in the midline along the nasofrontal suture line. In the surgical, if not the strictly anatomical, sense, the skeletal surface above this line of disjunction constitutes the **base of the skull**.

In this description of the Le Fort 2 and 3 fractures, the fractured segment as described is carrying the nasal segment with it. In the clinical situation, the nasal bone may be fractured independently in any of the ways already described. The Le Fort 2 and 3 fractures also appear to differ from one another, depending on whether or not the zygomatic complexes are part of the fractured maxillary segment. Just as with the nasal bones, the zygomas may be independently fractured in any of the recognised patterns.

Clinical picture

Although isolated fractures of the maxilla do occur, the fracture occurs sufficiently often along with fractures of the zygomas and nose that the clinical picture will be discussed under the heading of **middle third fractures**. In any case it is only after clinical examination that the fracture pattern in an individual instance can be separated from the hotch-potch of middle third fractures into the component fractures of maxilla, zygomas and nose.

It is often possible to diagnose a middle third fracture on inspection alone, the face as a whole, but predominantly its middle third, being diffusely swollen, with oedema of cheeks and eyelids, and looking 'like a rugby football'. (Fig. 12.25).

When the fracture is severely displaced backwards, there is an obvious 'dish-face' deformity despite the masking effect of the oedema. The teeth fail to occlude properly when the patient closes his mouth, the upper incisors, instead of occluding in front of the lower incisors, as they do in most patients, occluding behind, or failing

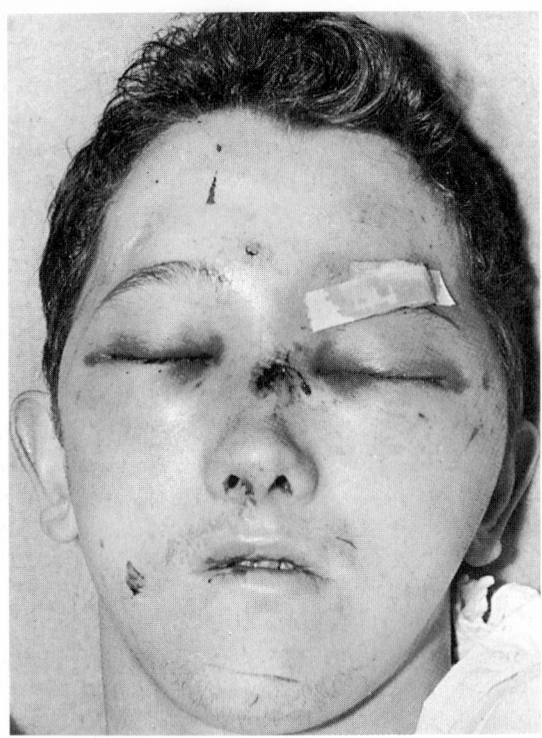

Fig. 12.25 The diffusely swollen face, 'like a rugby football', typical of the patient with a middle third fracture.

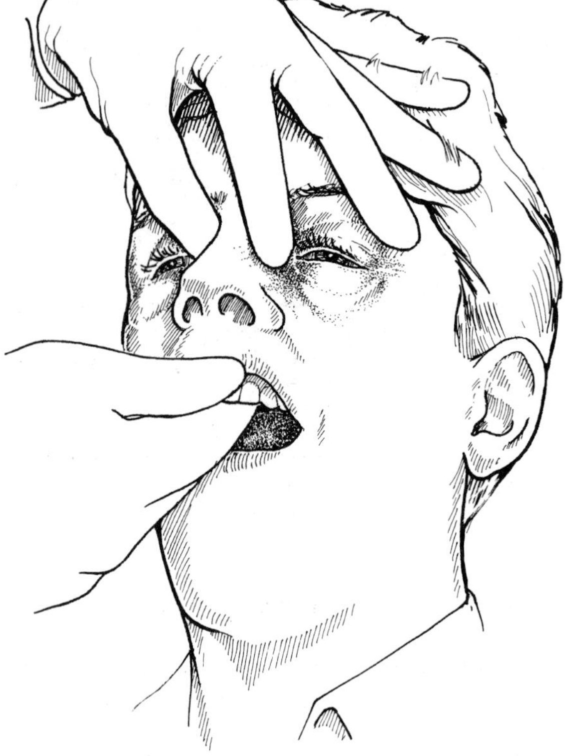

Fig. 12.26 Testing for mobility of the maxillary complex in a suspected middle third fracture.

to occlude at all because of the presence of an open bite.

Mobility of the maxillary complex is tested for (Fig. 12.26) by grasping the maxilla just above the incisors between the index finger and thumb of one hand, while the finger and thumb of the other hand feel across the bridge of the nose and hold the head steady. The maxilla is 'rocked' carefully backwards and forwards while feeling for independent movement of the maxilla. Movement of the maxilla associated with detectable movement at the nasal bridge suggests that the fracture is of the Le Fort type 2 or 3 while movement of the maxilla without detectable movement at the nasal bridge suggests a Le Fort 1 fracture.

As already stressed, middle third fractures may include fractures of either or both zygomas and/or nose, and the presence of these must be independently looked for by the methods already described.

X-ray diagnosis

The diagnosis can often be made largely on clinical examination. The interpretation of the X-ray is frequently very difficult but the views most likely to be helpful are the 30° **occipitomental projection** and the **lateral projection**. A CT scan can be of considerable help.

Management

The zygomas to a considerable extent, and the nose completely, are supported by the maxilla, and they can only be properly built on a solid foundation of maxilla reduced and fixed in position. Reduction and fixation of the maxillary fracture is therefore the first step in treatment. If the maxilla is floating or only slightly impacted, it may be possible to reduce it by finger manipulation, failing which it is necessary to disimpact

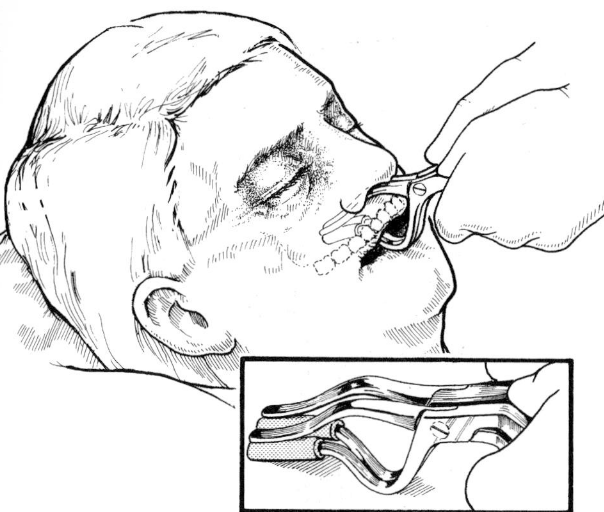

Fig. 12.27 Disimpaction of the maxilla, using downward leverage with Rowe's disimpaction forceps.

it with Rowe's disimpaction forceps (Fig. 12.27).

The methods of management which were previously standard involved final fixation to the skull, and the currently used methods of controlling the dentition, such as arch bars, cannot readily be adapted to allow this. This has contributed to the increased use of internal fixation, and today most middle third fractures are treated in this way.

With Le Fort 1 and 2 fractures, the orbital area is minimally involved, the fractured maxillary segment being essentially confined to its tooth-bearing element, and the key to effective reduction is the establishment and maintenance of satisfactory dental occlusion. Using an incision around the upper buccal sulcus, the soft tissues of the cheek on each side are elevated from the bony skeleton up to the infraorbital ridge and orbital floor. The maxilla is disimpacted, reduced on to the mandible and fixed using arch bars and intermaxillary fixation. Stabilised in this way, plates are used to fix it to the unfractured elements of the facial skeleton. Any residual comminuted bony fragments are reduced to the main maxilla, and fixed in their reduced position with plate-and-screws. The intermaxillary fixation can then be removed.

Stabilisation of the maxilla allows the zygoma and nasal fractures to be reduced and fixed, in the case of the zygoma with plate-and-screws or wires if the fracture is unstable, in the case of the nose with plaster of Paris or a through-and-through suture depending on the type of displacement.

Le Fort 3 fractures are fortunately rare, for they tend to be part of the more severe and extensive injury patterns, and the typical lateral displacement of the medial canthal areas is extremely difficult to correct completely. It is this fracture above all which has benefited from the application of internal fixation methods. The fracture sites around the skull base are exposed by combining bicoronal frontal flap exposure of the orbital area with upper buccal sulcus exposure of the infraorbital ridge and orbital floor, as already described. The various bony fragments are reduced and fixed with plate-and-screws, any dural defect being repaired at the same time. The orbital floor is reconstituted, and where necessary the bony fragments which are providing attachment for the medial canthal ligaments are restored to their original sites by transfixion wires passing through the glabellar bone. The lower maxilla is restored to proper occlusion with the mandible, and fixed also with plate-and-screws.

Despite the magnitude of the surgery involved, the combination of accurate fracture reduction and the effective fixation which plate-and-screws provides results in remarkably rapid resolution of swelling, surprisingly fast healing, and the settling of associated soft tissue injuries.

Index

WITHDRAWN
FROM STOCK
QMUL LIBRARY